Sound Changes

Sound Changes

*Improvisation and
Transcultural Difference*

Edited by Daniel Fischlin and Eric Porter

University of Michigan Press
Ann Arbor

For questions or permissions, please contact um.press.perms@umich.edu

Published in the United States of America by the
University of Michigan Press
Printed and bound by CPI Group (UK) Ltd, Croydon, CR0 4YY

First published May 2021

A CIP catalog record for this book is available from the British Library.

Library of Congress Cataloging-in-Publication Data

Names: Fischlin, Daniel, editor. | Porter, Eric (Eric C.) editor.
Title: Sound changes : improvisation and transcultural difference /
    edited by Daniel Fischlin and Eric Porter.
Description: Ann Arbor : University of Michigan Press, 2021. | Includes bibliographical
    references and index.
Identifiers: LCCN 2021003499 (print) | LCCN 2021003500 (ebook) | ISBN 9780472132423
    (hardcover) | ISBN 9780472128648 (ebook)
Subjects: LCSH: Improvisation (Music)—Social aspects. | Improvisation (Music)—
    Cross-cultural studies. | Music—Social aspects.
Classification: LCC ML3916 .S659 2021 (print) | LCC ML3916 (ebook) | DDC 781.3/6—
    dc23
LC record available at https://lccn.loc.gov/2021003499
LC ebook record available at https://lccn.loc.gov/2021003500

Contents

Digital materials related to this title can be found on the Fulcrum platform via the following citable URL: https://doi.org/10.3998/mpub.11 715165

Acknowledgments

This project began life during our conversations at the Lost in Diversity jazz studies conference at the Heidelberg Center for American Studies in November 2012. We thank Christian Broecking and the other conference organizers for making that connection. Our subsequent, 2013 call for papers for a "Sound Changes" volume elicited well over one hundred abstracts. Although we were able to include only a fraction of those proposed projects into what eventually morphed into this and two related volumes, the multifaceted response to the call confirmed our impression that scholars across disciplines and fields were pushing critical improvisation studies in important new directions, especially in relation to intercultural, transnational, and differential sites in which improvisation occurs. We appreciate the efforts of all who responded to our call for helping us understand the necessity of this and our other projects.

We are indebted and deeply grateful to our contributors for their profound insights and for their dedication to the substantive work required to take an emergent discipline forward. For some, dedication meant exhibiting tremendous patience during several stages of revision, as the volume's orientation shifted due to editorial input and through too-long waiting periods between our bursts of editorial activity as we carried on the necessary due diligence required for this work. Others demonstrated their dedication by responding affirmatively to eleventh-hour invitations to contribute and then revise pieces under strict time constraints. Collectively, the contributors helped us persevere and realize the stakes of this project.

The team at the International Institute for Critical Studies in Improvisation (IICSI) hosted by the University of Guelph was similarly dedicated through this process. We especially wish to thank our research assistants, Dr. Brian Lefresne and Rachel Collins, for their tireless work as liaisons with authors, careful readers and copy editors, project managers, and keepers of the files. Sam Boer, our wonderful Research Assistant funded by IICSI, provided invaluable assistance in completing the index to this volume. Justine Richardson, then IICSI project manager, and Ajay Heble, IICSI director, were unstinting in their support, providing much-needed assistance throughout the process. We acknowledge the Social Sciences and Humanities Research Council of Canada for its ongoing, significant contributions to both the Improvisation, Community and Social Practice (ICASP) and IICSI projects.

Mary Francis of the University of Michigan Press was supportive and encouraging when we presented the project to her and provided valuable advice for refocusing the volume as we finalized it. Sara Cohen, also at Michigan, inherited the project and was similarly supportive in shepherding the volume through the review process and into production. We also benefited from the work of editorial assistant Flannery Wise, project manager Melissa Scholke, and copyeditor Jessica Hinds-Bond. Two anonymous readers affirmed the integrity of the volume we have collectively produced and provided excellent, constructive suggestions for fine-tuning.

Last but not least, we are grateful to our families, friends, and colleagues for giving us their support and the time to work. And we thank those who improvise, as always, for the ways they have reimagined human sociability across various modes and spaces of difference. As Yusef Lateef proposed, succinctly and wonderfully, on the calling card he gave us at the Heidelberg conference: "LOVE FOR ALL. HATRED FOR NONE."

Preface

Field Notes on Cultural Difference
in Improvised Music

JOHN CORBETT

In high springtime, 1986, I presented the second gig under my own steam.

As an undergrad at Brown University, I'd spent three years apprenticing for other presenters who were organizing concerts of creative music, mostly Americans out of the jazz tradition—Marion Brown, Byard Lancaster, Dennis Charles, Steve McCall—and folks from the downtown New York scene, like John Zorn and Butch Morris. I'd learned by example from the elder organizers, and when they left school I eagerly picked up the baton. Most of what I did from then on I figured out on my own. My specialty, forged early in the process, was European free improvisation, often presented in the context of, or in combination with, American improvisers.

At that time, European improvised music had almost no profile in the United States except among super-specialists. I'd been fortunate to meet the main agents for European improvisers wanting to play in the States, Hope Carr and Larry Stanley, with whom I collaborated extensively for several years. After a failed attempt to book Swiss pianist Irène Schweizer—timing didn't work out with my exams—I managed to secure a date in Providence for Peter Brötzmann and Han Bennink. I knew the Dutch drummer Bennink only from his explosive and surprising recordings, but I'd been a fan of Brötzmann for a few years, and I'd heard the German saxophonist in concert already.

I knew Brötzmann liked to drink. His music was expressive, voluble, could be violent. He wore his handlebar mustache long in his beard, very nineteenth century. Working inductively, I'd formed an image of his personality based on some combination of the way he played and a battery of cultural stereotypes. Armed with these knuckleheaded ideas I decided that the best thing to do when they hit town a day before the gig, hospitality-wise, would be to treat them to a night of hardcore barbecue.

In this act was revealed the first great intercultural stupidity of my presenting career.

I'd imagined some sort of meat orgy. Something out of a Hermann Nitsch performance. A *Schlachtfest* or ritual slaughter. Tearing of flesh. Elbows deep in pork. Lubricated whiskers. Beer with schnapps chasers.

I was right about beer.

Except for Bennink, who immediately ordered a glass of milk. The server at the barbecue joint was confused. "You want *milk* with your ribs?" I wondered to myself: is this a Dutch thing? Bennink insisted, but they had no milk, so he settled for water. Brötzmann ordered a beer and some ribs. And more beer. Both musicians seemed put off by the fact that I ate my food with my fingers. Davey Williams and LaDonna Smith, the duo I'd booked to open the concert, were of course very familiar with American etiquette for the eating of barbecue, as they were from Birmingham, Alabama, by way of Chattanooga, Tennessee. Brötzmann and Bennink preferred forks and knives, even made of plastic. There was constant daubing of napkins and light dipping in sauce, but no bestial digging in, nothing remotely bacchanalian. I observed little that night that my twenty-two-year-old American brain pictured as Germanic.

These were northern European gentlemen.

They complained that the ribs were too greasy.

Which in fact they were.

* * *

1. A premise of freely improvised music is that all people can play together, regardless of their cultural background.
2. Japanese people can play with Germans.
3. Germans can play with Dutch.
4. Flemish musicians can get into this mix.
5. Supposed aversions or antipathies are no inherent impediment.
6. African American players can work with white musicians from France.

7. Successful music can be made by a British *shakuhachi* virtuoso in collaboration with a Korean *kayagum* player and a Norwegian who plays electronics.

8. In that sense, the music is utopian.

9. It is not reliant on geography.

10. It has a circumspect relationship to cultural tradition.

11. Such utopianism may be founded on differing notions of what exactly happens to one's cultural background when one plays improvised music.

12. Perhaps—one wing of practitioners imagines—culture is overcome by improvising. Could be suppressed. Could be sublimated. Superseded. Ignored. Disappeared.

13. These practitioners believe in an international style of improvised music. It should bear no established markers of the cultural, but should instead exist as a hermetic language of its own, a kind of instantly invented Esperanto.

14. These players are particularly on the lookout for jazz licks, samba rhythms, and folk-song quotations—any residual indigenous musical sensibilities—which they might discourage by cringing and frowning disapprovingly. The discipline of this music, so they say, resides in avoiding the most familiar parts of our psychological makeup and ideological identity, hence a desire to reduce cultural place markers to nil.

15. Alas, this can produce vividly ethnocentrist music.

16. As if nothing else in the wide world of sound exists but the approved lexicon of free improvisation.

17. Another wing of practitioners imagines the status of culture in improvised music differently.

18. One never escapes one's cultural conditioning, they figure, even in the deepest moments of meditative introspection, so how would we expect to elude it while improvising?

19. In free improvisation, all those cultural identities well up.

20. Performance with others is a place where difference is negotiated.

21. Or learned from.

22. Celebrated.

23. At least respected.

24. Culture is an aspect of the music, not an obstacle to it.

25. Taken to its extreme, this position can also produce extreme results.

26. A parade of cultural stereotypes.
27. Folkloric tropes, the specialties of one's tribe demonstrated for one another in real time.
28. Collages of ethnographic music and popular music and anything that can justifiably be called "the music of my people."

* * *

Like most international art forms, improvised music provides a platform for cultural exchange and productive misunderstandings. Improvised music was one of the first committedly international art forms, in which people from far-flung communities sought to collaborate.

We know the short-form history.

In the late 1960s, musicians from Europe teamed up regularly with musicians from other European countries. Brötzmann began to invite British, Dutch, and Belgian musicians to join his bands. Americans continued visiting Europe, as they had since early in jazz history, and some, like the Art Ensemble of Chicago, Steve Lacy, and Frank Wright, settled there for a spell, collaborating with local folks. A racially mixed group of South African musicians expatriated to London in 1965, palpably changing the scene there. Pianist Alexander von Schlippenbach founded Globe Unity Orchestra in 1966, though the globe in question, at that point, was quite contained, involving musicians from northern Europe only; later, the scope of global unity stretched much further to include musicians from the United States, Canada, southern and eastern Europe, and Japan. As the improvised music scene expanded, musicians from Japan, Australia, and countries behind the Iron Curtain were all invited to play together with improvisers in American and European contexts, and vice versa.

But in its initial phases, the music had been more or less exclusively regional. It had germinated on a local level. Chicagoans fostered the Association for the Advancement of Creative Musicians (AACM) while holed up in Chicago; there were equally exclusive local scenes in London, Amsterdam, Wuppertal, and Berlin. These scenes had their own identities, which, it is said, reflected certain inbuilt cultural traits. Americans were omnivorous, incorporating jazz and blues into their sensibility. Brits were fussy and analytical, and this temperament resulted in diffuse "insect music" built of little sounds that eschewed overt musical reference. The Germans were volatile and eruptive, Wagnerian. The Dutch were funny, absurd, and theatrical. But these supposed cultural markers of identity were quickly left behind as players began to actively collaborate, and in fact they were always somewhat misleading, based on little but the hollow stereotypes they seemed to confirm. Certain scenes that formed later, like the one in Stockholm, seemed willing to pick and choose elements from any of those historical precedents, actively mixing them all together. By the mid-1970s, exceptions were more common than the rule when it came to cultural markers in improvised music. It was thoroughly heterodox, and a player like British pianist Steve Beresford was a perfect example—in certain ways quite British, but always asking, by means of his playing, *what* that might mean.

* * *

Midway through the first concert I organized at Brown (a quintet led by trombonist Craig Harris), drummer Ronald Shannon Jackson—who'd agreed to a short midset duet with poet Michael S. Harper—took me aside, asking how much extra he'd be paid for this performance. A marquee star in this context, he was already making more than the rest of the band put together. When I told him there was no additional money, as he knew from the contract he'd signed, he said: "Come on kid, don't bullshit me. I worked with Cecil Taylor, man, I know the score. You're a rich white college student. You know you can ask for some money somewhere."

This was a shakedown, but one based on a long history of African American musicians being ripped off by white people, a painfully learned skepticism about presenters, their motives, and their means. In retrospect, it reminds me that cultural exchange never occurs in a bubble, but inevitably involves a political context, all the good deals and misdeeds that led up to it, shaped it, gave it substance. When Jackson got onstage with Harper a few minutes later, as he did, I understood his complex polyrhythms, Texas shuffles, and boogie beats a little differently.

* * *

What are we invoking when we say "culture" in relation to improvised music?

National identity?
Regional or local identity?
Ethnic identity?
Hybridism?

If we refuse "culture" in that context, what are we invoking?

Universalism?
Homogenization?
Individual persona?

* * *

Hanging out in the late-night downstairs after-fest dance party at a festival in Nickelsdorf, Austria, one year, I was chatting with drummer Hamid Drake. The room was crowded, the music was loud, and everyone was pretty drunk. An Austrian woman inserted herself between Drake and me, grabbing onto his arm and whispering into his ear loudly enough that I could plainly hear. "You are so beautiful. Come show me the secrets of your Black rhythms." Scandalized, I made a face. Hamid shook his head, his ever-present air of generosity extending even to this creepy person, from whom he politely disengaged. "Happens all the time," he said later. "You wouldn't believe."

* * *

Aside from the cultures that make up improvised music, there is a culture *of* improvised music listeners. Quite a normal kind of subculture, like *Star Wars* aficionados, football fans, and comic book collectors. Anyone who's gone to a festival of improvised music has witnessed it. You can feel it in the audience of most of the music's concerts, really. It transcends national and ethnic identity, though those categories are certainly superimposed on it and make it that much more diverse, when, indeed, it is diverse at all. Participants in this culture enjoy its rituals—making trips to and from the bar, conversing between sets about favorite records and the performance at hand, taping the music and sharing it via a vast network of tape traders, buying merchandise off the stage or from the merch tent, acquiring a festival T-shirt with which to proclaim one's cultural affiliation, perhaps wearing it right there, at the same festival, as if to give the event a positive review or to remind ourselves where we are and with which tribe we belong.

* * *

Sitting in the audience at a concert I've organized, listening to a brilliant quartet led by cellist Tomeka Reid, with guitarist Mary Halvorson, bassist Jason Roebke, and drummer Tomas Fujiwara, thinking: *maybe nowadays*

there is something like an intercultural style of improvised music—not interna-
tional, fuck nationalisms anyway—but one in which the voices of the culturally
conditioned individual and some sort of universal spirit mingle freely, are permit-
ted to coexist, but are not forced to demonstrate themselves or experience utopian
acculturation, instead are living components of an unfixed narrative.

* * *

At my apartment one night after a concert, eating pizza, a musician from
California seated himself on my kitchen counter and, in the middle of
telling a story, without any attempt to hide it or embarrassment over
it, cocked his hips and passed gas. "Hey! We cook on that surface," I
complained. He told me to chill out. Ten years later, in a similar situation at a subsequent apartment, a German musician, having failed in
a momentary search for a bottle opener, used the kitchen counter to
pound off the cap of his beer, chipping the countertop in the process.
I asked him to leave. Were these moments of cultural dissonance? Was
I just the uptight Chicago-born presenter and they the relaxed Californian and the pragmatic German? Or were they just rude?

* * *

There's a well-known scene in Sun Ra Arkestra lore in which John Coltrane races to the front of the stage, saying something like: "He's got it,
he's got it! Gilmore's got the concept!" Tenor saxophonist John Gilmore
told me that the "concept" that so impressed Trane was the result of
a difference in sensibility between Gilmore's laid-back Chicago timing
and the rhythms of the band he was working with—not only a more on-
top-of-the-beat New York ensemble, but one led by Willie Bobo, whose
Puerto Rican rhythms exaggerated the difference. Against this background, Gilmore's solo apparently sounded visionary. What, if anything,
was typically "American" about this encounter? Was it an intra-American
cultural encounter? Chicago culture versus New York culture? New York
culture amplified by San Juan culture? And what are all these signifiers?
Do they reach back from the sound of music through the player to some
other underlying reality? Some secret cultural dimension, archetypes
of Puerto Rico, New York City, and Chicago revealed by means of their
expression as different approaches to time? As different as two notions
of punctuality—one flexible, often a little late, the other always on time,
pushing everyone to stay on schedule, sometimes arriving early?

* * *

Speaking of timing, I adore the way that John Zorn and Michihiro Sato deal with it on their album *Ganryu Island.* They play together and apart at once. Distance is as important as proximity. Is this a recording of traditional shamisen with improvised accompaniment on alto saxophone and game calls? Is it the other way around, with shamisen performing its conventional accompanist role to the main narration by Zorn, as it might in the context of *nagauta* songs or Kabuki and Bunraku theater? At what point do the instruments cross? Zorn and Sato leave voluptuous space around each other, avoiding the most obvious kinds of interaction. It makes me think also of soprano saxophonist Steve Lacy's noninteractive dialogue with traditional Japanese percussionist Masa Kwate on *Shots,* Cyro Baptista's approach to traditional Brazilian percussion with guitarist Derek Bailey on *Cyro,* and Bailey's conversational duets with *pipa* player Min Xiao-Fen on *Viper.* Each of these duets, functioning as an intensive encounter, articulates a complex understanding of the flaws of dichotomous thinking, the line drawn between tradition and avant-gardism (or modernism or postmodernism), between different forms of cultural expression, between traditional culture and personal voice.

* * *

One night, postgig, after a late listening session spent sipping single malts and distinguishing the playing of London jazz saxophonists Tubby Hayes and Ronnie Scott from that of their American contemporaries, I returned from our kitchen with a bowl of ice cream for Evan Parker. A nightcap. The British saxophonist had a big smile on his face. He was leaning all the way back in our large lounge chair, which cranked into several reclining positions. "You Americans are so precise in your language," he said, pushing one position forward to accept the dessert. "*Lazy . . .*" slurp of ice cream ". . . *Boy.*"

Introduction

Sound Changes:
Improvisation and Transcultural Difference

DANIEL FISCHLIN AND ERIC PORTER

Sounding Contingency

Sound Changes begins with an understanding of improvisational music as a global, multivalent, socially situated set of practices found within and across different cultural and historical contexts, different national spaces and traditions. The book's title, with "changes" oscillating between its function as verb and as noun, speaks to the differential contexts in which improvisatory sounds occur. Contexts and practices change a sound's meaning. These contexts and practices have histories tied both to specific sites and to the ways sounds migrate and intersect with other soundings and relations where differential traditions and systems are in place. And sound itself is productive of changes that have an impact on wider spheres of human being. While sound is contingent on the contexts in which it is produced, echoing forward potentially across glocal and intercultural sites, the challenge of understanding what makes such contexts specific emanates from the aural experiences and histories of interpretation, social function, and affect associated with them.

Sound Changes, then, examines how transcultural processes are, in general terms, often improvisational—that is, products of real-time, creative decision-making. Spontaneous creation with the tools at hand has produced remarkable new directions in intercultural musicking. This book explores some of these new directions with a focus on the complex dynamics and potentialities of such transformative musical encounters. The specificities of sonic spaces, intermixed with the local social geographies of improvised sound, are coproductive and in dialogue with global sonic realities, as are breaks with those traditions—resistances and hybridizations that result from unexpected contingencies and encounters—improvisations against the ground of what has come before, what has laid the ground for the play of sounds yet to come. Ethnomusicologist Bruno Nettl observes, "There is, clearly, in the world at large and even in the culture of certain small societies, a wide spectrum of improvisation."[1] The vast array of practices, contingencies, and expectations that influence how sounds change, not only in musical contexts but also in terms of the wider social practices that music affects, is a focus throughout this book. The interplay of intercultural sites of transmission, experimentation, and dissonance this book studies suggests an emergent global network of soundings—built on a foundation of previous networks of soundings of various scales—that have much to teach us.[2]

Through a series of case studies drawn from Africa, Asia, the Americas, and Oceania—as well as musicians', sonic technologies', and ideas' travels among these regions—*Sound Changes* showcases the transcultural coproductivity of improvisatory practices across a variety of sites where the social utility (or not) of improvisation is subject to vastly different performance situations, historical circumstances, and social contingencies. Taken together, these chapters demonstrate that autonomy and reliance, hybridity and cocreativity, resistance and mutation, unpredictability and orthodoxy, emergent and discarded technologies all contribute to the composite event horizon of the possible, in which improvisatory practices materialize, reconstitute themselves, and also disappear. This volume traces some of these permutations and attends to what they convey about transcultural improvisatory practices that extend our vocabulary and knowledge of the discipline of critical studies in improvisation. Difference-producing practices mark improvisatory discourses as sites of dissonance and resistance, troublesome spaces that undermine facile notions of musical and cultural consonance and normative musicking.

As an extension of the Improvisation, Community, and Social Practice (ICASP) and now the International Institute for Critical Studies in Improvisation (IICSI) projects, this book's exploration of extant and potential sonic realities continues to chart a critical trajectory committed to understanding musical improvisation as a model, not without challenges and caveats, for political, cultural, and ethical dialogue and action—for imagining and creating alternative ways of knowing and being known in the world. It assumes value in the creative risk-taking imbued with the sense of movement and momentum that makes improvisation an exciting, unpredictable, ubiquitous, and necessary endeavor, one that extends human agency in cocreative contexts. But this volume also pushes beyond some of the cultural and political assumptions animating the ICASP and IICSI projects, asking whether the assumptions driving the work therein—and, more specifically, some of our own work there and elsewhere—may obscure the complexity of dialogue and action that becomes increasingly evident when one examines improvisatory musical practices globally, across a range of intercultural contexts.

In that regard, *Sound Changes* is part of a series of interventions that builds from a call for papers we issued in 2013 and that also includes "Improvisation and Global Sites of Difference" (a special issue of *Critical Studies in Improvisation / Études critiques en improvisation*) as well as our coedited collection *Playing for Keeps: Improvisation in the Aftermath.* As we developed our call for papers, we were keenly aware that critical studies in improvisation, which advance connections between musical practice and other forms of social practice, must do a better job of addressing the extraordinary diversity found in and across musical and cultural locations, especially those involving intercultural dialogue. While the discipline, which we remind people has only truly come into focus in the early part of the twenty-first century, has been building a lexicon of key terms and developing assumptions about core practices, the full breadth of improvisatory practices—in which music is a defining element in human creative and social expression—has remained a vexed if not impossibly ambitious subject of study. The staggering wealth of bio-/sono-diversity and of creative expressions found in local and site-specific improvisatory practices the world over is a sobering counterweight to hegemonic discursive strategies that mainstream any given form of practice as a singularity with significant idiomatic and nonidiomatic variations. This volume is a small, incremental step forward in the larger countervailing movement away from critical tendencies that homogenize and reduce practices and vocabularies in the name of the familiar.

The comparative study of improvisational projects situated across the globe may be found in foundational works from the 1960s and beyond.[3] These include Nettl's 1974 article "Thoughts on Improvisation: A Comparative Approach" and Derek Bailey's influential and widely read 1980 volume, *Improvisation: Its Nature and Practice in Music* as well as his 1992 four-part miniseries *On the Edge,* made for British TV Channel 4, which relied heavily on global comparisons of improvised musics. *Sound Changes* proposes that there is value in reanimating such discussions in light of recent trends in the field of improvisation studies. The field's musical and other cultural referents are significantly broader than they were four decades ago, a reflection of the disciplinary influence of ethnomusicology, the new musicology, improvisation studies, and interdisciplinary formations such as feminist studies, critical race and ethnic studies, cultural studies, and American studies. For example, significantly more attention is now devoted to "popular" artistic practices and to a wider range of experimental musical expressions, and a far more significant understanding exists of diverse practices, whether intercultural or not, of both traditional and nontraditional music across the globe. Also making the time right for such investigation is a range of newer work that insists on attention to the complex interpenetration of improvisation and the social, of the ways, as George E. Lewis and Benjamin Piekut put it, "that improvisation not only enacts such [social and political] formations directly but also is fundamentally constitutive of them."[4]

We take this exploration on with yet another cautionary tale in mind: the challenge for anyone not *of* a specific context to speak to that context or to address the vast gaps that open up in inter- and transcultural understanding. John Randolph LeBlanc, in a discussion of Edward Said's thoughts on the prospects of peace in Palestine and Israel, says, "Palestinian life is filled with improvisation."[5] An outsider might recognize that a young mother in Al Amari refugee camp, too poor to afford an actual percussion instrument, is nonetheless playing sophisticated rhythms while beating on the pots and pans in her kitchen and therefore improvising within a very particular set of oppressive circumstances and limited access to resources. But just how clearly does the reader wholly removed from the material realities subsumed in such an observation understand the meaning and function of such percussive sounds, so utterly specific to context?

We must be aware of the limitations of vision stemming from our lack of immersion in such contexts as well as of the obfuscating assumptions of anthropological difference. Here, it is worth examining Cuban ethnomusicologist Fernando Ortiz and his notion of transculturation—the deep permutations of history, chance, migration, hybridization, power, and resistance that forged complex Cuban social realities—and the creative expressions thereof:

> transculturation [is] . . . the highly varied phenomena that have come about in Cuba as a result of the extremely complex transmutations of

culture that have taken place here . . . without knowledge of which it is impossible to understand the evolution of the Cuban folk, either in the economic or in the institutional, legal, ethical, religious, artistic, linguistic, psychological, sexual, or other aspects of its life.

The real history of Cuba is the history of its intermeshed transculturations. First came the transculturation of the Paleolithic Indian to the neolithic, and the disappearance of the latter because of his inability to adjust himself to the culture brought in by the Spaniards. Then the transculturation of an unbroken stream of white immigrants. They were Spaniards, but representatives of different cultures and themselves torn loose, to use the phrase of the time, from the Iberian Peninsula groups and transplanted to a New World, where everything was new to them, nature and people, and where they had to readjust themselves to a new syncretism of cultures. At the same time there was . . . the transculturation of a steady human stream of African Negroes coming from all the coastal regions of Africa along the Atlantic, from Senegal, Guinea, the Congo, and Angola and as far away as Mozambique on the opposite shore of that continent. All of them snatched from their original social groups, their own cultures destroyed and crushed under the weight of the cultures in existence here, like sugar cane ground in the rollers of the mill. And still other immigrant cultures of the most varying origins arrived, either in sporadic waves or a continuous flow, always exerting an influence and being influenced in turn: Indians from the mainland, Jews, Portuguese, Anglo-Saxons, French, North Americans, even yellow Mongoloids from Macao, Canton, and other regions of the sometime Celestial Kingdom. And each of them torn from his native moorings, faced with the problem of disadjustment and readjustment, of deculturation and acculturation—in a word, of transculturation.[6]

Ortiz's notion of transculturation emphasizes "extremely complex transmutations of culture" and their ineluctable effect on virtually all intermeshed components of a site, in this case precolonial and colonial Cuba. His observations, notwithstanding the anachronistic racial language and inattention to the material dimensions of racial-colonial violence, are fair warning when it comes to critical studies in improvisation as they cast their attention beyond African American, North American, and European moorings. As the emergent discipline inevitably confronts its initial assumptions and begins the work of critically revising these assumptions transnationally, it is important to remember the lessons learned from scholarship that sits across the abyssal line from North American and European voicings.

Other volumes associated with ICASP and IICSI have taken us partway into this revisionist project, whether through the interface of gender and agency or through civil rights and social justice. Building significantly from feminist interventions in critical improvisation studies, then, Gillian Siddall and Ellen Waterman's *Negotiated Moments: Improvisation, Sound, and Subjectivity* (2016) moves significantly outside of the jazz idiom and "focus[es] less on moments of improvisational liberation and more on processes of improvisational negotiation in which agency is understood to be hard won, highly contingent, and relational."[7] Their volume, moreover, ultimately "refus[es] any singular theory about improvisational agency."[8] With the exception of a few chapters, however, *Negotiated Moments* remains primarily rooted in North American performance and interpretation scenes. Similarly, Daniel Fischlin, Ajay Heble, and George Lipsitz, in *The Fierce Urgency of Now: Improvisation, Rights, and the Ethics of Cocreation* (2013), focus primarily on African American improvisatory music in relation to struggles for rights and ongoing struggles to articulate new resistant social practices in the face of systemic racism, oppression, and disenfranchisement. An expansion of our understanding of improvisation as both a musical and a social practice across a wider range of geographic contexts, many of which inevitably necessitate intercultural dialogue, is a much-needed outgrowth from the foundational work we cite above, and perhaps something already implicit but unrealized in that scholarship.

By beginning to understand the particular, material experiences of sonic realities that are asymmetrical to our own, we can address the host of other factors that are imparted or sublimated via performance. These factors are varied and can range from the intimate affect associated with a performer's capacity to generate a distinctive "voicing," to the aleatoric addition of an unexpected sonic intervention only possible with that one configuration of players in that specific space and time. Sound changes in an improvised context are unthinkable without attending to these multiple constituents that improvisation instantiates. One underlying thesis of this book, then, is that as these contexts proliferate across global permutations of extant and potential sonic realities, so too do the dimensions of what we understand by improvisation as a creative imperative that underlies and defines human experiences. What this imperative means and how it is exercised across multiple realities are the topics of this book, balanced as it is between what Bailey has referred to as the ubiquity of improvisation as a global creative practice and the manifestations of difference in sites and contexts that challenge unifying theories about improvisation to go further.

Improvising Beyond Points Already Traversed

The chapters that follow explore what improvisation means in specific cultural contexts and how such meaning varies across an enormous spectrum of usage and enactments that require we think beyond "points already traversed."[9] The essayists in this book amply show that improvisation—as a form of adaptation, creative expression, problem solving, ludic risk-taking, reciprocal engagement, pedagogy, resistant politics, or utterly conventional expectation that variations occur—traverses a great many denotative and implied circumstances and differential meanings. This vast array of circumstances and meanings helps us better understand the diverse ways that improvisation continues to be—and will in the future be, in ways we cannot yet fathom—a vital site for the production of emergent social relationships and meanings. While the primary focus of these essays is music, we invite readers whose interests lie in other forms of improvisational activity—dance, theater, performance art, folklore, community organization, and so on—to engage with this book's breadth of sociabilities, cross-disciplinary potentials, and meanings produced in those expanding spheres of activity as well.

John Corbett's preface, "Field Notes on Cultural Difference in Improvised Music," drawn from his experiences as a presenter, performer, critic, and scholar, offers a creative approach to writing the ethnographic, historical, and performative experiences associated with transcultural improvisations. Corbett playfully disrupts some of the expectations people bring to improvisational encounters across various forms of difference. His text opens our eyes to the array of elements of musicking (performing, listening, thinking, wage working, curating, drinking, bullshitting, and so on) that inform such encounters, onstage and off, reminding us, sometimes humorously, that the potentials of cultural exchange and productive (or unproductive) misunderstandings sit in gravitational relation to one another, each ready to be activated at a moment's notice. Corbett asserts that "performance with others is a place where difference is negotiated," his text highlighting the remarkable ways in which improvised musicking brings together differential voicings of the hyperlocal and the global to enact transcultural exchange.

Jason Robinson's "Grooving with the Gnawa: Jazz, Improvisation, and Transdiasporic Collaboration" illustrates the connection between the ecstatic and improvisation as a cocreative form of concerted sounding. Recognizing that "transdiasporic collaborations" among African American jazz musicians—Randy Weston, Pharoah Sanders, and Archie Shepp—and different complements of Gnawa musicians exhibit distinct qualities of exchange, he offers the concepts of *juxtaposed* improvisations ("collaborations in which the constituent traditions and their respective improvisational approaches are superimposed on each other with relatively few changes to either approach") and *articulated* improvisations (those in which "the distinct improvisational and musical practices of the constituent traditions give way to new, emergent, or hybrid musical approaches"). Robinson's chapter demonstrates the potential in, if not the absolute need for, developing new terminology to better describe the sonic and theoretical specifics of the music that emerges from such sono-divergent encounters.

Robinson's chapter is foundational to this volume in how it attends to transcultural encounters' capacity to generate new critical approaches to improvisation studies' familiar objects of study, namely, jazz as Afrodiasporic expression. By contrast, Kirstie Dorr's "Improvisation and the Politics of *Nueva Canción* Activism" shows how improvisation studies' paradigms may be applied productively to musical forms less familiar to the field—and thus suggest new directions for transforming the field. Dorr traces the development of the *nueva canción* (new song) movement in 1960s Chile and then again in the San Francisco Bay Area in the 1980s and 1990s. Her work insists, in ways crucial to the project of this volume, that site-specific attention to the political geographies of improvisational encounter, to the multiple, overlapping publics that shape aesthetic activism, is critical to understanding changes to sounds' meanings. By emphasizing the improvisational practices of encounter that defined this movement, both in Chile and in the United States, Dorr opens our ears to the transformative potential in activities beyond the extended solo or locked-in improvisational groove. She explores those subtle, unscripted, makeshift, and ephemeral improvised expressive practices within *nueva canción* as a multifaceted movement of songwriting, performance, community activism, and concert promotion that developed in response to state violence.

Beverley Milton-Edwards's "'We Are the Ones Who Are Impatient': Improvising Resistance and Resilience in Jordanian Hip-Hop and Rap" is similarly attentive to the particulars of sounds and place and bodies in space as she moves the discussion from the "performance geographies" of Chile and Northern California to refugeeism in Jordan. Her essay, based on fieldwork, studies a youth movement that developed in an authoritarian Arab state and occupied Palestine. Focusing on the musicking of The Synaptik, a Jordanian Palestinian performer, composer, artist, and producer, Milton-Edwards examines his journeys (physical and metaphorical) into spaces that address power and its contingencies in Jordan. She contextualizes her chapter against the wider situational geostrategic and ideological place Jordan holds in the Middle East, not only as the space in which some two million Palestinian refugees live, but also as a liminal site between the Occupied Territories and other states. Her analysis necessarily engages with politics, identity, diaspora, statelessness, refugeeism, belonging, nation, transculturation, and occupation, and it also demands careful listening to sounds that gather new meanings as they travel across national and territorial borders and as they move from and between neighborhoods in Amman.

Sally Macarthur and Waldo Garrido provide something of an alternative to Dorr's and Milton-Edwards's emphasis on political geographies in their chapter, "Nomadic Improvising and Sites of Difference," although they are no less attentive to movement. Drawing on the work of social theorists Gilles Deleuze and Félix Guattari, they explore the itineracy of the nomad, defining nomadic thought as existing "in a place of potentiality, thereby enabling improvisation to always occupy that potentiality, to open onto something that exceeds the bodies that create it." Macarthur and Garrido argue that while improvisational practices may well be structured by the socially imposed, cultural politics of encounter, the embodied, nomadic identities that emerge from improvisational collaborations exceed the limits imposed by structural conditions or by the expected resistances to them stemming from fixed social positionalities. Instead, nomadism, immigration, and border-crossing—voluntary and involuntary—are all profoundly generative of improvisatory voicings and new soundings based on kinetic flows of cultural energy that are remapping local and global relations. Like Corbett's preface, Macarthur and Garrido's chapter suggests the possibility of reimagining improvisation studies through cocreative research that blurs the lines between scholar and performer. Garrido, himself a practicing improviser, is both author and interview subject of the piece, and the insights of another practitioner-interviewee, Jessica Arlo Irish, further help shape the chapter's conceptual apparatus.

Jemma DeCristo also draws deeply from critical theory and artist theorizing in "'That Which Exceeds Recognition': Sound and Gesture in

Hassan Khan's *Dom Tak* and *Jewel*." Examining how Egyptian sound artist and theorist Hassan Khan's sound installations incorporate and automate improvisational techniques from the Shaa'bi genre of street and festival music, DeCristo traces the inextricability of improvisatory practices within traditional/classical musical forms across multiple cultures. DeCristo argues that these installations, designed by an artist-theorist versed in phenomenology and decolonial aesthetics, "depart from that formal opposition between genre and improvisation, automation and improvisation," in the process critiquing models of improvisational freedom that rely on the singularity of a Western, liberal, artistic subject. Part of the contribution of DeCristo's piece, then, lies in how it draws on US- and European-oriented Black aesthetic theory while also showing how Khan deploys the same in both philosophical and practical senses, thus demonstrating the analytical possibilities in the transcultural movement of intertwined theoretical-improvisational conjunctures.

Mike Heffley's "Improvising Mythoi and Difference in the Asian/Woman More-Than-Tinge," too, focuses on the movement of music and ideas about music across space, and on the way that performers often balance their commitments to tradition and their openness to creative risk-taking in the dynamic present. Heffley analyzes the work of four Asian women expatriates who have helped shape contemporary improvised music scenes in North America. These musicians synthesized traditional and hybridized musical forms while developing improvisatory practices in their countries of origin, and then they changed things up again as they encountered new forms of experimental music and a substantially different politico-critical discourse in North America. Heffley is attentive to the wildly fluctuating meanings improvisation has in the constantly evolving, combinatory practices of his subjects. Along the way, he makes a compelling case for how an "Asian/woman more-than-tinge," pace Jelly Roll Morton, is transforming the "creative music" scene in North America in the twenty-first century, somewhat under the radar of the racial and gendered logic often brought to bear in analyses of this scene. Again, sound changes as differential practices born of collided circumstance and hybrid engagements emerge.

Also addressing transformations in meaning when Asian-based improvisatory forms travel to the United States is Monica Dalidowicz's "*Upaj*: Improvising within Tradition in Kathak Dance." Dalidowicz describes how both the practice and the status of this North Indian art form change as kathak dance moves from the Indian subcontinent to the San Francisco Bay Area, where one of its key practitioners, Pandit

Chitresh Das, was inspired to balance both "traditional" and "modern" elements of the practice in relationship to the shifting expectations of multiple audiences. Key to the argument is how the concept of *upaj*, which can loosely be translated as improvisation but which also connotes, paradoxically, close adherence to rules of performance, was increasingly foregrounded in the art form in its new Californian context during the late twentieth century. Effectively, Dalidowicz shows how the demands of audiences and practitioners predisposed to see, hear, or practice a liberating improvisation as they were familiar with it in North America helped reshape kathak. Yet, conversely, even as this shift happened, an emphasis on "improvisation in tradition" reemerged in the Bay Area during the twenty-first century, as an increasing number of South Asians, invested in maintaining connections to their assumed home culture, began studying and practicing the art form with an eye on the long-standing spiritual practices that have helped shape it.

The Bay Area is also home to Hafez Modirzadeh, whose "Ode B'kongofon," is a powerful meditation in mixed verse and prose on the relationships among rubber harvesting, the birth of the saxophone, and the imperialist legacies of violence in the Congo. Modirzadeh's provocative text, then, born of his experiences as a musician, theorist, and cultural traveler, returns us to the foundational violence of transcultural exchanges (pace Ortiz). But it also taps into the stunning array of emergent potentials that continue to be expressed via improvisatory manifestations of the liberatory "B'kongofonic spirit" breathed through the instrument. As Modirzadeh concludes, "climbing to tremendous heights, others' interpretations of the original idea are propagated / while shoots of fruit begin to flower at younger ages, feathering beats / even before life has grounded their sound." Modirzadeh's genre-defying text calls on scholarship to auto-poeticize its too often stale aesthetics, to enter into intersectional historical dialogues that attend to the material transpositions that generate new soundings, and to remake itself in the name of plurivocal forms of sounding/thinking. Arising from a profound knowledge of saxophonic history and the transcultural material realities the sax embodies, Modirzadeh's text explodes conventional academic discourses. But it also suggests alternative ways of sounding the invisible histories of putatively familiar objects—objects with vexing material origins that traverse and transpose multiple voices, cultural realities, and often violent historical intersections.

Modirzadeh's piece, along with all the other ways these chapters express, animate, and draw on musicians' theorizations of their own practices, thus sets the stage for our own afterword, "Sound Changes: The Future Is Dialogue." There we offer thoughts about future directions in improvisation—as a constellation of expressions and fields of study—that might propagate their own "shoots of flower and fruit." We describe "an improvisation without end" growing out of "our contingent relation to one another, to difference, and to the environments in which we act and sound" as a potential way out of the abyssal thinking (pace Boaventura de Sousa Santos) that is currently guiding human societies quickly toward their own destruction. What form cocreative and improvisatory responses to our collective crises might take, and how effective, if at all, they will be, remains to be seen. We suggest, however, a potentiality along the transmodern trajectory, mapped out by Enrique Dussel, with its emphasis on intellectual and cultural work developing in "shadows." While recognizing the capacity for alternative political and cultural expressions to be incorporated into, and made an agent of, hegemonic apparatuses, we continue to see in improvisational exchanges across a range of musickings, especially as theorized by practitioners, a remarkably resilient counternarrative to a modernity defined by industrial, imperial, and technological realities of subordination, alienation, and violence.

How these exchanges play out, how much they are defined by productive or unproductive misunderstandings, how exploitative they are—all these questions remain to be seen. The stochastic permutations of human interaction in the intersectional, transmodern moment in which we live are too various and complex to be assimilated or described comprehensively, whatever the Google and Facebook AI data reapers might imagine. Too much of this interaction flies below the radar, lives in the margins, shuns self-annunciatory and narcissistic social media, all the while forging new alliances and sounding new changes to the human condition. In a world where questions of authenticity and purity of origin have become symptomatic of populism, white nationalism, racism, and anti-immigrant sentiment, transcultural differences continue to assert their realities through encounter, hybridization, experimentation, and improvisatory agency. As we note at the end of our afterword, "the future, or ongoing coda to the historical contingencies we have arrived at in this moment, resides in the improvised dialogues yet to be made across the differences that sustain new ways of knowing the magic that 'even the magician does not fully comprehend,'" quoting there at the end lyricist Iola Brubeck talking about Louis Armstrong's playing. We invite, then, readers of this volume to explore the remarkable range of performance practices and social contexts that provide definitive clues as to how this multiplicity of stories of sound changes will play out in a world shaped by transcultural encounters and the sonic contingencies that give us agency, meaning, and the capacity to speak of, and across, difference.

Notes to the Introduction

1. Nettl, introduction, 6.
2. Gabriel Solis points to how "studying traditions of music making and listening, looking at the ways those traditions work . . . and the ways they are similar and different" enables a deeper understanding of very different forms of music tied to specific histories and sites of cultural production, which "can each influence the ways we understand the others." Solis, introduction, 10.
3. Lewis and Piekut, introduction, 1–2.
4. Lewis and Piekut, 13.
5. LeBlanc, *Edward Said*, 130.
6. Ortiz, *Cuban Counterpoint*, 98.
7. Siddall and Waterman, *Negotiated Moments*, 4.
8. Siddall and Waterman, 9.
9. Tim Ingold sees improvisation as a way of following "the ways of the world, as they unfold, rather than to connect up, in reverse, a series of points already traversed." See Ingold, "Bringing Things to Life," 10.

Works Cited

Bailey, Derek. *Improvisation: Its Nature and Practice in Music.* Ashbourne, England: Moorland, 1980.

Bailey, Derek. *On the Edge: Improvisation in Music.* Four-part miniseries. Channel 4, 1992.

Fischlin, Daniel, Ajay Heble, and George Lipsitz. *The Fierce Urgency of Now: Improvisation, Rights, and the Ethics of Cocreation.* Durham, NC: Duke University Press, 2013.

Fischlin, Daniel, and Eric Porter, eds. "Improvisation and Global Sites of Difference." Special issue, *Critical Studies in Improvisation / Études critiques en improvisation* 11, nos. 1–2 (2016). https://www.criticalimprov.com/index.php/csieci/issue/view/204

Fischlin, Daniel, and Eric Porter, eds. *Playing for Keeps: Improvisation in the Aftermath.* Durham, NC: Duke University Press, 2020.

Ingold, Tim. "Bringing Things to Life: Creative Entanglements in a World of Materials." NCRM Working Paper Series no. 15, ESRC National Centre for Research, University of Manchester, July 2010. http://eprints.ncrm.ac.uk/1306/1/0510_creative_entanglements.pdf

LeBlanc, John Randolph. *Edward Said on the Prospects of Peace in Palestine and Israel.* New York: Palgrave Macmillan, 2013.

Lewis, George E., and Benjamin Piekut. "Introduction: On Critical Improvisation Studies." In *The Oxford Handbook of Critical Improvisation Studies*, vol. 2, edited by George E. Lewis and Benjamin Piekut, 1–35. New York: Oxford University Press, 2016.

Nettl, Bruno. "Introduction: An Art Neglected in Scholarship." In *In the Course of Performance: Studies in the World of Musical Improvisation*, edited by Bruno Nettl and Melinda Russell, 1–23. Chicago: University of Chicago Press, 1998.

Nettl, Bruno. "Thoughts on Improvisation: A Comparative Approach." *Musical Quarterly* 60, no. 1 (January 1974): 1–19.

Ortiz, Fernando. *Cuban Counterpoint: Tobacco and Sugar*. Translated by Harriet de Onís. Introduction by Bronislaw Malinowski. Durham, NC: Duke University Press, 1995.

Siddall, Gillian, and Ellen Waterman, eds. *Negotiated Moments: Improvisation, Sound, and Subjectivity*. Durham, NC: Duke University Press, 2016.

Solis, Gabriel. Introduction to *Musical Improvisation: Art, Education, and Society*, edited by Gabriel Solis and Bruno Nettl, 1–20. Urbana: University of Illinois Press, 2009.

ONE | Grooving with the Gnawa

Jazz, Improvisation, and Transdiasporic Collaboration

JASON ROBINSON

For more than forty years, jazz pianist Randy Weston nurtured a musical and personal relationship with the Gnawa of Morocco, a concatenation of families of Islamic Sufi healers who, through the trans-Saharan slave trade spanning the eighth to twelfth centuries, trace their ancestry to sub-Saharan African cultural systems.[1] Organizing performances for and with the Gnawa since the early 1970s, Weston helped pioneer a theoretically and musically rich articulation of African American and continental African *interculturality*. Their work together first appeared as a commercially released recording in 1994, on *The Splendid Master Gnawa Musicians of Morocco*, for which Weston played with an ensemble that comprised musicians from throughout Morocco. Subsequently, in 2000, Weston's full African Rhythms jazz group appeared with a Gnawa ensemble on *Spirit! The Power of Music*, a configuration that performed several concerts over the two decades since this recording.

Weston's work with the Gnawa inspired others to follow suit. The year 1994 also saw jazz saxophonist Pharoah Sanders visit Essaouira, Morocco, for a Bill Laswell–produced project pairing Sanders with the Gnawa in an impromptu musical encounter that resulted in the album *The Trance of the Seven Colors*. Conceived by Laswell, the Sanders encounter involved an ensemble led by Mahmoud Ghania, a well-known m'alem (master musician) from a prominent Gnawa family in Essaouira. By all accounts, the project was a success: critics praised the music for both its intensity

15

and its intriguing confluence of Gnawa tradition and Sanders's incendi-
ary improvisational approach.

In 2007, the Archie Shepp Quartet, led by saxophonist Archie
Shepp, released *Kindred Spirits*, vol. 1, recorded with Dar Gnawa, a
Tangier-based ensemble led by m'alem Abdellah El Gourd, a longtime
associate of Weston's. The recording has since served as the basis for
a number of festival appearances that feature Dar Gnawa and Shepp's
jazz quartet. Shepp's approach to working with the Gnawa was initially inspired by Weston's piece "Blue Moses," which appeared on
the 1972 recording of the same name.[2] Indeed, "Blue Moses," written
nearly thirty years before Weston's first recorded collaboration with
the Gnawa, serves as an important touchstone for much of the music
described below; it is no coincidence that Pharoah Sanders was a featured soloist on the 1992 version of the piece included on Weston's
album *The Spirits of Our Ancestors*.

These three projects—with Weston, Sanders, and Shepp—reveal how
musical improvisation and experimentation work together, acting as
modes through which African American and continental African musicians theorize their connections to each other. Musical strategies drawn
from these modes are revealed in the actual sounds of such collaborations and serve to link different musical traditions and diasporic locations. I describe these projects as *transdiasporic collaborations*, projects that
activate and explore diasporic connections and generate diasporic formularies through musical collaboration. More specifically, improvisation
serves a central and complex role in each of these projects, revealing
differential and sometimes hybrid forms of itself. As such, I introduce
the concepts of *articulated* and *juxtaposed* improvisation to delineate the
processes through which different traditions interact within the musical
moment. In addition to being located in the music itself, these analytical understandings of improvisation are also exhibited in the ways that
musicians, producers, critics, and audiences make sense of the intricate
intercultural work accomplished in these projects. "These collaborations," notes anthropologist Deborah Kapchan, have "transfigured racial
identities in the public sphere on both sides of the Atlantic."[3] Through
a rich combination of improvisation, traditional repertoire, and musical
experimentalism, these projects activate critical transcultural perspectives on diasporic belonging and difference and reveal novel understandings of diaspora and pan-Africanism and the transnational linkages
sounded through musical improvisation.[4] These transcultural encounters illustrate how sound and improvisation serve as links between dif-

ferent traditions, and how, in so doing, sound itself takes on new inter-cultural meanings—the sounds change. As we will discover, differential uses of improvisation signify varied aesthetic approaches to mediating musical and cultural difference. While Weston's long engagement with the Gnawa provides a chronological beginning, we will first turn—after briefly contextualizing the Gnawa, improvisation, experimentalism, and diaspora—to Sanders's 1994 collaboration with the Gnawa, which precedes any similar recordings made by Weston.

The Gnawa

Etymologically connected to the Berber word *gnawi*, *gnawa* has, since at least the twelfth century, roughly meant "black people," in acknowledg-ment of the phenotype that distinguishes the Gnawa from other domi-nant racial groups of the Arabo-Berber cultures of the North African Maghreb.[5] In Morocco, since the 1960s, Gnawa identity has taken on larger national and international symbolism. Gnawa music was adopted into postindependence popular music in Morocco and "became Morocco's link to the African diaspora and international struggles for racial equality."[6]

Today, Gnawa musical and spiritual practices are present in Morocco in two primary ways. The first, and most public, consists of vocal and instrumental performances for tourists at large markets and other tour-ist destinations. Such performances usually include call-and-response vocals, as well as the use of *krkabas* (large handheld crotales or castanet-like instruments) and the *guimbri*,[7] the iconic Gnawa three-stringed lute, similar to a plucked bass. The more traditional context for Gnawa prac-tice usually occurs beyond the purview of the public sphere and coalesces around the *lila*, an intricate, multisectioned, trance-oriented ceremony meant to placate various spirits (*jinn*) and heal people afflicted with spirit possession.[8] Most *lila* ceremonies occur over the duration of a single night, although some can last for several days and nights. A *lila* is usually guided by two important figures, the *mqaddema*,[9] an experienced female initiate of the tradition whose task it is to assist and direct participants as they progress through various stages of the ceremony and spirit posses-sion, and a mʿalem, a male master musician and initiate who usually plays the *guimbri* and sings and directs the other musical performers (vocalists and *krkabas* players) through the repertoire and stages of the *lila*.

Written accounts of the Gnawa's intersection with others of the African diaspora trace back to at least the 1930s, when Claude McKay, the Jamaican-born writer and key figure in the Harlem Renaissance, witnessed what was likely a Gnawa *lila* during his travels in Morocco.[10] One might consider McKay's account to be the beginning of a long series of interactions between the Gnawa and African diasporic peoples of North America and the Caribbean. The transdiasporic collaborations that are the subject of this chapter take shape through the convergence of different musical practices. In these intercultural encounters, differences *and* diasporic connections are activated and imagined through differential uses of improvisation.

Improvisation, Experimentalism, and Diaspora

Parsing improvisation within transdiasporic collaboration requires a nuanced understanding of the ways that improvisation coexists with other modalities of creative expression. Improvisation's close conceptual association with jazz, and with African American music more broadly, reflects a historical discourse shaped by issues of race, power, and exclusionary conceptions of musical experimentalism. For some, improvisation is the sine qua non of jazz. Yet the compositional output of Edward Kennedy ("Duke") Ellington, Charles Mingus, and others suggests that a more nuanced and expansive understanding of jazz will by necessity take into account a wide variety of compositional approaches, the relationship between music and community (social and political movements, for example), and, of course, various approaches to improvisation, all of which hold some relationship to experimentation. And it is more interesting to see how these trajectories—improvisation, composition, and experimentalism—coexist, interact, and fold into one another, rather than operate as fixed, separate modes within African American music making.

Following the lead of scholars who have challenged the exclusion of African American and other African diasporic musicians within the discourse of experimentalism, I emphasize experimentalism as a particularly rich framework for parsing the improvisatory and intercultural aspects of collaborations between African American and continental African musicians.[11] For Tamar Barzel, experimentalism—and by extension improvisation—"discursively contests received traditions (plural) by using musical language in unprecedented, extreme, confounding, unconventional, or illegitimate ways . . . [and does so] by engaging *any* musical material that tends toward a truly sui generis, expressive end."[12] In my view, improvisation *signifies* the experimental in transdiasporic collaboration; it exposes, mediates, and emphasizes musical and cultural differentiality; it is "the modality through which performance is articulated."[13]

In transdiasporic collaboration, improvisation generates and manifests conjunctural and disjunctural points of contact between performers of different social, cultural, religious, and other backgrounds. Improvisers embody and extend culturally specific improvisational practices that are given meaning both within and beyond the communities from which they emerge. Thus, collaborations between Gnawa and African American musicians act as a coming together of different improvisational practices and understandings about improvisation; their work together highlights multiplicity, difference, and cocreation.

Since at least the late 1990s, such collaborations have been described as *intercultural*.[14] This label, however, risks relativizing difference while eschewing the power dynamics that configure global cultural economies. Daniel Fischlin, Ajay Heble, and George Lipsitz offer an important warning to those of us theorizing the intercultural: "Too often the term *intercultural* is used to delineate (simplistically) different ethnicities' coming together, or passing exchanges that are strategic or tentatively explored."[15] Facile celebrations of difference hark back to the shortcomings of "multicultural" policies in the Unites States, Canada, and Great Britain during the 1980s, in which celebrations of cultural difference often relied on problematic, reified images of cultural identity.[16]

As with other analyses of interculturalism, my aim here is to avoid shallow celebrations of sameness and difference; instead, this essay provides a more detailed understanding of the necessarily complex moments within which intercultural encounters occur. To help with this discussion, I offer a hermeneutic framework for thinking about the role of improvisation in transdiasporic collaborations. I use the term *juxtaposed improvisation* to refer to collaborations in which the constituent traditions and their respective improvisational approaches are superimposed on each other with relatively few changes to either approach. I offer the term *articulated improvisation* to describe instances when the distinct improvisational and musical practices of the constituent traditions give way to new, emergent, or hybrid musical approaches. As we will see below, articulated and juxtaposed improvisation commonly occur within the same collaborations, and it is sometimes difficult to distinguish between the two. This hermeneutic framework can help generate questions about the dynamic, complex cultural codings embodied in each collaboration, thus revealing what and how improvisation signifies in transdiasporic collaboration.

As we turn our attention to three case studies, I contend that improvisation in collaborations between African American musicians and continental African musicians evinces a special kind of transdiasporic theorizing. Such collaborations investigate and forward concepts of diasporic "sameness and difference"[17] through musical choices made during collaboration—on stages, in recording studios, during rehearsals, through dialogue—during which improvisation may serve a central role. A number of preexisting concepts can be used to help us understand these musical manifestations of diaspora, including the concepts of pan-Africanism, Black globalism, transnationalism, and diaspora itself.[18] I offer the neologism *transdiasporic collaboration* not so much as a corrective than as a magnification: to emphasize the manners in which collaboration is a conscious enactment of diasporic connection. Transdiasporic collaboration offers a particularly furtive way to think about collaborations between musicians of Africa and its diaspora, bringing into greater relief the ways that musicians imagine their connections to one another, explore their differences, and find a path forward in their novel musical encounters. It is in these moments that a kind of "rifference," following Fischlin, Heble, and Lipsitz, is emphasized: "the capacity of improvised music to invoke differential ways of being in the world across multiple contingencies that include politics, ideology, history, spirituality, ethnicity, and alternative forms of social and musical practice."[19]

"I Play Avant-Garde": Improvisation and Encounter

Pharoah Sanders (born Ferrel Sanders on October 10, 1940, in Little Rock, Arkansas) likely had a brief musical encounter with Moroccan musicians when he lived in Oakland, California in the late 1950s.[20] The passing encounter, however, played little to no role in his collaboration with the Gnawa of Essaouira. As he explained in 1998, he was drawn to the Gnawa because, "instead of looking at music as notes, they [the Moroccans] were looking at it as a feeling they were trying to project through the notes."[21] Sanders sensed in their music something similar to his own philosophical orientation to sound, which he had tried to emphasize with various collaborators since the 1970s: "I hear that in a lot of music around the world—in India, in Japan, in Africa."[22] For Sanders, the expression of an intentional "feeling" through music has been a fundamental aspect of his approach since his early exposure to the blues during his formative years in Arkansas, where he played with Bobby Bland and toured with a regional rhythm and blues group called the Thrillers.

Sanders was catapulted to prominence after joining saxophonist John Coltrane's group in 1965, at the beginning of Coltrane's so-called "late period." Like Coltrane's late works, Sanders's music, on albums such as *Journey to the One, Rejoice,* and *Elevation,* demonstrates a strong proclivity for spiritualism. While Coltrane's late music adopted freer, less groove-oriented rhythmic structures, much of Sanders's music marries ecstatic, free-blowing improvisation with an underlying groove. An iconic example of this approach is found on "The Creator Has a Master Plan," from his 1969 album *Karma.* After a rubato opening phrase, the piece revolves around a repeated bass ostinato that oscillates between two chords. Used as a vehicle for collective and solo improvisation, such a structure approximates what occurs during his work with the Gnawa.

Sanders's 1994 recording with mʿalem Mahmoud Ghania, other Gnawa musicians, and a small ensemble from the Hamadcha ethnic group in Essaouira, Morocco, was conceived by bassist and producer Bill Laswell and was released as *The Trance of the Seven Colors.*[23] The album consists of seven traditional Gnawa pieces, plus a piece with the Hamadcha and one ("Peace in Essaouira") composed by Sanders in homage to his then recently deceased longtime collaborator and guitarist Sonny Sharrock. The project coalesced Laswell's ongoing interest in Gnawa music—he had produced a 1991 album of traditional Gnawa music called *Night Spirit Masters*—with his longtime desire to work with Sanders (he would later produce other Sanders recordings).[24]

Laswell's introduction to Moroccan music came from listening to the 1971 album *Brian Jones Presents the Pipes of Pan at Joujouka.* He subsequently encountered the Gnawa while visiting Marrakech, where he began collecting cassette releases of their music. Like others, he was fascinated by their relationship to the trans-Saharan slave trade and saw a parallel between Gnawa and African American history, a kind of diasporic echoing.[25] A chance encounter with Canadian musician Eric Rosenzveig provided connections to Ghania and the Gnawa of Essaouira. Rosenzveig lived in Essaouira from 1989 through 1991, during which time he developed a close relationship with the Ghania family. Because of this, Rosenzveig was brought on as coproducer of *The Trance of the Seven Colors,* providing crucial logistical support for the three-day recording session, which took place in an interior courtyard of a house in the medina of Essaouira.[26]

Sanders arrived in Morocco with little understanding of the Gnawa, but he quickly forged a musical connection with them. As Laswell explains, "He naturally played well with them. Even in the hotel, he was practicing a theme and I was telling him that he should bring that to the session. We recorded in a house outdoors, in the courtyard of a big house. . . . When [Sanders] arrived in the courtyard, [the Gnawa] were playing pretty much the same thing. It was weird, and then he just started playing it as well and it worked. He claimed that it's a song he learned from Seminole Indians in Arkansas and they say it's a few thousand years old."[27] Laswell's account details the creation of the opening track of the album, "La Allah Dayim Moulenah" (Allah [God] is always our supreme leader).[28] The piece begins with an improvised pentatonic phrase by Sanders. Ambient sounds of children and birds fade in, likely from the courtyard where the recording took place. The ensemble of *krkabas* enters briefly and then fades out. Then a single *guimbri* enters, playing an elongated version of the melody that repeats throughout the duration of the piece.

"La Allah Dayim Moulenah" features several improvisations by Sanders, alternating with sections of call-and-response vocals. According to Laswell, the piece was created on the spot, was largely improvised, and was the result of an uncanny similarity between different preexisting musical ideas brought to the session by Sanders and the Gnawa. As a result, not only are the saxophone solos improvised, but the overall piece was also the product of an improvised process. How, then, might we characterize such an improvised, collaborative process? How might the heuristic framework of articulated and juxtaposed improvisation offer insights into the nature of the music as a transdiasporic collaboration? And is it possible to hear moments of articulated or juxtaposed improvisation in the recording?

Laswell's explanation suggests that a certain degree of articulated improvisation is present: Sanders "played well" with the Gnawa, and "La Allah Dayim Moulenah" arose from a combination of pieces by Sanders and the Gnawa. Yet the encounter also required Sanders to find a way into the music of the Gnawa. The album, like many collaborations between Gnawa and non-Gnawa musicians, consists primarily of a specific, well-established Gnawa repertoire of pieces drawn from *lila* ceremonies. The Gnawa play a set repertoire with clearly defined expressive features, while their collaborators find a way into the music. Thus, one might expect that juxtaposed improvisation would characterize such collaborations.

Laswell and Rosenzveig corroborate this analysis. Laswell explains that very little rehearsal occurred before each track was recorded. "No, not so much," offers Laswell. "[The Gnawa] would play a piece and [Sanders] would listen and pretty much straightaway improvise with them."[29] In part, this practice reflects the fact that Ghania and the other Gnawa are deeply ensconced in their musical tradition; for them, to record is to perform a repertoire embodied through years, decades, and generations of enculturation. The same may be said for Sanders, whose performance on the project reflects his long musical development from rhythm and blues to the jazz avant-garde of the 1960s, to his contemporary repertoire. In this sense, juxtaposed improvisation serves as the link between Sanders and the Gnawa, thus bringing together their constituent musical traditions in the moment of performance.

Rosenzveig offers a more candid description of the encounter: "Mahmoud and his band just pumped out what they knew and Pharoah stood there in front of a Neumann [microphone] and was supposed to deal with it. Come in where you want, when you want, go in when you want, with what you want."[30] Such an unscripted approach allowed Sanders to negotiate a way in that drew on his personal musical vocabulary. He developed a way to perform within the structures of the Gnawa repertoire, with each song consisting largely of an ostinato on the *guimbri*, with sections of call-and-response between a lead vocalist and a chorus, and with interspersed sections of instrumental music. One might expect that Sanders's contribution to the musical moment would affect the performance practices of the Gnawa, nudging the musical forms in novel directions through improvisational interactions. Sanders, however, adopted an approach that closely adhered to the forms offered by the Gnawa. "[Sanders] stayed pretty close within repetition and melody," explains Laswell.[31] While such decisions may appear to be a practical solution to musical differences, they reveal the complex intercultural codings that take place in transdiasporic collaborations, where musical styles speak across cultural boundaries while simultaneously reinforcing and foregrounding cultural and musical differences.

These connections and disjunctures can occur at the same moment; sounds may reveal intercultural slippages, differences in understandings of language and music. "[The Gnawa] do not like dissonance or arrhythmic sounds," explains Laswell. "If you say, 'I'm bringing a jazz musician to play with you,' they will not like that idea because to them jazz is a very nervous, detached, fractured, confused, sick kind of music. So when I said I'm bringing Pharoah Sanders, [they ask] what's his background, ah well, he's known in the jazz area but I wouldn't say he's a jazz musician necessarily. They were kind of not that interested. I brought him and one of the guys who spoke with him said, 'Are you playing jazz? Because we don't like that.' And he said, 'No, no, no, I play avant-garde.' And they said 'that's okay, that's just fine.'"[32] Of course, there is a certain humorous irony to the fact that, for the Gnawa, avant-garde is an acceptable alternative to jazz. If the Gnawa see jazz as a "nervous, detached, fractured, confused" form of music, then what did they understand avant-garde to mean? According to Laswell, they had "no idea. What it meant is that it wasn't jazz."

Sanders's collaboration with the Gnawa provides a good example of encounter, of those moments in which difference is negotiated intercorporeally, through face-to-face interaction. We find evidence of both articulated and juxtaposed improvisation in the project, but the latter appears to far outweigh the former. While Laswell imagined very real connections between the musicians, anecdotes from the recording session nevertheless illustrate what Fischlin, Heble, and Lipsitz describe as "differential ways of being in the world across multiple contingencies." The slippages caused by these differences appear in playful confusions of the signifiers "jazz" and "avant-garde," but they are also manifest in the role that juxtaposed improvisation serves in mediating significant musical traditions and vocabularies. As we turn our attention to Randy Weston's extensive relationship with the Gnawa, we will see how different ways of thinking about tradition affect the nature of transdiasporic collaboration.

"Our Hands and Our Bodies": Presenting Tradition through Improvisation and Collaboration

In the liner notes to his self-released 1964 recording *African Cookbook*, pianist and composer Randy Weston (born April 6, 1926, in Brooklyn, New York, died September 1, 2018, also in Brooklyn, New York) explains that the "album, especially the composition 'African Cookbook,' is in very heavy debt; to Africa." For Weston, the "melody evokes North Africa and the rhythms come from all over Africa."[33] Composed in a six-eight meter and adopting melodic and harmonic forms that evoke North Africa, the piece reflects Weston's compositional imagination and the broad ways in which jazz musicians from the United States have activated ideas about Africa in sound.

While many of Weston's peers looked to Europe in the 1950s and 1960s for performance opportunities and a more genial environment toward the arts, Weston was instead drawn to Africa.[34] His first trip to Africa took place in December 1961, when he was invited by the American Society of African Culture (AMSAC), a US-African cultural exchange program founded in 1956, to visit Nigeria as part of a cultural attaché that included Nigerian percussionist Babatunde Olatunji (then living in the United States), author Langston Hughes, bandleader and vibraphonist Lionel Hampton, saxophonist Booker Ervin, percussionist and dancer Scoby Stroman, painter Hale Woodruff, choreographer Geoffrey Holder, vocalist Nina Simone, bassist Ahmed Abdul-Malik, and a number of other important African American artists and intellectuals.[35] Weston visited Nigeria under the auspices of AMSAC again in 1963, and he then undertook a US State Department–sponsored tour of fifteen countries in Africa and the Middle East in 1967, a year that proved to be a turning point for Weston's relationship with Africa.[36]

Shortly after returning from the tour, Weston received an encouraging letter from the US embassy in Rabat, Morocco, explaining that enthusiasm for his music had continued to grow since his performance there.[37] At the same time, Weston's discontent with the jazz scene in the United States was steadily increasing. In Weston's words, "the vibrations and the spirits were just right," so in 1967 he moved himself and his two children to Morocco.[38] They lived for a year in Rabat, and then, in 1968, they moved to Tangier so that Weston's children could attend an American school. But Weston was also likely drawn to the city because of its international and cosmopolitan reputation.[39] Weston lived in Tangier until 1972, during which time he co-owned a music venue called the African Rhythms Club and produced a musically successful but financially catastrophic music festival.[40]

Weston's relationship with the Gnawa began in 1968, shortly after he arrived in Tangier, when he was introduced to Abdellah El Gourd by a teacher at his children's school. At the time, El Gourd was working for Voice of America radio in Tangier, and although he was already deeply ensconced within the local Gnawa community, he was not yet a m'alem.[41] El Gourd introduced Weston to Gnawa history, beliefs, and music, and in 1969 he facilitated Weston's first attendance at a *lila* ceremony.[42] During the *lila*, Weston experienced a particularly strong draw toward the color blue, which is associated with Sidi Musa, a saint (*salihin*) in the pantheon of Gnawa spirits related to the prophet Moses from the Old Testament of the Bible.[43] Weston's relationship to the Gnawa has since been shaped by his connection to Sidi Musa. After he attended this first *lila*, Weston wrote a piece inspired by one of the devotional songs that celebrated Sidi Musa. He called his new composition "Blue Moses," a reference to the color associated with the saint combined with the translation of "Musa" as "Moses." Upon sharing this news with the m'alem that performed the *lila* in Tangier, however, Weston was asked not to perform the song in public because of its spiritual nature. Weston honored the request, but he continued to ask the mʿalem for permission to perform the new song in public, eventually receiving this permission about a year later. The piece was subsequently recorded as the title track of Weston's 1972 large ensemble recording *Blue Moses,* and it remained in his repertoire.

As with the other Gnawa collaborations discussed in this chapter, the shared relationship to slavery possessed by the Gnawa and their African American collaborators serves an important role in the way that the participants imagine their historical and musical connections to each other. "Randy Weston's music is related to Gnawa music," explains mʿalem Ahmed Boussou; "the exodus of Black people during the age of slavery transported Gnawa ritual both to America and to the North African Maghreb. Such ritual, after its development in America, was lost in concentration on sheer rhythm, while the influence of the Church gave rise to the 'Negro Spiritual.'"[44] While tracing the exact connections shared by Gnawa and African American musical practices to specific sub-Saharan cultural origins proves difficult, it is nevertheless apparent that such historical imaginaries deeply influence the ways in which Gnawa and African American musicians understand their connections to each other. While a shared relationship to slavery is often invoked in discourses surrounding these collaborations, El Gourd nevertheless emphasizes the different form that slavery assumed in Morocco, where sub-Saharan slaves were granted more self-determination and an earlier freedom than their American counterparts. In El Gourd's conception of Gnawa history, these differences help account for the confluence of diverse sub-Saharan African influences into a codified set of Gnawa practices.[45] Indeed, El Gourd's group Dar Gnawa—and his home, as we see below—embodies this nuanced understanding of Gnawa history while also reflecting the transatlantic linkages so central to his collaborations with African American musicians.

In Arabic, *dar* translates to "house"; hence the group's name means "House of Gnawa." The title of Dar Gnawa hangs above the entrance to El Gourd's home in the medina of Tangier, which operates as a kind of Gnawa museum, ancestral shrine, and place of worship.[46] A wall of the house is adorned with numerous photos of influential African American jazz musicians—Shepp, Weston, Rahsaan Roland Kirk, Eric Dolphy, Dexter Gordon, Thelonious Monk, Milt Hinton, Roy Eldridge, Johnny Copeland, and Ben Webster—surrounded by other photos of Gnawa musicians of the past.[47] Referring to the jazz musicians as "ancestors,"

El Gourd playfully rearranges common understandings of the diasporic timeline; embodying a "younger" tradition, African American musicians are celebrated as ancestors by those on the African continent itself. El Gourd's photos of jazz musicians act as tangible representations of imagined and real connections between Gnawa and African American musicians, between the histories of African American culture and Gnawa culture, connections often articulated through shared historical relationships to slavery and West Africa.

While the chronological and diasporic relationships of the Gnawa and Weston to the African continent vary, so too do their relationships to ritual and performance. As Kapchan astutely observes about El Gourd and Weston's relationship, "El Gourd, a ritual musician, became more of an artist or *fannan*, while jazz artist Randy Weston's career veered toward ritual music."[48] Gnawa participation in festivals and in collaborations with non-Gnawa musicians is a shift away from the ritual performance context of the *lila*. Inversely, Weston's performances with Gnawa musicians almost always invoked a kind of rituality that is not normally associated with jazz improvisation.[49] Part of this rituality comes from the way that Weston often structured his performances as educational opportunities. Between numbers or as an introduction to specific songs, for instance, he frequently offered short, well-rehearsed lectures about the relationship of jazz to music of the African continent and diaspora.

Even though Weston began performing with the Gnawa as early as 1970, his first album-length recording with Gnawa musicians did not occur until 1992.[50] "It was kind of a dream of Abdellah El Gourd and myself of getting the masters [m'alem] together to record," explains Weston, "because a lot of the elders were dying. A long time ago we had talked about that and we finally had the possibility to do it."[51] The opportunity occurred when Verve approached Weston about making a solo piano recording, eventually to be released in 1994 as *Marrakech in the Cool of the Evening*. Weston leveraged Verve's interest in the solo recording to strike a two-album deal. The resulting *The Splendid Master Gnawa Musicians of Morocco* was a turning point in Weston's future collaborations with Gnawa musicians. Both *The Splendid Master Gnawa Musicians of Morocco* and *Marrakech in the Cool of the Evening* were recorded at the luxurious Mamounia Hotel, a short walk from the souk (open-air market) of Marrakech. Working with French producer Jean-Philippe Allard of Polygram Jazz France and El Gourd, Weston released *The Splendid Master Gnawa Musicians of Morocco* in 1994.

Along with Weston on piano, the recording features eleven Gnawa musicians, including nine m'alem, from Casablanca, Essaouira, Marrakech, Rabat, Sale, and Tangier. Each m'alem is featured as a lead vocalist at least once, plays *guimbri* (listed as *hag'houge* in the liner notes), sings backing vocals, and provides clapping in the style of the *krkabas* (*krkabas* are also present on the recording). The album is organized into three pieces, "La Voix Errante," "Sound Playing," and "Chalabati." The first two pieces are long suites of traditional songs, each featuring a different m'alem in the varying styles of the Gnawa traditions of the families and cities from which they come. The final piece, "Chalabati," is a well-known Gnawa song that references their enslavement and ancestors and serves as a prayer to God.[52]

While *The Splendid Master Gnawa Musicians of Morocco* is sometimes cited as an example of pan-African jazz, commentators rarely mention Weston's limited performance role on the recording. Serving more as producer or facilitator, Weston plays piano only on "Chalabati," the shortest and final track of the recording. An important piece within the Gnawa repertoire, the song features call-and-response lyrics that address the enslavement of the Gnawa by the Berber. Weston is silent for the first forty seconds of the piece; when he enters, the piano is nearly a quarter step sharp in relation to the *guimbri*. For the next five minutes, Weston improvises between vocal phrases, suggesting a tonality centered on F dominant seventh. After the vocals conclude, Weston then solos for the remaining two minutes of the track. Jason Stanyek observes that "the mere presence of the piano in an ensemble of *guimbris* and *krkabas* is not typical and could be read as a kind of ironic postcolonial retort to European hegemony,"[53] and he emphasizes that Weston views the piano as a harp or zither-like instrument (which are common in various African musical traditions). The juxtaposition of piano and Gnawa instruments and Weston's limited performance role on the album, however, offer a minimal blending of jazz and Gnawa music; indeed, the project evidences minimal juxtaposed improvisation.

A more recent recording with the Gnawa, Weston's *Spirit! The Power of Music*, captures a live performance from September 24, 1999, at Lafayette Presbyterian Church, less than a mile from Weston's Brooklyn residence.[54] Like other later performances with Weston and the Gnawa, the concert features Weston's long-standing jazz group the African Rhythms Quintet, with Weston on piano, alto saxophonist and flutist Talib Kibwe, the late trombonist Benny Powell, bassist Alex Blake, and percussionist Neil Clarke. They are joined by six Gnawa musicians: El Gourd, Abdenebi Oubella, and Mostafa Oubella from Tangier, and

M'Barek Ben Othman, Ahmed Ben Othman, and Ahmed Saassaa from Marrakech. Both El Gourd and Saassaa sing lead vocal parts and perform on *guimbri*, wherein most traditional contexts would only have one such instrumental performer. The other Gnawa play *krkabas* and sing vocal response parts as a chorus. As with many Weston performances, the recording has a kind of educational, celebratory feel, and it features the Gnawa trios performing separately, together as one large Gnawa ensemble, and finally together with Weston's group in varying configurations.

The pieces that combine Gnawa musicians and Weston's ensemble most clearly embody the transdiasporic potential of the project. For example, "Introduction to Hag'Houge and Strings Bass" consists of a duo improvisation by El Gourd on *guimbri* and Alex Blake on contra bass, accompanied by Neil Clarke on congas. At the beginning of the piece, El Gourd offers an ostinato figure on the *guimbri*, while Weston gives a brief verbal introduction, describing the piece as a "musical trip" between the different musicians and their instruments. Weston's remarks frame the improvised piece as a relationship between performers, instruments, and movement across distance and time, while the sounds and musical roles of the instruments, presented in these new configurations, suggest transnormative positionalities that redraw diasporic linkages in unexpected but natural ways.

This metaphor of movement emphasizes transdiasporic aspects of the collaboration through novel improvisatory encounters. The history and presence of different African and non-African instruments, both of which have important relationships to movements of African diasporic peoples within and beyond the African continent, reflect for Weston a deep sense of continuity across space and changing historical epochs. Weston elaborates in the liner notes: "Seeing the Moroccan instrument, the *hag'houge [guimbri]*, which is a very ancient African instrument that came out of ancient Egypt, travelled, [was] carried by different people, changed a bit . . . , and the European string bass played by a Panamanian bassist, Alex Blake, and the way they create this introduction together. *It shows that we can capture that Africa, musical spirituality through anything at all—could be a piano, or a trombone, could be a matchbox, could be our hands and our bodies.*"[55] The side-by-side presentation of *guimbri* and bass is intended to reveal to the audience the similar sounds and musical functions of the instruments. Weston employed a similar strategy as early as the 1972 festival that he produced in Tangier, during which he had jazz flutist Hubert Laws perform with three Berber flute players. "The purpose," explains Weston, "was to show the connections between our people."[56] Although the connections manifest in similar performance practices distributed across different instruments, these musical moments nevertheless move beyond any specific instruments to "our hands and our bodies," therefore enacting diasporic connections and articulating diasporic imaginaries.

The album also includes performances of "Chalabati" and "Who Know Them?" (a new Gnawa piece likely written for the occasion), and it concludes with a two-part rendition of "Lalla Mira," a staple of the Gnawa repertoire that is related to the color yellow and the playful, dance-oriented spirit of the same name. Part 1 of "Lalla Mira" begins with both El Gourd and Saassaa playing *guimbri*. They are joined by the *krkabas* and Clarke on percussion, followed by lead and background vocals. The texture of the music shifts as the two horn players gradually enter with an arranged line, giving way to extended solos by both Kibwe and Powell. Weston also takes a brief solo, providing a transition for the return of the vocals. Behind the horn lines and each of the solos, Weston's piano accompaniment (or "comping") serves as a "sound bridge" between the soloists and the Gnawa musicians.[57] The percussiveness of Weston's rhythmic placement creates relationships between the *krkabas*, Clarke's percussion, and the soloists, and the harmonic choices offered in Weston's piano voicings bring together the jazz language of the soloists with the harmonies implied by the *guimbri* and bass. Stoking excitement among the audience and performers, the piece comes to an abrupt halt, only to begin again with a slightly faster tempo and with more active and intricate interplay between Clarke and the Gnawa before gradually coming to an end. In each of these moments, intricate improvisatory decisions draw together the different musical traditions of the performers, thus repositioning sounds in new diasporic formularies.

The album concludes with part 2 of "Lalla Mira," a reprise of the fast section of the first version of the piece. After a fade in, it begins with another impassioned solo offering by Kibwe, with Gnawa vocals entering and exiting, increasing the overall excitement of the piece. At the end of Kibwe's solo, Powell joins him briefly to play the horn line and then takes another solo of his own. Weston's comping during Powell's solo becomes more angular and harmonically suggestive, thus illustrating the influence of pianist Thelonious Monk on Weston. These harmonic shifts also reveal that Weston's group moves from what I hear as a space of articulated improvisation to one that is more juxtaposed: a more modern, chromatic, and angular harmonic vocabulary is juxtaposed against the traditional practices of the Gnawa. Toward the end of Powell's solo,

Kibwe rejoins him to again state the horn line, but by this time the track begins to fade out. The album concludes with a fade.

While both articulated and juxtaposed improvisation are used to great effect in Weston's recordings with the Gnawa, it is also clear that no one issue propelled his transdiasporic collaborations. Since the late 1950s, Weston emphasized various diasporic relationships between jazz and African music. This trope has carried over into the ways that he structured performances with the Gnawa. Both *The Splendid Master Gnawa Musicians of Morocco* and *Spirit! The Power of Music* illustrate a great reverence for tradition; the Gnawa musicians are given ample space to present their music in its traditional form without participation by Weston or his ensemble. This space is especially evident on *The Splendid Master Gnawa Musicians of Morocco*, in which Weston only plays on a portion of the final track. But this reverence for tradition also appears in the ways that Weston framed the connections between jazz and Gnawa music. He provided information to audiences that explained the relationships between, for example, the bass and the *guimbri*. As a result, moments of articulated improvisation were presented as *expressly diasporic*. Of course, transdiasporic collaborations are by their very nature expressly diasporic, but Weston's emphasis on tradition and his four-decade relationship with the Gnawa make him unique. In the next section, we will see how Weston inspired Archie Shepp to imagine his own improvisatory collaboration with the Gnawa in a broad diasporic formulary that includes music from the Caribbean and South America.

Kindred Spirits: Trance and Broadening the Diaspora

Iconic saxophonist Archie Shepp first encountered the Gnawa in 1999 at Le Festival Gnaoua et des Musiques du Monde d'Essaouira, in Essaouira, Morocco. He was invited to perform an improvised set with an ad hoc group that included El Gourd and jazz bassist Reggie Workman, among others. Intrigued by the event, Shepp and his partner, Monette Rothmuller, set out to re-create the experience in France. Just a few months later, in December 1999, the French organization Entrop'Art sponsored performances that brought together Shepp's quartet and Dar Gnawa at two Paris venues, Institut du Monde Arabe and Le Trianon, as part of Le Temps du Maroc, a festival that celebrated Moroccan culture and France's long historical relationship with Morocco. The success of these initial performances led to an ongoing collaboration between Shepp and the Gnawa. The project is captured on a live recording from a 2003 performance in Évry, France, which was subsequently released as *Kindred Spirits*, vol. 1, in 2005 on Shepp's label, Archie Ball Records.[58] It features Shepp's quartet (including pianist Tom McClung, bassist Wayne Dockery, and drummer Steve McCraven), along with El Gourd on vocals and *guimbri*, and Abdeljabar El Gourd, Abdelkador Khlyfy, Khalid Rahhali, and Noureddine Touati on *krkabas* and vocals.

Kindred Spirits, vol. 1, consists of six pieces: "Main Street Medina," "Suite Blue," "Middle Passage," "Groove Mosso," "Dawn of Freedom," and "Kindred Spirits." Each piece follows a similar emergent form: El Gourd begins an ostinato on *guimbri*, the four *krkabas* players join in, and then the rhythm section of Shepp's quartet (piano, bass, and drums) enters, before the piece picks up with alternating sections of vocals and saxophone solos. Harmonically, the pieces generally consist of a repeated one- or two-chord vamp. After an introductory improvisation by Shepp on either soprano or tenor saxophone, El Gourd usually sings the lead vocal part, which is answered by vocal responses, sung in unison, by the four *krkabas* players. This moment then gives way to more extended improvised offerings by Shepp, all the while a continuous, usually building accompanying groove is supplied by the rest of the ensemble. These interchanges of improvisation and tradition dramatically recast the aesthetic strategies of both sides in the collaboration, thus modulating the function and context of improvisation and musical meaning.

Shepp recalls how he experienced certain difficulties when he first encountered the music of the Gnawa: "I must confess: the first time I played with them I wasn't quite sure what was going on. I didn't feel that I was part of the mix, because they play a very specific kind of rhythm using the . . . [*krkabas*]. Yeah. A sort of six-eight groove that they have. But it was my first meeting with them. I wasn't so happy with what I did. Though I really enjoyed what they did."[59] In preparation for the rehearsals that preceded the project's performances in Paris in 1999, Shepp listened repeatedly to Weston's piece "Blue Moses," noticing an underlying six-eight meter that in turn catalyzed his own conceptions of how his quartet would play with the Gnawa.[60]

> I listened over and over again and I was at the piano. And finally I, sort of, heard a connection between what I was doing and the rhythms they were doing. In fact, I could see a relationship between that rhythm and the rhythms that come from South America. Samba, salsa. . . . And it's bizarre, because, in fact, perhaps because they're playing in triple meter, that the triplets actually fit very comfortably.

What I was doing began to meld with what they were doing. I found
that if I had my rhythm section play kind of a salsa rhythm, . . . that's
where I found that—you could say Afro-Cuban rhythms—fit very well
into the traditional six-eight that they were playing on.[61]

That Shepp used Weston's recording as a point of reference for his own
collaboration with the Gnawa, something we've already encountered
with Sanders, attests to Weston's important historical role in such projects.

Shepp's response to Weston's recording also evidences a decidedly
diasporic imagining of the relationship between African American
and Gnawa music. For Shepp, recognition of an underlying six-eight
meter provided tangible connections between Gnawa musical practices and those of other African diasporic expressive cultures, including
Afro-Cuban and Afro-Brazilian musics. This recognition, for example,
accounts for the *montuno* approach (what Shepp calls a "salsa rhythm")
used by McClung on "Middle Passage."[62] Shepp encouraged McClung to
use *montunos* throughout the collaboration.[63]

While Shepp drew on African diasporic musics in the Caribbean and
South America to bridge the gap between the performance practices
of his quartet and the Gnawa, he also imagined more direct connections. "The 'blues people,'" writes Shepp in reference to early African
Americans, "are not so far removed from the Gnawi. In some ways I
can say that our experiences were very similar: loves lost forever, lives
irreplaceably destroyed, memories of family and ancient friends indel-
ibly erased," an analysis perhaps similar to that of Laswell, mentioned
above.[64] Indeed, as we have seen in the collaborations with Sanders and
Weston, such a shared relationship to slavery acts as a pivot on which the
musicians imagine historical connections to each other.

A direct relationship between African American and Gnawa cultures
also manifests in specific musical practices. "Sometimes Abdellah [El
Gourd] will sing during part of our performance," explains Shepp. "He
sings a solo. . . . No dancing. And then I'll sing or chant some kind of a
spiritual motif. It's amazing when I hear them back. They seem to . . . over-
lap."[65] Shepp's example can partially be found just over two minutes into
the album's title track, "Kindred Spirits" (the final track of the album).
Shepp offers an improvised vocal solo, whose timbre and melodic shapes
resemble the sounds of El Gourd's *guimbri*. Shepp's blues-infused phrasing evokes the spirituals, while the sinewy sounds of El Gourd's *guimbri*
signify Gnawa tradition.

Other connections in the collaboration also draw the musical practices offered by Shepp's group and those of the Gnawa closer together. In
Gnawa *lila* ceremonies, extended *guimbri* ostinatos and call-and-response
vocals are used to induce trance states for participants. Shepp's performances with the Gnawa emphasize similar trance or spirit possession
characteristics. This trait is principally found in the extended solos taken
by Shepp and the accompaniments provided by McClung, Dockery, and
McCraven. McClung offers a near constant background of piano chords
with rapidly alternating rhythms that closely follow the ebb and flow of
intensity of Shepp's improvised solos. Dockery similarly evolves his bass
lines to support the shape of Shepp's solos, but he does so in a more
complex dialogue with the *guimbri* ostinatos offered by El Gourd. And
McCraven's drum set accompaniment mirrors and enhances the building tensions and the unfolding resolutions that occur throughout improvised sections in each piece. Shepp's wailing, searching solos and the
driving, gradually intensifying accompaniment provided by his quartet
and the Gnawa create an ecstatic quality in each piece. For the Gnawa,
repetition, intensification, and incremental changes through improvisation are intended to provoke trance states in participants, reflecting
possession by various spirits (*jinn*) associated with different songs and
segments of the *lila*.

Indeed, the phenomenon of spirit possession provides an important link between Shepp and the Gnawa. "I entered into Dar Gnawa's
aura," explains Shepp, "girded up by my own perceptions as an erstwhile
'Baptist.' I heard as a young man the shouting spirituals, revivals and
ring dances of my own people."[66] Shepp remembers attending church
services when he was a child in Florida, during which people would be
taken by the spirit, sometimes crying and dancing, a kind of spirit possession common in some Baptist, Pentecostal, and other African American
churches of the time. He connects this phenomenon—what he calls
"getting happy"—to spirit possession in Gnawa ritual performances.[67]
Similar kinds of possession may in fact take place during performances
by Shepp's quartet and Dar Gnawa. It is common, for example, for one
or two of the Gnawa to step in front of the other musicians and begin
dancing with more abandon during some of Shepp's solos, as if physically manifesting the rising intensity of the solo and accompaniment.[68]

It is perhaps this connection to trance that most distinguishes
Shepp's collaboration from the others explored in this chapter. The phe-
nomenon of spirit possession provides tangible links between African
American spiritual practices and those present in the Gnawa *lila* cere-

mony. But Shepp's musical vision for the project further distinguishes it from the other collaborations. Inspired by Weston's "Blue Moses," Shepp encouraged members of his quartet to draw from Afro-Caribbean and Afro-Brazilian musical forms to activate links between Gnawa music and the African diaspora. An experimental approach, the resulting music is rich with diasporic resonances and simultaneously illustrates both juxtaposed and articulated forms of improvisation. The use of various diasporic musical practices thus generates a new improvisational approach that moves beyond the constituent musical practices of the participants, even if the articulated form is more pronounced.

The collaborations of Sanders, Weston, and Shepp with Gnawa musicians from Morocco illustrate various ways that improvisation serves as a cocreative, intercultural, corporeal realization of what I have called transdiasporic collaboration. Through a complex combination of articulated and juxtaposed forms of improvisation and traditional Gnawa repertoire, a combination that is inherently experimental, these projects activate important transcultural perspectives on diasporic belonging and difference. Sanders's collaboration with Mahmoud Ghania and other Gnawa from Essaouira, captured on the album *The Trance of the Seven Colors*, reveals how such projects can model an encounter that highlights ways in which difference sometimes generates intercultural slippages. Weston's long history with the Gnawa, on the other hand, demonstrates how a deep reverence for tradition and a keen sense of connections between African American and African musical forms might influence the shape of transdiasporic collaborations and performative modes used within them. Finally, Shepp's project with Dar Gnawa demonstrates how music from elsewhere in the African diaspora may catalyze linkages at the intersection of Gnawa and African American musical practices, and how spirit possession in African American Christianity and Gnawa practice offers a form of articulated improvisation that produces an ecstaticism within the music. Through varied and fundamentally experimentalist uses of improvisation, these three projects offer remarkably rich examples of how African American and continental African musicians theorize their connections to each other.

Notes to Chapter 1

1. The author thanks many friends and colleagues who have offered invaluable support at various stages of this essay, including Bob Weiner, Michel

Moushabeck, Mohamed Mejaour, Glenn Siegel, Monette Rothmuller, Adam Rudolph, Ian Stahl, Jamie Sandel, and colleagues in the Department of Music at Amherst College. For more on the relationship between the Gnawa and West Africa, see Kapchan, *Traveling Spirit Masters*, 17; and Ennaji, *Serving the Master*. Not all Gnawa, however, trace their ancestry to West Africa. Abdellah El Gourd, for example, traces his ancestry to Kenya. El Gourd, personal interview, September 19, 2015.

2. Archie Shepp and Monette Rothmuller, personal interview, June 5, 2014.

3. Kapchan, *Traveling Spirit Masters*, 22.

4. Two recent books that explore the relationship between jazz and Africa are worth noting: see Kelley, *Africa Speaks, America Answers*; and Feld, *Jazz Cosmopolitanism in Accra*. For an interesting overview of references to Africa within the work of jazz musicians, see Weinstein, *A Night in Tunisia*.

5. El Hamel, *Black Morocco*, 273–74. For the sake of consistency, I have chosen to adopt the capitalized version of "Gnawa" throughout this essay. It serves as both noun and modifier.

6. Kapchan, *Traveling Spirit Masters*, 21.

7. The three-stringed lute of Gnawa music goes by three common names: *guimbri*, *sintir*, and *hag'houge*.

8. Aidi, *Rebel Music*, 117.

9. Kapchan, *Traveling Spirit Masters*, 243–44.

10. Aidi, *Rebel Music*, 128; and McKay, *The Long Way Home*, 228. McKay compares the Gnawa *lila* to the Maroon Kumina ceremony of Jamaica, a tradition that similarly involves trance-oriented music intended to induce spirit possession.

11. See Barzel, "Subsidy, Advocacy, Theory," 162; Lewis, *A Power Stronger Than Itself*, xiii; and Piekut, *Experimentalism Otherwise*. See also Nyman, *Experimental Music*.

12. Barzel, "Subsidy, Advocacy, Theory," 163 (italics in the original). "Illegitimate" may also be taken as a mode of relegitimizing aesthetic practices and traditions that have been marginalized in historically dominant narratives about musical experimentalism.

13. Lewis, "The Condition of Improvisation," 4.

14. See Slobin, *Subcultural Sounds*; Stanyek, "Diasporic Improvisation"; and Stanyek, "Transmissions of an Interculture."

15. Fischlin, Heble, and Lipsitz, *The Fierce Urgency of Now*, 59.

16. See Taylor, "The Politics of Recognition."

17. See Radano and Bohlman, introduction, 31.

18. See Stanyek, "Transmissions of an Interculture"; Monson, *The African Diaspora*; Falola, *The African Diaspora*; Rahier, Hintzen, and Smith, *Global Circuits of Blackness*; Hamilton, *Routes of Passage*; Manning, *The African Diaspora*; Johnson, *Black Globalism*; and Robinson, "Dubbing the Reggae Nation."

19. Fischlin, Heble, and Lipsitz, *The Fierce Urgency of Now*, 58.

20. Sanders moved from Little Rock, Arkansas, to Oakland in 1959, where he lived with relatives for two years and attended Oakland Junior College (and also acquired the nickname "Little Rock"). The only known reference to his encounter with Moroccan musicians during this time in the Bay Area occurs in Prater, "Pharoah Sanders."

21. Quoted in Himes, "Sanders."

22. Quoted in Himes.

23. The album's name refers to the colors of the Gnawa *lila* ceremony.

24. Bill Laswell, personal interview, July 22, 2013. See Sanders, *Message from Home* (Verve, 1996); and Sanders, *Save Our Children* (Verve, 1998).

25. Laswell, interview.

26. Eric Rosenzveig, personal interview, July 24, 2013; and liner notes to *The Trance of the Seven Colors.*

27. Laswell, interview.

28. Thanks to Mohamed Mejaour for help with the translation from Moroccan Arabic to English.

29. Laswell, interview.

30. Rosenzveig, interview.

31. Laswell, interview.

32. Laswell, interview.

33. Weston, liner notes to *African Cookbook.*

34. Weston explains: "[Europe was] not for me, I always preferred to go to Africa." Weston, *African Rhythms,* 210.

35. Weston, 102–3.

36. Weston, 107. The State Department tour was an immense success and created a foundation for further connections to Africa. Weston was particularly excited by the response his music received from local audiences: "I knew the rhythms were African, of course, but I didn't realize how universally African they were until the 1967 tour when Africans in nearly every country we visited claimed the rhythms in [the song African] Cookbook as their own, as typical of Ghana or Gabon or Upper Volta or Morocco or wherever. That's pretty heavy!" Weston, liner notes to *African Cookbook.* For an excellent analysis of the racial and political dimensions of US State Department–sponsored tours during the Cold War, see Monson, *Freedom Sounds,* 107–51. See also Von Eschen, *Satchmo Blows Up the World.*

37. Weston, *African Rhythms,* 138–39.

38. Weston, 139.

39. Weston, 142–43. Writers Paul Bowles and William S. Burroughs are among the most celebrated American expatriates to have lived in Tangier.

40. Weston, 194–203.

41. Weston, 172–73.

42. Weston, 175–76.

43. For more about the role of Sidi Musa during the *lila,* see Kapchan, *Traveling Spirit Masters,* 182–83. For El Gourd's account of the significance of Weston's connection to Sidi Musa, see Kapchan, "Dar Gnawa," 6.

44. Quoted in McNeill, liner notes to *The Splendid Master Gnawa Musicians of Morocco.*

45. El Gourd, interview.

46. See Kapchan, "Dar Gnawa."

47. Kapchan, 5. Also see Kapchan, *Traveling Spirit Masters,* 218.

48. Kapchan, "Dar Gnawa," 3.

49. Travis A. Jackson also draws connections between jazz and ritual practices throughout the African diaspora. See Jackson, "Jazz Performance as Ritual."

50. A photo from 1970 in Tangier appears in Weston's autobiography and includes Weston, flutist Mohamed Zain, El Gourd on *guimbri*, and a dancer. See Weston, *African Rhythms*. Recordings (with photos) and chronology of performances are available at Weston's website, Randy Weston African Rhythms. Weston had planned to record *The Spirits of Our Ancestors* in 1991 on location in Morocco, but the outbreak of the first Gulf War that year prevented the recording from proceeding as planned; it was recorded in New York without the participation of the Gnawa. McNeill, liner notes to *The Spirits of Our Ancestors*.

51. Quoted in McNeill, liner notes to *The Splendid Master Gnawa Musicians of Morocco*.

52. McNeill.

53. Stanyek, "Transmissions of an Interculture," 113.

54. The liner notes to the album indicate that the concert took place on September 22, 1999, while the album credits indicate the date of September 24, 1999. I have chosen to list the date according to the album credits.

55. McNeill, liner notes to *Spirit! The Power of Music*.

56. Weston, *African Rhythms*, 201.

57. See Chude-Sokei, "Dr. Satan's Echo Chamber."

58. Rothmuller, liner notes to *Kindred Spirits*; and Shepp and Rothmuller, interview. The concert took place at the Théâtre de l'Agora d'Evry, as part of New Morning à Paris and the Festival de Vaulx-en-Velin. See Les Allumés du Jazz, "Kindred Spirits."

59. Shepp and Rothmuller, interview.

60. Shepp and Rothmuller.

61. Shepp and Rothmuller.

62. The *son montuno* is one of several Afro-Cuban popular music forms. Shepp makes the connection explicit in the liner notes to the album: "It is interesting to ponder that a group like the Dar Gnawa might provide an interesting link to the evolution of performance styles in the new World [*sic*]." Shepp, liner notes to *Kindred Spirits*. For an interesting take on the connection between Afro-Cuban music and African music, see Shain, "Roots in Reverse." Also see Dessen, "Improvising in a Different Clave."

63. Shepp and Rothmuller, interview.

64. Shepp, liner notes to *Kindred Spirits*.

65. Shepp and Rothmuller, interview.

66. Shepp and Rothmuller.

67. Shepp and Rothmuller.

68. Shepp and Rothmuller.

Works Cited

Aidi, Hisham D. *Rebel Music: Race, Empire, and the New Muslim Youth Culture*. New York: Pantheon Books, 2014.

Barzel, Tamar. "Subsidy, Advocacy, Theory: Experimental Music in the Academy, in New York City, and Beyond." In *People Get Ready: The Future of Jazz Is Now!*, edited by Ajay Heble and Rob Wallace, 153–65. Durham, NC: Duke University Press, 2013.

Chude-Sokei, Louis. "'Dr. Satan's Echo Chamber': Reggae, Technology, and the Diaspora Process." *Emergences* 9, no. 1 (1999): 47–59.

Dessen, Michael. "Improvising in a Different Clave: Steve Coleman and Afro-Cuba de Matanzas." In *The Other Side of Nowhere: Jazz, Improvisation, and Communities in Dialogue*, edited by Daniel Fischlin and Ajay Heble, 173–92. Middletown, CT: Wesleyan University Press, 2004.

El Hamel, Chouki. *Black Morocco: A History of Slavery, Race, and Islam*. New York: Cambridge University Press, 2013.

Ennaji, Mohammed. *Serving the Master: Slavery and Society in Nineteenth-Century Morocco*. Translated by Seth Greebner. New York: St. Martin's Press, 1999.

Falola, Toyin. *The African Diaspora: Slavery, Modernity, and Globalization*. Rochester, NY: University of Rochester Press, 2013.

Feld, Steven. *Jazz Cosmopolitanism in Accra: Five Musical Years in Ghana*. Durham, NC: Duke University Press, 2012.

Fischlin, Daniel, Ajay Heble, and George Lipsitz, eds. *The Fierce Urgency of Now: Improvisation, Rights, and the Ethics of Cocreation*. Durham, NC: Duke University Press, 2013.

Hamilton, Ruth Simms, ed. *Routes of Passage: Rethinking the African Diaspora*. East Lansing: Michigan State University Press, 2007.

Himes, Geoffrey. "Sanders: From Coltrane to a Spiritual Plane." *Washington Post*, April 24, 1998.

Jackson, Travis A. "Jazz Performance as Ritual: The Blues Aesthetic and the African Diaspora." In *The African Diaspora: A Musical Perspective*, edited by Ingrid Monson, 23–82. New York: Garland, 2000.

Johnson, Sterling. *Black Globalism: The International Politics of a Non-State Nation*. Aldershot, England: Ashgate, 1998.

Kapchan, Deborah. "Dar Gnawa: Creating Heritage and the African Diaspora through Sound, Image and Word." Paper presented at the Conference on Music in the World of Islam. Assilah, Morocco, August 8–13, 2007.

Kapchan, Deborah. *Traveling Spirit Masters: Moroccan Gnawa Trance and Music in the Global Marketplace*. Middletown, CT: Wesleyan University Press, 2007.

Kelley, Robin D. G. *Africa Speaks, America Answers: Modern Jazz in Revolutionary Times*. Cambridge, MA: Harvard University Press, 2012.

Les Allumés du Jazz. "Kindred Spirits." Accessed August 30, 2019. https://www.lesallumesdujazz.com/produit-kindred-spirits,444.html

Lewis, George E. "The Condition of Improvisation." Keynote talk, International Society for Improvised Music (ISIM), Santa Cruz, California, 2009.

Lewis, George E. *A Power Stronger Than Itself: The AACM and American Experimental Music*. Chicago: University of Chicago Press, 2008.

Manning, Patrick. *The African Diaspora: A History through Culture*. New York: Columbia University Press, 2009.

McKay, Claude. *The Long Way Home*. Edited by Gene Andrew Jarrett. New Brunswick, NJ: Rutgers University Press, 2007. Originally published 1937.

McNeill, Rhashida E. Liner notes to Randy Weston, *The Spirits of Our Ancestors*. Verve 511 857-2, 1992. Two compact discs.

McNeill, Rhashida E. Liner notes to Randy Weston, *Spirit! The Power of Music*. Verve/Gitanes 543 256-2, 2000. Compact disc.

McNeill, Rhashida E. Liner notes to Randy Weston, *The Splendid Master Gnawa Musicians of Morocco.* Verve 521 587-2, 1994. Compact disc.

Monson, Ingrid, ed. *The African Diaspora: A Musical Perspective.* New York: Garland, 2000.

Monson, Ingrid. *Freedom Sounds: Civil Rights Call Out to Jazz and Africa.* Oxford: Oxford University Press, 2007.

Nyman, Michael. *Experimental Music: Cage and Beyond.* New York: Schirmer Books, 1981.

Piekut, Benjamin. *Experimentalism Otherwise: The New York Avant-Garde and Its Limits.* Berkeley: University of California Press, 2011.

Prater, David. "Pharoah Sanders (1940–)." *The Encyclopedia of Arkansas History & Culture.* Updated September 18, 2013. https://encyclopediaofarkansas.net /entries/pharoah-sanders-3614/

Radano, Ronald, and Philip V. Bohlman. "Introduction: Music and Race, Their Past, Their Presence." In *Music and the Racial Imagination*, edited by Ronald Radano and Philip V. Bohlman, 1–54. Chicago: University of Chicago Press, 2000.

Rahier, Jean Muteba, Percy C. Hintzen, and Felipe Smith, eds. *Global Circuits of Blackness: Interrogating the African Diaspora.* Urbana: University of Illinois Press, 2010.

Randy Weston African Rhythms (website). Accessed July 3, 2020. http://www.ra ndyweston.info

Robinson, Jason. "Dubbing the Reggae Nation: Transnationalism, Globalization, and Interculturalism." In *International Reggae: Current and Future Trends in Jamaican Popular Music*, edited by Donna P. Hope, 284–310. Kingston, Jamaica: Pelican, 2013.

Rosenzveig, Eric and Peter Wetherbee. Liner Notes to Maleem Mahmoud Ghania, with Pharoah Sanders. *The Trance of the Seven Colors.* Axiom/Island 314–524 047-2, 1994. Compact disc.

Rothmuller, Monette. Liner notes to Archie Shepp Quartet with Dar Gnawa, *Kindred Spirits*, vol. 1. ArchieBall ARCH0501, 2005. Compact disc.

Shain, Richard M. "Roots in Reverse: *Cubanismo* in Twentieth-Century Senegalese Music." *International Journal of African Historical Studies* 35, no. 1 (2002): 83–101.

Shepp, Archie. Liner notes to Archie Shepp Quartet with Dar Gnawa. *Kindred Spirits*, vol. 1. ArchieBall ARCH0501, 2005. Compact disc.

Slobin, Mark. *Subcultural Sounds: Micromusics of the West.* Hanover, NH: University of New England Press, 1993.

Stanyek, Jason. "Diasporic Improvisation and the Articulation of Intercultural Music." PhD diss., University of California, San Diego, 2004.

Stanyek, Jason. "Transmissions of an Interculture: Pan-African Jazz and Intercultural Improvisation." In *The Other Side of Nowhere: Jazz, Improvisation, and Communities in Dialogue*, edited by Daniel Fischlin and Ajay Heble, 87–130. Middletown, CT: Wesleyan University Press, 2004.

Taylor, Charles. "The Politics of Recognition." In *Multiculturalism: Examining the Politics of Recognition*, edited by Amy Gutman, 25–73. Princeton, NJ: Princeton University Press, 1994.

Von Eschen, Penny. *Satchmo Blows Up the World: Jazz Ambassadors Play the Cold War.* Cambridge, MA: Harvard University Press, 2004.

Weinstein, Norman C. *A Night in Tunisia: Imaginings of Africa in Jazz.* Metuchen, NJ: Scarecrow Press, 1992.

Weston, Randy. *African Rhythms: The Autobiography of Randy Weston.* Arranged by Willard Jenkins. Durham, NC: Duke University Press, 2010.

Weston, Randy, with Willard Jenkins. Liner Notes to *African Cookbook.* Atlantic SD 1609, 1972. LP.

Audio Recordings

Archie Shepp Quartet, with Dar Gnawa. *Kindred Spirits*, vol. 1. ArchieBall ARCH0501, 2005. Compact disc.

Ghania, Maleem Mahmoud, with Pharoah Sanders. *The Trance of the Seven Colors.* Axiom/Island 314–524 047–2, 1994. Compact disc.

Gnawa Music of Marrakech. *Night Spirit Masters.* Axiom/Island 314–510 147–2, 1990. Compact disc.

Sanders, Pharoah. *Karma.* Impulse!/GRP 153, 1995 (1969). Compact disc.

Sanders, Pharoah. *Message from Home.* Verve 314 529 578–2, 1996. Compact disc.

Sanders, Pharoah. *Save Our Children.* Verve 14 557 297–2, 1998. Compact disc.

Weston, Randy. *African Cookbook.* Atlantic SD 1609, 1972. LP. (Originally released as *Rabap!! Beep Boo-Bee Bap*, Bakton BRS-1001, 1964, LP.)

Weston, Randy. *Blue Moses.* CTI Masterworks Jazz CTI6016, 2011 (1972). Compact disc.

Weston, Randy. *The Spirits of Our Ancestors.* Verve 511 857–2, 1992. Two compact discs.

Weston, Randy. *Spirit! The Power of Music.* Verve/Gitanes 543 256–2, 2000. Compact disc.

Weston, Randy. *The Splendid Master Gnawa Musicians of Morocco.* Verve 521 587–2, 1994. Compact disc.

TWO | Improvisation and the Politics of *Nueva Canción* Activism

KIRSTIE DORR

This essay explores the political and aesthetic work of improvisational performance practices within the Latin American *nueva canción* (new song) movement between the 1960s and the 1990s.[1] Scholars within various fields of social and cultural inquiry have taken up improvisation as a lens for analyzing connections between spontaneous creative acts and "critical issues in politics, social organization, alternative community formation, and human rights."[2] Indeed, as histories of new song activism demonstrate, the improvisational constitutes a crucial domain of aesthetic innovation and oppositional action for those who are precluded access to institutionalized artistic resources or sanctioned venues of political expression. What follows contributes to this line of inquiry via a discussion of the unscripted, makeshift, and ephemeral expressive practices that defined grassroots repertoires of *nueva canción* cultural activism in two unexpectedly linked geohistorical contexts: Cold War Santiago de Chile, a site of underground, leftist agitation in the wake of neofascist and neoliberal political transformations; and post-1980 new nativist San Francisco, California, where anti-immigrant xenophobia has coexisted with progressive local politics. Specifically, the chapter examines how and to what end Latinx artists of this cultural current improvised innovative mobilization techniques in the interanimating social realms of the sonic and the spatial to circumvent both vertically and horizontally imposed structural constraints. I argue that for feminist and queer cultural workers the improvisational served as a performance-based pedagogy of

42

encounter that enabled the address of ideological conflict, social difference, and political exclusion within an ostensibly "unified" popular movement. The integration of improvisational spatial practices such as siting, staging, and repurposing with improvisational aural practices such as jam sessions, sonic experimentation, and audience participation enabled these *nueva canción* artists and activists to emplace unique performance geographies of social encounter, cultural exchange, and political mobilization.

To explore these queries and claims, this essay proffers two case studies of prominent cultural centers that, though separated by three decades and two continents, were veritably connected improvisational cultural enterprises: La Carpa de la Reina, established in the outskirts of Santiago de Chile in 1965, and La Peña del Sur, founded in San Francisco circa 1992. Networks of migration and exile—and consequently, of cultural and economic exchange—linking these Pacific urban centers were first formalized in the 1840s, when thousands of Chilean merchants, miners, and entrepreneurs arrived at the Port of San Francisco during California's gold rush.[3] Maritime trade routes that were established to provision this expanding city served as transport passages for subsequent waves of Chilean migrants who settled in San Francisco's sizable pan-ethnic Latinx neighborhoods such as Chilecito (Little Chile), Rincon Hill, and, later, the Mission District.[4] Geohistorical links between Santiago and San Francisco were further entrenched in the mid-1970s, when thousands of South Americans fleeing the Dirty Wars in the Southern Cone chose to relocate to "San Pancho," owing to its enrooted Spanish-speaking Latinx barrios and its international reputation as a locus of artistic experimentation and political activism. These exiled cultural workers, most of whom had been active in the South American leftist art scene of the 1960s–1970s, would go on to found two of the most prominent Latinx cultural centers in the San Francisco Bay Area: Berkeley's La Peña, founded in 1974, and La Peña del Sur.

In addition to—and in fact because of—these geohistorical ties, La Carpa de la Reina and La Peña del Sur were comparable creative endeavors, in that both were imagined and actualized according to what we might call a "politics of improvisation." Their ongoing realization relied not on bureaucratic entrenchment and institutional expansion, but rather on the spontaneous, adaptive, and transient practices that so often defined *nueva canción* repertoires of artistic expression. The leftist artists and activists that materialized these projects integrated two sets of improvisational techniques to actualize their ideological goals:

improvisational practices of musicking, spontaneous artistic collaborations rooted in political solidarities rather than in national or regional genres; and *improvisational practices of encounter,* the organization of spontaneous grassroots events that transformed domestic spaces such as the home and the neighborhood into vibrant places of public encounter and political convocation.[5] *Nueva canción* practitioners mined popular musical practice for tactical strategies. Rejecting conventional divides between high and low culture, audience and performer, text and context, they adopted the art of improvisation as a technique for staging popular *encuentros* (encounters) that conjoined diverse artistic traditions and aesthetic repertoires to manifest undisciplined expressive vernaculars and modes of convocation. Recognizing the mobility, adaptability, and reproducibility of sonic texts, new song activists also used spontaneous encounters of musical production and exchange to popularize oppositional struggles, articulate leftist agendas, and express political solidarity.

My interest in historicizing the improvisational politics of performance and place that defined these experimental sites of *nueva canción* activism is twofold. Despite its aesthetic dynamism, multigenerational duration, and geographic reach, *nueva canción* has received scant attention within US-based Latinx, cultural, and sound studies scholarship. This scholarly neglect is perhaps due to the intercultural movement's deliberate capaciousness and refusal to be bound by the national(ist) imaginaries and generic scripts that most often frame musical study in the Americas. Rather, *nueva canción* references an artistic affiliation that straddles the particularism of geographic emplacement and the dynamism of cultural exchange. Eschewing fixed or stable notions of sonic origin or musical destination, its practitioners embrace the alchemic capacity of aural encounter to produce, contest, or reimagine individual and collective perceptions of and claims to social space. Thus, it is precisely the movement's geocultural fungibility—that is, its ability to express pan-American solidarities while connecting these to immediate political agendas and local aesthetic traditions—that makes *nueva canción* a dynamic terrain of social contest worthy of scholarly consideration.

This unique cultural formation raises fertile questions about how attention to improvisational performances and practices can enrich our understanding of both quotidian and enduring forms of social contest. Within social movement scholarship, there is a tendency to privilege institutionalized sites and forms of contest over those places and practices deemed spontaneous, temporary, or ephemeral. The small body of work on *nueva canción* activism gravitates toward this trend, most often chronicling the instrumentalization of new song repertoires in the service of nationalist revolutionary propaganda in Cuba or in support of Unidad Popular and the Allende administration in Chile.[6] Conversely, this essay adopts improvisation as a lens for theorizing the political import of *nueva canción*'s organic function within informal and quotidian spheres of cultural (re)production and exchange. As scholars of improvisation studies have persuasively demonstrated, unscripted moments and makeshift milieu of political expression hold the potential to raise oppositional consciousness, mobilize aggrieved publics, and effect political change.[7] This essay gives focus to such moments and milieu. In drawing our analytical and aesthetic attention to improvised scenes and sounds of *nueva canción* performance, I aim to expand our scholarly mappings of oppositional sonic action in general and new song activism in particular, demonstrating how these likewise reshaped both conditions and terrains of social struggle throughout the Americas.

My discussion of the improvisational sonic and spatial politics that defined repertoires of *nueva canción* activism in San Francisco and Santiago likewise raises a number of generative theoretical and methodological questions that are explored herein: How might we develop an interpretative framework that attends to the dynamic interplay of the performance and place-making within quotidian practices of social contest? How might such an analytic engender or require new approaches to the study of cultural politics, approaches that emphasize the performative logics and improvisational strategies of political organizing? And, in our current political moment, what might we learn from previous community struggles that have leveraged improvisational modes of social and sonic encounter to confront multiscalar socioeconomic abandonment, relish moments of leisure and pleasure, and envision and territorialize new modes of transnational, multiracial, and multiethnic community formation?

Performance Geography

A central proposition of this essay is that within the *nueva canción* movement, improvisation figured as both pedagogy and practice for cultural workers who adapted their musical activism to the contingencies of immediate, unstable conditions of struggle. To theorize the improvisational as an ever-evolving organizational tactic, I use the concept of *performance geography*. Elsewhere, I have extended this phrase first introduced by Caribbean feminist geographer Sonjah Stanley-Niaah to describe the range of situated and imagined places at and through which the collective cultural task of materialization—from embodiment and mobility to attachment and speculation—collides with the physical and ideological constraints of context.[8] For scholars of improvisation studies, performance geography proffers productive theoretical tools for materializing analyses of the oft unruly and unscripted interplay of performance, text, and place; it avers that geographies of creative production rooted in spontaneous, ephemeral, and improvised forms of encounter perform the crucial political work of disrupting the coherence and function of imposed spatial hierarchies that seek to bound and fix relations of imagination, labor, sociality, and belonging.[9]

In this sense, performance geography signals an analytical departure from ethnomusicological approaches to the study of Latin American musical traditions. As I have previously argued, US-based ethnomusicological research about South American aural expression, for example, has tended to rely on anthropological constructs of a static, bounded "field" that desires localized, invariable modes and forms of cultural production. Such a research model invariably provincializes aural forms of the Global South by emphasizing rootedness and continuity over movement and dynamism. Conversely, performance geography is a mode of analysis scaffolded by performance cultures rather than capitalist scales, positing the site/sound relationship as an entangled, often impromptu negotiation between social text and spatial context. As such, performance geography destabilizes binaries—orthodox versus abyssal, individual versus collective, impromptu versus institutional, or fleeting versus stable—instead theorizing collective improvisation as an organizing tactic intentionally grounded in immediate, impermanent, and anti-institutional terrains of contest.

In the case studies that follow, I use performance geography as a lens to examine contexts in which *nueva canción* cultural workers mobilized improvised sonic and spatial encounters to promote and territorialize their ideological goals. At a moment when the neoliberal values of individual entrepreneurship and authorship, scripted and sanctioned encounter, and unfettered market expansion have transformed contemporary landscapes of artistic production and collective action, my aim is to highlight the urgent work and radical possibilities that improvisational modes of political encounter and artistic exchange have historically enabled. As I detail below, improvisatory practices of encounter that defined *nueva canción* activism often blurred gendered and classed boundaries between the public and private spheres. Places conventionally coded as domestic and idle—personal homes, vacant lots, neigh-borhood streets, and anterior alleys—were reconstituted as critical sites of aesthetic innovation, popular education, and political activism. This embrace of the unscripted encounter, in turn, disrupted normative divides between audience and performer, *gestor cultural* (cultural cura-tor) and artistic innovator, making room for novel modes of intercul-tural collaboration and exchange. It is to a brief historical overview of this vibrant movement that I now turn.

The Origins of *Nueva Canción*

Popularized throughout Latin America beginning in the 1960s, the *nueva canción* movement strategically adopted and adapted the power of song to mobilize listening publics across regional, national, ethnic, cultural, and linguistic divides.[10] The roots of new song can be traced to the confluence of two political trends: the spread of socialist ideals and anti-imperial activism throughout the Americas during the early Cold War period, and folkloric revival projects that took place, particularly in South America, from the late 1950s to the early 1960s.[11] Rather than constituting a particular musical style, *nueva canción* is best defined as a pan-American musical alliance that varies in sonic expression among individual artists and across national, regional, and historical contexts. Revolutionary artists ranging from Chile's Violeta Parra, Victor Jara, and Inti-Illimani, to Mexico's Amparo Ochoa and Los Folkloristas, to Cuba's Silvio Rodríguez and Pablo Milanés, to Argentina's Atahualpa Yupanqui and Mercedes Sosa were among the hundreds of *nueva canción* artists that fused political poetry with regional and pan–Latin American and Caribbean rhythms, melodic structures, and instrumentation to sound trenchant critiques of and transnational solidarities against Western imperialism and racial capitalism.

In this sense, the aurality of *nueva canción* as an artistic formation has been, since its inception, deeply improvisational; repudiating the bounds of nation and genre, its myriad forms and ferments intentionally broke with established lyrical, generic, and instrumentational scripts. The sonic cultures of *nueva canción* were born of *improvisational practices of musicking*—that is, unscripted intercultural collaborations rooted in political solidarities rather than in bounded geographic or sonic reg-isters. "La canción comprometida" (politically committed song) was a guiding refrain of the movement, as cultural workers fused political poetry with popular forms to express dissent and mobilize *el pueblo* (the village).[12] With an eye toward the racial, ethnic, and class diversity of potentially politicized listening publics, artists embraced rhythmic, instrumentational, and generic promiscuity; this experimental intermixture of, collapse of, and sampling across musical conventions was often actualized through spontaneous jam sessions and extemporaneous performances held at street and house parties, clubs, and festivals.

The work of Inti-Illimani, who performed at three of the four *peñas* discussed herein, exemplifies the intercultural politics of sonic experimentation and extemporization that came to define new song expression. Over the course of its thirty-year musical career, the renowned Chilean group performed and recorded a remarkable breadth of rhythmic traditions, including Ecuadorian *san juanitos*, Afro-Andean *sayas*, and Peruvian *huaynos*, as well as Colombian *cumbias*, Bolivian *takiraris*, and Mexican *rancheras*.[13] Inti-Illimani's interpretation of these tracks varies across geohistorical moments and performance contexts, evincing the group's artistic commitment to improvisation as a method of artistic activism; its vocal, percussive, and instrumentational arrangements of staple sonic texts shift according to the contingencies of a given performance and are determined by spontaneous collaborations with other artists and interactive exchanges with audiences. In this sense, Inti-Illimani epitomizes the improvisational practices of musicking that have consistently defined *nueva canción*; the group, like its musical comrades, privileges in its creative vision the collective, collaborative cultivation of pan-American musical repertoires that mobilize dynamic aesthetic alchemies to express solidarity across sites of and among subjects in struggle.

In some cases, these improvised departures from established cultural norms and generic registers enabled new song cultural workers to expose and challenge commonsense geocultural divides between high and low, traditional and modern, political and aesthetic, and so forth. In turn, this embrace of improvisational sonic repertoires, and the contradictions that they revealed, impelled the adoption of impromptu techniques for cultivating listening publics, establishing networks of cultural exchange, and carving out strategic sites of convocation. As *nueva canción* cultural workers consistently affirmed, the emplacement of alternative communication networks and practices was crucial to addressing the political and economic effects of ever-expanding music industries from the Global North, as foreign-owned conglomerates rapidly displaced local and national media platforms and strategically marketed US and European popular musics throughout the southern Americas.[14] These alternative media channels could be exploited to popularize neo-folkloric protest musics. Famed cantor and theater director Victor Jara remarked in the liner notes of his 1970 studio album *Canto Libre,* "Our duty is to give our people weapons to fight against [the North American commercial music industry]; to give our people its own identity" and "to make our people understand their reality through the protest song."[15] Artists and activists such as Jara astutely observed that the respatialization of performance networks across the hemisphere could challenge the effects of US imperialism while fostering transregional connections across and between aggrieved constituencies within Latin American nations and their diasporas. Here, I use the term *respatialization* to refer to the negotiation and remapping of dominant sociospatial orders in a manner that activates distinctive relations of race, gender, economy, and place—from relations of attachment and emplacement to those of mobility and boundary transgression. Among *nueva canción* cultural workers, such practices of respatialization were often manifest via the organization of spontaneous grassroots events that transformed factory floors, community centers, and public parks into vibrant places of public encounter and political convocation.

The hemispheric proliferation of the *nueva canción* movement was made possible through interconnected improvisational practices of encounter: the organization of international festivals, often hosted in public venues such as parks and plazas; public radio programming, which artists used to popularize their work both at home and abroad; and informal networks of sonic exchange, such as street performance and record sharing. A crucial site of quotidian, popular encounter among South American cultural workers and audiences was the *peña.* Politically oriented *encuentros* where artists gathered to perform or display their work for local audiences, *peñas* were popularized throughout Latin America beginning in the 1960s. In response to the industrialization of Western mass media, these neighborhood cultural centers were heralded as alternative, grassroots forums for the instruction, development, and showcasing of regional Latin American artistic and musical practices. Although the character and function of these organizations differed across regional contexts, the *peña* was arguably the emblematic institution through which the *nueva canción* movement sought to attain its musical goals: to foment political dialogue and solidarity across racial, regional, national, and class divides, and ultimately, to create a broad-based anti-imperial, anticapitalist movement in the Americas.

In the sections that follow, I juxtapose two *peñas* that, although staged nearly thirty years and six thousand miles apart, can be understood as

performance geographies that relied on similar improvisational sonic
and spatial techniques to mobilize aggrieved populations within surprisingly linked geotemporal contexts: Cold War Santiago de Chile and post-
1980 new nativist San Francisco, California.

La Carpa de la Reina

On an early summer evening in December 1965, renowned Chilean composer, songwriter, folklorist, and celebrated progenitor of the Chilean
new song movement Violeta del Carmen Parra Sandoval inaugurated La
Carpa de la Reina, an experimental cultural center located in a residential borough on the outskirts of urban Santiago. La Carpa was neither
the first nor the most renowned of the various *peñas* founded that year,
but it was certainly the most unique. In both imagination and design,
La Carpa was to be enrooted as a distinctive kind of place: housed in
an enormous, hand-hewn canvas tent nearly sixty-five feet in diameter,
the semipermanent venue was sited in a vacant, tree-lined municipal lot
ceded to Parra by La Quintrala Park district mayor Fernando Castillo
Velasco. Parra had acquired the tent, designed for use at agronomical
events, in exchange for a free vocal performance at the international
agricultural fair La Fisa.[16] The rustic pitched pavilion was anchored by a
central post around which Parra fashioned a circular adobe stove. Facing
its open-air fire was a stage of wood and stone that could accommodate
an ensemble of ten. At La Carpa's opening, Parra and her collaborators
distributed brochures detailing the scheduled activities. By day, painting
and craft workshops would be offered by local artists and artisans. And
at night, La Carpa would be transformed into a *peña* that could hold up
to five hundred people.

As Chilean journalist Mónica Garrido notes, "*Peñas* were *the* place in
which artistic manifestations of the era were proliferated, propitiating
the development of writing, painting, sculpture, and, above all, music—
primarily of the bohemian left."[17] By the end of 1965, these unique venues had become commonplace features in urban centers throughout the
nation, such that Parra's son, Ángel, quipped that "*peñas* had become
an epidemic," as constituencies ranging from youth organizers to union
leaders "sought the strength of art as a form of expression."[18] While the
peña scene no doubt galvanized the rising national prominence of *canto
popular* (popular song), Violeta became a vocal critic of the increased
formalization of these venues and expressed disdain for the middle-
class hipsters that increasingly patronized them. Her vision of the *peña*

was that of a place that intentionally broke with sanctioned forms and scripted norms of encounter, instead fostering organic relationships, meaningful political debate, and spontaneous moments of artistic collaboration and exchange. In response to the increased trendiness of *las peñas* in urban Santiago, where, in her view, the middle-class left dominated the artist-activist scene, Parra envisioned and erected La Carpa de la Reina to serve as an alternative performance geography: a hub of education, arts, and politics that would attract artists and audiences of the rural working class living in the city's unincorporated periphery. With time, it was her hope that La Carpa would become a destination that attracted and featured the creative work of the nation's proletariat and peasantry. In a leather-bound personal diary, Parra recorded that "Here [at La Carpa] we will hear the unknown songs, those that spring from the peasant women, the laments and joys of the miners, the dances and the poetry of the islanders of Chiloé."[19]

Parra's creative vision of La Carpa reflected the early influences of her artistic formation and her fierce commitment to organic, spontaneous modes of encounter that signaled the culmination of her activist career. Parra was born in 1917 in San Fabián de Alico, a small village in the rural foothills of southern Chile.[20] Her interest in the arts was cultivated from an early age; Parra's father, Nicanor, was an elementary school music teacher, and her mother, Clarisa, a seamstress by vocation, was also a talented vocalist and guitarist. Clarisa, a self-described *campesina*, taught Violeta and her siblings to interpret the Chilean folk songs and other popular ballads that she had grown up with, and soon the Parra children began performing covers of boleros, *rancheros*, and Mexican *corridos* in nightclubs and other popular venues on the outskirts of Santiago. In 1934 Parra married Luis Cereceda, a railway driver and militant communist, and became involved in the Communist Party of Chile. She had two children with Cereceda, Isabel and Ángel. When the couple separated in 1948, Parra began touring with her children and her sister Hilda, performing at *carpas* (tent shows) and other provincial spectacles throughout Argentina.

In the early 1950s, with the encouragement of her elder brother, Nicanor, Parra began traveling throughout the Chilean countryside, culling and collating Chilean folk musics.[21] This pedagogical project signaled a decisive shift in Parra's musical politics; she abandoned her staple repertoire of "música repetida, estereotipada" (mainstream, stereotypical music) and began composing original songs that combined the popular rhythmic, generic, and instrumentational traditions that she encountered during her travels with powerful, poetic lyrics detailing the violence of imperialism and capitalism and the transformative power of song.[22] Parra's pioneering practice of integrating distinctive musical styles and forms with poignant lyrical arrangements became a hallmark of *nueva canción* expression. The fervor with which her protest music was received inspired Parra's interest in the politics of musical dissemination, most particularly as it related to the forging of anti-imperial and anticapitalist solidarities. In 1954, Parra began hosting an incredibly successful radio program titled *Sing Violeta Parra*, which transmitted live performances in rural venues across national public airwaves. *Sing Violeta Parra* presented a popular alternative to Western genres and media outlets, which in her view further entrenched colonial and capitalist relations between Global North and Global South.

In the early 1960s, following a brief stint in Europe, Parra joined forces with like-minded Santiagan cultural workers of the emergent *nueva canción chilena* movement in the siting and establishment of alternative platforms for musical performance and popularization. In collaboration with her children, she helped found La Peña de los Parra, widely recognized as Chile's first and most acclaimed *peña*, in early 1964. Located in central Santiago in the spacious home of painter and vocalist Juan Carpa, this *peña* began as an intimate exhibition space for local artists but quickly transformed into a "true academy of music and arts."[23] Within months, the vibrant cultural center featured exhibition space, classrooms, dining areas, a patio performance venue, and a small store that sold handwoven goods. The space was wildly popular among Santiago's bohemian left. Attendees and artists recall La Peña's candlelit ambiance and its homespun decor, with ceilings dressed in trained vines and fishing nets, rustic wooden tables and chairs adorned with abalone shell ashtrays, and a large empanada oven that infused the space with the scent of baking meat pies.

Following La Peña de los Parra's overwhelming success, *la peña* emerged as a pivotal institution for the development and dissemination of *nueva canción chilena*.[24] La Peña de los Parra remained the most reputed and, as some opined, the most esoteric of this growing type of venue; many of Chile's most renowned *nueva canción* artists graced its stage, including Rolando Alarcón, Tito Fernández, Victor Jara, Patricio Manns, and Osvaldo Gitano Rodríguez. Buoyed by the project's popularity among Santiago's bohemian left, the Parra siblings Ángel and Isabel set their sights on expanding the center's institutional programming and reach. Famed Chilean poet Osvaldo Rodríguez recalls: "The great house [where La Peña de los Parra was housed], which was once a simple workshop for various artists, went on to grow like the legendary casas of the Latin American novel, and was transformed into a true academy of song and folk art. It began with two small rooms, but with time it boasted a mezzanine, dining rooms, a grill, a recording studio, a store that sold handwoven items, and classrooms for study and instruction."[25] As the siblings' investment in expanding La Peña deepened, however, conflict arose within the Parra family; Violeta disapproved of what she dubbed their "forma de vida aburguesada" (bourgeois lifestyle) as she began to embrace an increasingly divergent artistic and political vision.[26] While many *nueva canción* cultural workers, including the Parra siblings, celebrated the gradual formalization of movement venues and event calendars, Violeta mourned the decline of less scripted spectacles such as the tent shows of her youth, which mobilized spontaneous, makeshift techniques to adapt to local contexts, connect with rural audiences, and bring together diverse listening publics. Of concern for Parra was that the increasingly formal structure of the urban *peña*—specifically its institutional organization and geographic location—prevented artistic connection with *el pueblo chileno*: the popular masses that, owing to enduring cultural and class divides, were relegated to the physical outskirts and artistic margins of the modernizing city.

For Parra, *una peña* would ideally function as a staging ground for critical convocation, where impromptu practices of creative exchange might activate solidarities across a diverse range of publics. In founding La Carpa de la Reina only a year after La Peña de los Parra, then, she fashioned a physical and social space to promote these political imperatives. For example, La Carpa was sited in the unpaved, unincorporated foothills of outer Santiago, facing the Andes rather than the urban metropolis. As Ángel Parra explained, "My mother had reached a culminating point [in her life]. . . . she just wanted to be close to her people and to live, literally, with her feet on the earth."[27] And Violeta did just that. She lived in La Carpa's compound with her daughter Carmen Luisa in a two-room adobe structure built by her brother Roberto. In this sense, La Carpa's intentional collapse of public and private space— from its function as both private home and public venue to its pairing of performance stage and domestic hearth—drew on modes of feminist organizing that politicized the domestic sphere as a rich, untapped site of potential movement building. La Carpa's unique emplacement— from its peripheral geographic location, to its impermanent structure, to its collapsing of public and private spheres—promoted improvisational encounter so as to attract a broad cross section of constituencies and, ultimately, to "make space" for the organic fomentation of political solidarities across ethnic, gender, and class lines.[28]

Scholar of Latin American cultural studies Catherine Boyle has described La Carpa de la Reina "as a place for the realization of the goals of Violeta's life work, a space for creativity and apprenticeship, for teaching and learning, and for bringing dignity, recognition and renewal to the folk music, dance and art of Chile."[29] Indeed, in both aspiration and design, Parra's La Carpa was dramatically different from La Peña de los Parra and other mainstream *peñas* of the era. La Carpa was mounted in a makeshift circus tent rather than a permanent colonial structure; it was located in the unincorporated rural periphery rather than the modern city center; it was proclaimed a pedagogical hub—a "Universidad Nacional de Folklore" in the making—rather than a professional exhibition space or boutique record label; and it was considerably less "accessible" to urban Santiagans, who favored the convenient proximity of downtown venues over negotiation of the unruly, semipublic transport networks that serviced denizens of the capital's periphery. La Carpa's fundamental structural elements, which we might describe as organized around *improvised* rather than *institutionalized* modes of encounter, earned Parra the skepticism of some and the scorn of many. Rather than prioritizing institutional permanence and expansion (naturalized markers of "success" within a capitalist economy), and rather than privileging the attraction of predictable, niche audiences through the marketing of predictable, niche spectacles, La Carpa de la Reina defiantly broke with extant social and aesthetic conventions. Yet, the important political work that La Carpa performed as a site of immanent critique and alternative imagination within the broader *nueva canción* has received little public or academic attention. Few scholars and activists have contemplated the extent to which La Carpa's makeshift, improvisational structure was an intentional—and in fact ideological—territorialization of Parra's artistic and activist vision.

Parra gestured toward her fierce commitment to improvisational encounter and performance in a 1966 interview with Chilean folklorist René Largo Farías, in which she stated:

> I believe that all artists should aspire to have interpenetration as a goal, the interpenetration of their work in direct contact with the public . . . I am okay with maintaining La Carpa and working at this moment with live elements, with the public close to me, which I can

feel, touch, speak with, and incorporate into my soul. (Author's translation) [30]

Boyle is one of few to rightly aver that Parra's unique enterprise was designed to circumvent "the national and domesticated structures that had, in her experience, failed to recognize and act on the importance of the folk and the popular art of the country as a deep expression of national letters and history."[31] As Parra's daughter Isabel recalls, "su decisión de vivir en la carpa era un rechazo absoluto a lo convencional" (her decision to live in the tent was an absolute rejection of the conventional).[32] In contrast, Parra's bold rejection of gendered and class scripts of respectability, modernity, and advancement have consistently been described as the source of her individual demise rather than as an enduring critique of *nueva canción* institutions and practices that reproduced, rather than uprooted, structures of colonial-capitalist oppression. Read through a colonial-capitalist lens, La Carpa failed to achieve the markers of economic success: institutional permanence, marketability, and expansion. Indeed, La Carpa's former patrons and artists have noted at length the project's shortcomings: the establishment was inhospitable during the winter months and impossible to access by road amid periods of heavy rain. The impermanent structure likewise required vigilant maintenance: Parra's daughter Carmen Luisa recalls a severe winter storm that upended a portion of La Carpa's roof, causing her to look on in horror as her aging mother wrestled the unmoored structure amid howling winds and freezing rain. The rural locale was difficult to promote, and over time it failed to attract even steady crowds, much less the "salt of the earth" audiences that Parra craved for improvisational interaction. Unlike the traveling tent shows with which Parra toured during her youth, La Carpa did not attract Chile's working class and rural peasantry. Given this, Parra's unique performance geography has been consistently dismissed as the tragic antithesis of the "vibrant, successful, and accessible music venue" that was La Peña de los Parra.[33] As Boyle poignantly concludes, "La Carpa de la Reina was the culmination of [Parra's] development as an artist; that it failed is also the tragedy of her life's final labour."[34]

But did La Carpa in fact "fail"? Parra undoubtedly felt the emotional and logistical effects of La Carpa's unmaking. Friends and family recount that the daily battle to keep it going was exhausting, and the lack of support from neighboring communities reportedly left the artist profoundly saddened and disillusioned. These challenges were further compounded by a recent separation from her longtime companion, Gilbert Favre, and tension with her adult children. All these factors have been cited for her tragic death in February 1967, when she took her own life at her La Carpa residence. For Parra, a passionate artist and committed activist, the fact that La Carpa did not build the political, pedagogical, and performance space that she envisioned was nothing short of devastating.

The contradictions and controversies that color Parra's national repute—her rejection of "modern" urban life in Santiago, her eschewing of gendered codes of respectability and decorum, her critique of cultural and class divides, and her investment in engaging folklore as anticolonial episteme rather than colorful tradition—have been sutured together via dominant popular and academic accounts of her life's work that narrate La Carpa as her fall from public grace, descent into madness, and inability to provide respectable maternal leadership. Alternatively, I want to suggest that the internal political critiques and improvisational tactics that La Carpa aimed to address and spatialize proffer invaluable insights into both the limits and the possibilities of *nueva canción* activism, as embodied in her earlier endeavor of La Peña de los Parra. For example, what of the fact that most *nueva canción* vocalists and nearly all *nueva canción* musicians of that generation were men? And, given that many of Chile's most renowned *nueva canción* artists were also educated professionals living in Santiago, how "successful" were institutions such as La Peña de los Parra at generating and sustaining dialogue and solidarities across cultural, class, and regional constituencies? In posing these questions, I do not aim to minimize the crucial geohistorical import of La Peña de los Parra and other institutions of its kind; rather, I want to suggest that we likewise contemplate the crucial, often pathbreaking political work performed by artistic endeavors that are by design contingent, fleeting, improvised. The value of La Carpa lies not in what it achieved but rather in what it proposed: a return to the improvisational as a means of re-sounding and respatializing the aesthetic and social barriers that persisted within the *nueva canción* movement and thus inhibited its transformative potential. Read this way, Violeta Parra's astute vision— that improvisational practices of encounter and musicking can potentially disrupt divides between high and low, urban and rural, traditional and modern—remains an unsung legacy of her creative enterprise. And though La Carpa de la Reina failed to attract the political and public support that its realization would have required, it nonetheless provided both a creative vision and a geographic template for future generations of cultural workers committed to sustaining the *nueva canción* movement while activating changes within it. It is to such an example—in which artists and activists, inspired by Parra, enrooted such an improvisational performance space—that I now turn.

La Peña del Sur, 1992–2001

On a crisp evening in the summer of 1992, an extended network of Bay Area–based artists and their friends convened in the backyard patio of queer Chilean artist Alejandro Stuart's basement apartment for a night of musical revelry. Hosted in an aging Victorian rental in the residential heart of San Francisco's largest Latinx neighborhood, the Mission, this seemingly provincial event signaled the establishment of the neighborhood's first permanent *peña*, La Peña del Sur. A grassroots neighborhood venue, La Peña del Sur was envisioned as a local hub for artists, activists, and audiences to gather and share sonic, visual, and performed art; to trade relevant news and resources; and mobilize around local and international political issues.[35] With founders representing at least three generations and four regions of Latin American and Latinx artists and intellectuals, this ambitious enterprise was the product of extensive imaginative and logistical community synergies. These included the conception of a cultural center capable of operating beyond the juridical and economic purview of local authorities, as well as its "do-it-yourself" (DIY) actualization through the collective recovery of secondhand tables and chairs, the construction of a makeshift stage, and the word-of-mouth recruitment of patrons. The institution born of these efforts would endure for nearly a decade, representing a remarkable convergence of overlapping political aspirations, hemispheric histories, and diverse practices of musicking.

La Peña del Sur was envisioned and inaugurated in the shadow of various Latinx and Latin American cultural centers that had thrived in the San Francisco Bay Area since the late 1970s. Perhaps the most influential of these was (and is) Berkeley's La Peña, which has continued to exist for more than forty years as a self-described "non-profit multi-cultural organization" that "promotes and supports Bay Area, California, nationally and internationally recognized music, dance, theater, film, inter-disciplinary and visual artists."[36] Berkeley's La Peña was incorporated on September 11, 1974, exactly one year after Augusto Pinochet's military coup in Chile, and it opened its doors in summer 1975. In keeping with the tenets of the *nueva canción* movement, its pronounced mission was "to make the necessary connections between art and politics."[37] Alejandro Stuart was among the handful of exiled activists who established the center, which operated in a small rented commercial storefront on South Berkeley's Shattuck Avenue.[38] Many of La Peña's founders had been active in the Chilean *peña* scene, and some had even patronized or performed at the historic La Peña de los Parra and La Carpa de la Reina.[39]

While initially focused on Chilean art and politics, Berkeley's La Peña became a haven for Central American artists during the Dirty Wars of the 1980s, as the center's cultural workers introduced programming that linked US militarism in the Middle Americas to other, overlapping histories of US imperial and anticommunist intervention in the hemisphere. As the center's constituency grew, its leadership opted to expand and formalize the locale. By the early 1990s Berkeley's La Peña was a registered nonprofit funded by numerous federal grants and private arts foundations, and its board of directors had successfully purchased the performance space, opened an adjoining restaurant and pub, and booked an impressive calendar of acclaimed international artists.

Strikingly, La Peña de Berkeley's growing institutionalism (including its ties to external funding agencies and its formalization as a nonprofit) directly motivated the 1992 founding of La Peña del Sur. California statist politics in the early 1990s was defined by a "new nativism"—including militarization of the US-Mexican border, the passage of California Propositions 187 and 227, and the burgeoning carceral industry—that dramatically constrained the sociospatial mobility of California's immigrant populations by designating the state's classrooms, hospitals, workplaces, and social service offices as serving English-speaking, middle-class white citizens only.[40] In this political climate, the founders of La Peña del Sur expressed concern about La Peña de Berkeley's ability to serve the region's most vulnerable populations. In particular, though invested in the *peña* as a leftist institution, the founders were unsettled by how the venue's institutional structure, location, and cost limited its management and patronage to primarily documented, bilingual, middle-class Latinxs and Anglos. For Stuart and his cohort, these structural limitations breached the grassroots spirit of the Latin American *peña*, an institution they associated with popular assembly, affordable fare, and improvisational encounter.[41]

In a statement published in honor of La Peña del Sur's two-year anniversary, its founders proclaimed that given "the absence of venues within existing cultural institutions for our artistic-cultural expression, we found it necessary to form our own center, which, owing to its geopolitical orientation, we decided to call La Peña del Sur."[42] Here, *la peña's* cultural workers draw astute connections among the politics of place, the policing of difference, and expressive cultures of dissent. First, they argued that the multiculturalist turn in mainstream US cultural politics had permeated local institutions such as Berkeley's La Peña, which they viewed as increasingly disconnected from the radical political agendas from which such institutions had emerged.[43] Next, they observed that the largely international focus of programming at institutions such as Berkeley's La Peña had eclipsed local agendas that were of concern to the Mission-based cultural workers: the new wave of anti-immigrant xenophobia and legislation, the soaring incarceration rates of Bay Area youth of color, and the gentrification of Bay Area neighborhoods of color. Finally, they linked institutional formation to questions of artistic and economic access. To address these concerns, this cadre of Mission District artists and activists established a neighborhood *peña* that prioritized improvisational performance and encounter over progressive institutionalization; echoing the political vision that inspired the foundation of La Carpa de la Reina, La Peña del Sur's founders envisioned a locale that could attract a broader range of publics, facilitate spontaneous, interactive encounter, and foment multiscalar networks of grassroots organizing. Following a series of informal gatherings and late-night brainstorming sessions, the group concurred that these aims would best be realized through the creation of a different kind of venue: a "Latin American cultural center that [functioned] independent of [state] authorities and official recognition."[44]

Throughout its near ten years of operation, circa 1992–2002, La Peña del Sur functioned outside of formal relations of publicity, commerce, and regulation. Its reproduction thus required innovative, improvisational strategies of emplacement and administration. While it remained under the directorship of its cofounder Alejandro Stuart, its ongoing management and maintenance were accomplished through the collaborative efforts of La Peña artists and supporters. A programming committee tasked with the visionary and logistical labor of the center met frequently to hammer out programmatic themes, artistic lineups, and other nitty-gritty details.[45] Initially made up of Stuart and La Peña's other four founders—Puerto Rican guitarist and singer Ronaldo Rosario, Chicano musician Enrique Ramírez, Nicaraguan vocalist and guitarist Ernesto Jiménez, and Ecuadorian musician and singer Elena Alvarado—the committee would see its membership change over time.[46] Subsequent participants would include Peruvian activist Samuel Guía and Ecuadorian artist and musician Galo Paz. Changes in leadership were often the result of internal committee strife, owing in no small part to ongoing debates and dissension over the structure, management, and future of the neighborhood nitery. Yet, an abiding avowal of at least three political imperatives—echoing key organizational strategies of the *nueva canción* movement—consistently shaped La Peña del Sur's uniquely improvisational institutional architecture: first, that improvisational musicking and intercultural exchange can function as a vital means of political dialogue and convocation; next, that extemporaneous moments of collective reflection, respite, and revelry can encourage the renewal of imaginative and organizational political energies; and finally, that a venue endeavoring to incite such activities must be socioeconomically, geographically, and logistically accessible to a wide range of publics.[47]

Despite its improvisational and makeshift operations, La Peña del Sur was active nearly every Friday through Sunday of its ten-year stint in the Mission. In contrast with other cultural centers in the area, La Peña del Sur was located in a residential sector of the district. By day, the rented basement apartment that housed it was indistinguishable from its neighboring, high-density Victorian flats; at night, its conversion into a clandestine nitery was signaled only by a small wooden sign fastened to the unit's gated entrance. Because many musicians and audience members were undocumented or exiled, and because it was designed to function as a nexus for *reuniones críticas* (critical encounters),[48] promotion for La Peña del Sur was accomplished through word-of-mouth invitations, the circulation of flyers, and ads in local bilingual newspapers.[49] Strikingly, while La Peña was located within fifty miles of the global epicenter of digital technological development, its cultural workers returned to *nueva canción* technologies of promotion that were by design spontaneous, informal, and analog.

Nightly proceedings at La Peña were equally informal. Event attendees were greeted at the door by Stuart, who, in an adorned coffee can, collected sliding-scale donations (typically $2 to $5) to compensate featured artists and to offset the costs of maintaining the locale. Children attended for free, as did those who were unable to contribute financially. Guests were shuttled through Stuart's apartment—the principal hallway of which served as a makeshift gallery for local artists—to an outdoor covered patio. Adorned with holiday lights, hanging plants, and trellised vines, the festive courtyard-cum-theater seated forty to sixty guests in a miscellany of secondhand folding chairs arranged at handmade wooden tables opposite a small wooden stage. Visitors could purchase Stuart's homemade empanadas and mulled Chilean wine, as well as, on occasion, tamales or floral bouquets from vendors, transactions that sustained the neighborhood's thriving informal economy. And although "bring your own beverage" was not an encouraged practice, it was also not uncommon for contraband flasks and bottles to circulate among audience members. La Peña's grassroots orientation and informal atmosphere in no way thwarted its popular appeal; within its first two years of operation, La Peña del Sur attracted over ten thousand participants and hosted more than twenty visiting Latin American cultural workers.[50]

During its near decade in existence as an underground cultural center in the Mission, La Peña featured an impressive range of artists and events. Fridays were reserved for poetry and *canto*, literary readings that spotlighted local and visiting authors. On October 21, 1994, for example, La Peña hosted "Un beneficio para La Cooperativa de Mujeres Centroamericanas, C.R.E.C.E." (A Benefit for the Cooperative of Central American Women, CRECE), which featured "una presentación de nuestro trabajo como cooperativa y un programa de música, poesía, y lectura sobre nuestras experiencias" (a presentation about our work as a cooperative and an evening of music, poetry, and lectures about our experiences).[51] The structure of this event, like others of its kind, was that of a *taller* (workshop) rather than a formal concert or presentation, and it privileged extemporaneous interaction and dialogue. Benefits such as this one were not uncommon at La Peña; accounting for at least two evenings of its monthly calendar, they afforded seed money for community publications and projects while granting oranizations and their staff free publicity and networking opportunities.

Of equal significance was the extent to which the informal and interactive logics of social and artistic encounter(s) expanded the discursive purview of *nueva canción* activism. As Parra and like-minded cultural workers of her era observed, the spirit of unification around a shared investment in anticapitalist and anti-imperial activism enabled cultural workers to stage and sound transnational solidarities, but at times this objective was achieved at the expense of addressing questions of power and difference within and among communities of the Global South. A primary function of La Peña del Sur was to promote unlikely, informal, and impromptu modes of social and artistic encounter that confronted global schematics of imperial expansion and capitalist development and that always cut across racial, gender, sexual, and class lines. Examples of such programming are abundant; La Peña organized exhibitions ranging from reports from Latina feminists who attended the 1995 UN international women's conference in Beijing, to annual celebrations honoring

El Día Internacional de la Mujer (International Women's Day), to tribu-
tive commemorations of famed Latina feminist artists such as Amparo
Ochoa and Gabriela Mistral, to concerts to raise money and supplies
for single mothers in the community. Themed performances were also
common. During the month-long festivities honoring La Peña del Sur's
two-year anniversary in June 1994, the center featured "De la Mujers,
por las Mujers, para las Mujers . . . y los Hombres" (About Women, by
Women, for Women . . . and Men), a night of poetry, music, theater,
and testimony exploring issues of gender and inequality in Latinx communities throughout the Americas. And to commemorate its seven-year
anniversary, the center sponsored "Desde Afuera del Closet: Encuentro,
lectura de poesía y foro con autores y activistas de la comunidad gay
latinoamerica" (From Outside of the Closet: Encounter, poetry, and
forum with authors and activists of the gay Latin American community).
Significantly, programming of this kind engendered a place of encounter
and potential connection for members of distinctive activist groups and
artistic communities. Echoing Parra's vision, La Peña del Sur articulated
cancion compretida in capacious terms, embracing contradictions within
the movement and faultlines among its various practioners. In doing so,
it "made space" for feminist and queer cultural workers to engage critically with patrons from the broader Latinx Mission community.

Both local and international musical talent headlined on Saturday
nights, which were by far the most well-attended evenings. In constrast
with the logistical arrangements of other local cultural centers and concert venues, La Peña's performances were often punctuated or followed
by improvisational collaborations of featured artists and audience members, thereby troubling spatiotemporal divisions between production
and consumption, and ideological divisions between artistic virtuosity
and popular appeal. At times, La Peña included surprise "after hours"
appearances from visiting international artists who were in town to
perform at mainstream Bay Area venues. For example, Alejandro dis-
patched La Peña supporters to recruit and transport musicians from
Los Folkloristas and Inti-Illimani following performances at Berkeley's
Zellerbach Hall, inviting them to "tocar y cantar con el pueblo" (to play
and sing with the people).[52] Nights such as these produced unusual and
often cherished artistic encounters, with emergent artists performing
alongside musical giants, the repertoires dictated by rowdy audiences
who clapped, sang, and danced. In this sense, La Peña del Sur actualized
what Parra could only envision several decades earlier: the emplacement
of a locale that, through improvisational encounter and musicking prac-

tices, "made space" for otherwise unlikely artistic collaboration, pedagogical exchange, and participatory engagement.

In keeping with the tenets of new song as a transnational, transgenic mode of musical expression rooted in political solidarities rather than in national or regional genres, La Peña del Sur's monthly programming featured a stunning array of musical genres, including *música andina, rock en español,* Mexican boleros and *corridos mexicanos, música tropical, son jarocho* and *huasteco,* samba, marimba, *bomba, música afroperuana, nueva canción* and *trova, cumbia,* merengue, *bachata,* reggae, salsa, rumba, bossa nova, and *música afrocubana.* What was both rare and innovative about La Peña del Sur's approach to programming is that these musics were staged not as representations of monolithic national cultures or unified national publics, but rather as collective moments of dialogue, exchange, experimentation, and pleasure. Rather than the calculated progression of scripted performances, event itineraries were organized around spontaneous encounter—between musical genres, instrumentational arrangements, unaquainted musicians, and participatory audiences. And they always included open mic interludes, which brought emergent artists and old friends to the stage, as well as community members wishing to introduce polemics, share news, or register dissent. Late Stanford professor and poet Fernando Alegría—an active *peña* participant—once remarked, "La Peña del Sur is a site of intense Latinoamerican cultural exchange, a bit of creativity and an opening to trans-American solidarities."[53] As Alegría observed, La Peña's staging of political and cultural *intercambio* (exchange) was structured around the forging of hemispheric solidarities through improvisational practices of encounter and musicking: dialogue and dance, singing and shouting, clapping, and foot tapping collectively performed by an international, intergenerational array of cultural workers. Recalling what distinguished this project from other cultural centers in the Bay Area, Stuart remarked, "[F]or me, a peña is more spontaneous, more experimental."[54] When asked the same question, co-founder Samuel Guía added that, in holding *peñas,* "the process itself is the most important, not the product."[55] Here, both Stuart and Guía acknowledge how the foundational principles of La Carpa de la Reina influenced the structure La Peña del Sur as a cultural and political enterprise.

Read through a performance geography lens, the establishment of La Peña can be understood as the strategic emplacement of a unique location that deployed improvisational logics to confront governing techniques of spatial differentiation and immobilization. To expand, geogra-

phers and cultural critics alike have demonstrated that the (re)produc-
tion of boundaries between the body, home, and nation, and between
the foreign and domestic, sovereign and settled, is an inherently political and highly contested process. Such distinctions sediment, naturalize,
and manage raced, gendered, sexualized, and classed divisions within
and among geographies of labor, desire, knowledge, and subjectivity. By
operating in the scripted space of the domestic, and by rejecting the purview of local and state authorities, La Peña defiantly reoriented reigning
distinctions between public and private space, residential and commercial spheres, and licensed and informal activities. For some, this refusal
to embrace institutional formalization and expansion may appear to be
imprudent or short sighted. Yet, the spatial politics and practices that
(re)produced this performance geography can alternatively (and more
accurately) be read as a critique of the co-constitutive regimes of state-
sanctioned emplacement and heteropatriarchal racial capitalist management. In other words, the emplacement of La Peña del Sur within
informal economic networks and the domestic sphere, coupled with its
flexible programming and grassroots popularization, signaled a refusal
to capitulate to the social norms and state regulations that constrained
coalition-building and cross-community encounter.

The establishment of La Peña del Sur as an informal economy within
the domestic sphere was the most expedient way to launch the project.
The process of securing business permits, liquor and food licenses, and a
commercial venue would have been lengthy and expensive, and it would
have required petitioners of a particular financial and legal status. But
for Stuart and his cohort, expediency was neither the sole nor even the
primary imperative informing La Peña's design. Rather, as *peña* collaborator Galo Paz put it, the goal of the project was to create a venue for
"critical assembly . . . oriented around music rather than economy."[56] For
Paz and other cultural workers, this act of privileging musical encounter over monetary logic, and critical assembly over consumer crowds,
demanded a circumvention of the territorial techniques through which
state power was exercised at the municipal scale. Siting, zoning, permit-
ting, licensing: these banal bureaucratic procedures figured at the center of the Mission's gentrification wars, as wealthy developers and white,
middle-class professionals exerted the force of legal authority to displace
Latinx renters, eliminate small businesses, criminalize informal employ-
ment, and police local youth of color. Moreover, as California's new nativism coalesced around legislative attacks on immigrant access to public
and bilingual education, hospital care, and social services, state agencies

were legislated into sites of immigrant policing and surveillance. Thus, this refusal to emplace La Peña del Sur within sanctioned geographies of encounter and exchange can be read as a trenchant critique of the ways in which racial capitalist mediations of social space protect the wealth, security, and interests of heteronormative, white, propertied citizen-subjects. And, at a moment when most of its participants were denied full or meaningful access to institutionalized artistic resources or sanctioned venues of political expression, this unique performance geography provides a vibrant example of how *nueva canción* cultural workers mobilized improvisational practices of social and sonic encounter in their alternative terrains of artistic activism.

The improvised acts of "respatialization" that defined La Peña's unique programmatic and institutional structure enabled moments of convocation that would have otherwise been foreclosed for most *peña* participants.[57] In turn, such moments of convocation engendered ideological alliances and political action that would have otherwise been implausible or unattainable. In redefining the terrains of public and private, residential and commercial, La Peña del Sur became a place where attendant scripts concerning leisure, culture, commerce, politics, and desire could be "queerly" renegotiated.[58] The nitery's location, hours of operation (opening in the evening, after eight o'clock, and closing after festivities ended, often the following morning), and all-ages policy made it accessible to an unusual cross section of publics. Swing-shift workers, care workers, children and youth, the elderly, the undocumented, and other constituencies constrained by conventional divisions of social space collectively performed, listened, danced, drank, sang, slept, argued, and applauded from late in the evening until dawn. This intergenerational comingling among community and kin effectively destabilized many of the geotemporal roles and rules that produce and preserve the heteropatriarchal nuclear family: distinctions between gay and straight space, between adult and familial activities, between men's and women's work, and between productive and reproductive labor. Through this unsettling of normative categories of emplacement and embodiment, La Peña del Sur cultivated vibrant political dialogue, artistic exchange, and (in the best of moments) nascent coalitions across inter- and intracommunity divides.

Central to the staging of these conversations and interactions was La Peña del Sur's strategic reconstitution of cultural production and community reproduction not only as habits of leisure but also, more importantly, as generative opportunities for activist work. The center's colocation of recess and rabble-rousing allowed working-class Mission residents with scarce free time to combine moments of political dialogue and organizing work with opportunities for respite and revelry. La Peña del Sur's cultural workers developed this unique programming structure with the practiced awareness that similarly structured *nueva canción* events had historically been held in local *peñas*, regional festivals, and international *encuentros populares* (popular encounters), where they were crucial to the recruitment of large and diverse crowds, the renewal of waning political energies, and the spontaneous formation of coalition. Central to the actualization of La Peña as an alternative performance geography was the mobilization of music as method: its deployment as both an organizing tool and, as Paz observed, an organizational schema.

While La Peña del Sur echoed many of the tenets of the *nueva canción* movement and its hallmark institution, the *peña*, the cultural center also adapted itself to the geopolitical contingencies of its context: its position in the urban Global North, its location in a neighborhood in transition, and its *pueblo* of diverse migrant subjects. As noted above, these differences of historical and geographic context enabled La Peña's cultural workers to confront some limitations of *nueva canción* discourse, which, in its privileging of particular "unities," failed to effectively grapple with how the colonial-capitalist system it so trenchantly critiqued is always already constituted through relations of racial, gender, and sexual difference. As a nexus for the performance of sonic and visual cultures, La Peña del Sur convened an impressive range of artists and media representing divergent political interests and affiliations, aesthetic techniques and concerns, and generational trends. Yet, its organizers embraced the fragility and unpredictability of such conventions. Whereas historical *nueva canción encuentros* had emphasized ideological continuity and presumed universal political agendas, La Peña del Sur was constituted and celebrated as a place of *(des)encuentro*: a site of convocation that, through musical performance and artistic exchange, embraced disorientation, discord, and disjuncture.[59]

As a place of *(des)encuentro*, La Peña del Sur became a site of both personal encounter and political fragmentation. It was a place where Farabundo Martí National Liberation Front (FMLN) poets collaborated with Mission Chicano youth to perform political rock *en español*; where Andean and Afro-Peruvian musicians came together to perform *huaynitos* and dance *festejo*; where internationally renowned musicians like Los Folkloristas and Inti-Illimani became the audience of "undiscovered" talent of Mission youth; where queer performance installations brushed up against photo exhibits of *iglesias católicas*; where prison abolitionists gabbed with immigration reformists; where the local homeless folks ate free empanadas and toasted with the self-proclaimed intelligentsia. My use of the word *(des)encuentro*, which can loosely be translated as a failed meeting, a temporary mix up, or an ongoing disagreement, signals the inherent, productive contradictions of such a "contact zone."[60] It acknowledges the inevitable losses, confusions, and failures of recognition that mark the "encounter" of socio-sonic differences, as well as the coalitions that can be built on the foundations of such unlikely, disorienting, often painful yet urgent confrontations. Through these improvised practices of social and sonic *(des)encuentro*, La Peña came to function as what cultural critic Josh Kun has called an "audiotopia": "identificatory "contact zones," . . . [that] are both sonic and social spaces where disparate identity-formations, cultures, and geographies historically kept and mapped separately are allowed to interact with each other as well as enter into relationships whose consequences for cultural identification are never predetermined."[61]

Some Conclusions

La Carpa de la Reina and La Peña del Sur were cultural institutions established at distinctive geohistorical junctures: the former, amid the pan–Latin Americanist struggles of the Cold War period, and the latter, in response to the new nativist era of border militarization and anti-immigrant revanchism in California. Yet, despite their distinct contexts, La Carpa and La Peña were both bound by and constituted through hemispheric histories of networked migration and displacement, transnational art and agitation. Taken together, these cultural collectives provide provocative flashpoints within the rich if understudied archive of *nueva canción* activism in the Americas, demonstrating how cultural workers have built, sustained, and critiqued this vibrant anticapitalist, anti-imperialist hemispheric movement that has persisted for six decades. Strikingly, despite the breadth and reach of this creative foment, its intercultural, transgenerational reproduction has often relied on unscripted, makeshift, and ephemeral expressive practices of social and aesthetic encounter. For some *nueva canción* cultural workers, as we saw in the cases of La Peña de los Parra in the 1960s and La Peña de Berkeley in the 1970s, improvisational modes of cultural activism were viewed as temporary tactics to be utilized only until more permanent and formalized institutions could be established. But for others, improvisational practices of encounter and musicking were the utopian premise and material lifeblood of this cultural current. For cultural workers such as Violeta Parra or Stuart and his cohort, improvisational convocation and *canto* (singing) were viewed as invaluable tools not only for expanding the *nueva canción* movement, but also for "making space" to address relations of power and difference within it by generating accessible terrains of aesthetic innovation and oppositional action.

La Carpa did not enjoy the popular support that its prolongation would have required, but it did provide a valuable model for how the growth of, and interventions within, the *nueva canción* movement night be improvised. La Peña del Sur is but one example of cultural centers inspired by Parra's vision, and the political and artistic work accomplished throughout its duration attests to how improvisational practices of social and artistic encounter could effectively diversify the movement and expand its artistic and political engagements. I want to conclude my discussion of these unique socio-sonic projects by highlighting the critical insights that they offer to future modes of cultural activism.

First, this history exemplifies the importance of cultural production as a means of combining localized sites and moments of leisure and play with urgent political and theoretical work. In the case studies historicized herein, improvisational practices of encounter made possible the blurring of labor and leisure time, eventually making the *peña* accessible to and engaging for a wider range of publics. The auditory *(des)encuentros* of La Peña del Sur, for example, persuasively demonstrate how improvised musical encounter can productively enable socio-sonic linkages between the global and the local, the written and the oral, the historical and the present, the dystopic and the imaginative.

A second important insight to be drawn from the history of La Carpa de la Reina and La Peña del Sur regards the importance of forging activist communities that do not assume stable or monolithic political affiliations but rather maintain a constant commitment to addressing the contingencies of heterogeneity, contradiction, and difference. For many *nueva canción* cultural workers, improvisation has served as a pedagogy of social and sonic encounter that has enabled this type of work within the broader movement, such that colonial and capitalist structures can be examined both horizontally and vertically, both within communities and nations as well as between Global North and Global South. As a site of *(des)encuentro*, La Peña del Sur persuasively illustrates that a popular cultural movement can only meaningfully be sustained through a return to the internal and external contradictions that edify and explain relations of power and difference.

A third important lesson to be gleaned from the history of La Carpa de la Reina and La Peña del Sur concerns how, when, and where various political agendas can and should be imagined and activated. Throughout La Peña's near ten years of operation, its organizers and participants engaged in heated debates over conceptions of sustainability as they relate to the limits and possibilities of institutionalization. On one side of the debate were those that viewed La Carpa's rapid demise as a cautionary tale and lobbied for the securing of a permanent, licensed locale in order to grow and expand La Peña del Sur. Proponents of La Peña's institutionalization argued that it would enable greater community participation and ensure the long-term sustainability of the venue. On the other side of the polemic were those who viewed La Peña del Sur's situatedness in the Mission District's informal economy as an opportunity to engage in modes of performance, dialogue, and exchange that circumvented disciplinary mechanisms of state power and the logics of racial capital accumulation and development. In the end, the latter constituency won out: *la peña* remained an ephemeral, extra-economic affair until it concluded its tenure on Harrison Street. Those who view expansion and permanence as markers of political success might argue that the closing of La Peña del Sur's doors in 2002 represented a failure or loss for San Francisco's Latinx community. But for activists like Stuart, this *peña* project was an overwhelming political victory in that it made physical and ideological space for convocation, conversation, creativity, and coalition. In this sense, informality, ephemerality, and improvisation can be viewed as La Carpa's greatest pedagogical legacies and La Peña del Sur's greatest political strengths. We might understand the failed fruition of the former and the closure of the latter as expressions or effects of shifting economic conditions and political urgencies. At the dawn of the new millennium, the demographics of the Mission District neighborhood dramatically shifted, owing to the combined effects of recession and gentrification. In that context La Peña del Sur achieved what La Carpa set out to accomplish: it provided a space of social and sonic encounter that embraced the *nueva canción* movement's genre-bending aesthetics while confronting its internal divides and contradictions. The spirit, solidarities, and insights that these experimental enterprises engendered live on in the innumerable creative projects that they spurred, the artists that they fostered, and the subsequent emplacements of cultural activism they seeded.

Notes to Chapter 2

Parts of this chapter appeared in *On Site in Sound: Performance Geographies in América Latina* published in 2018 by Duke University Press.

1. The term *nueva canción* first gained traction in Latin America at the end of the 1960s. As music scholar Jan Fairley rightly asserts, it is an "all-embracing term, an umbrella under which much music and many musicians shelter." See Fairley, "La nueva canción," 107. While the intellectual and artistic origins of the movement were rooted in earlier periods, this "countersong" movement combined traditional Latin American folk genres and with politicized lyrics to unite students and the urban working and rural peasant classes. *Nueva canción* spread across Latin America and the Caribbean in the 1960s and 1970s when musicians joined the Indigenous, mestizo, and African mass uprisings that called for an end to state militarism and US intervention; see Zolov, *Refried Elvis*. In this sense, as music scholar Jane Tumas-Serna puts it, "more than a musical style, [*nueva canción*] signifies an ideological stance." See Tumas-Serna, "The 'Nueva Canción' Movement," 139. For a discussion of the movement's origins in the Southern Cone, see Carrasco Pirard, "The Nueva Canción"; and Reyes Matta, "The New Song."

2. Heble and Caines, *The Improvisation Studies Reader*, 2.

3. These migrants established a vibrant ethnic enclave in the Telegraph Hill basin. Dubbed "Chilecito," it endured through the late 1880s, when white nationalist revanchism left the neighborhood in ashes and forced its inhabitants into other pan-Latino barrios, such as Rincon Hill. See Bevk, "Chilecito."

4. See Nasatir, "Chileans in California."

5. Musicking is a term developed by Christopher Small to describe musical production as a dynamic, interactive process. See Small, *Musicking*.

6. See, for example, Fairley, "La nueva canción"; Morris, "Canto porque es necesario cantar"; Reyes Matta, "The New Song"; Tumas-Serna, "The 'Nueva Canción' Movement"; and Carrasco Pirard, "The Nueva Canción."

7. Fischlin, Heble, and Lipsitz, *The Fierce Urgency of Now*; Heble and Caines, *The Improvisation Studies Reader*; and Lewis and Piekut, *The Oxford Handbook*.

8. Stanley-Niaah, *Dancehall.*

9. In addition to Stanley-Niaah's illuminating book, works that have influenced my thinking on the relationship between performance and space include Nash, "Performativity in Practice"; Thrift, "The Still Point"; and Houston and Pulido, "The Work of Performativity."

10. See Tumas-Serna, "The 'Nueva Canción' Movement"; and Fairley, "La nueva canción."

11. For an exhaustive history of the birth and spread of *nueva canción* throughout the Southern Cone and, later, to northern regions of Latin America including Brazil and the Caribbean, see Carrasco Pirard, "The Nueva Canción in Latin America"; Morris, "Canto porque es necesario cantar"; Tumas-Serna, "The 'Nueva Canción' Movement"; and Fairley, "La nueva canción." Most authors trace the roots of this movement to Argentina and Chile specifically, but as I have argued elsewhere activities in these countries were deeply influenced by Andean

folklore from Peru, Bolivia, and Ecuador, which circulated through radio air-waves in decades prior. See Dorr, *On Site, In Sound.*

12. See, for example, González, "Chile y los festivales."

13. For example, the discography of Inti-Illimani includes albums entitled *Si Somos Americanos* (1969), *A la Revolución Mexicana* (1969), *Canto de Pueblos Andinos,* vol. 1 (1973), and *Chile Resistencia* (1977).

14. Carrasco Pirard, "The Nueva Canción"; Moreno, "Violeta Parra"; and Reyes Matta, "The 'New Song."

15. Jara, liner notes to *Canto Libre.*

16. García, "En busca de la carpa de Violeta Parra."

17. All translations are the work of the author except where otherwise indicated. See Garrido, "La Peña de los Parra según Ángel" (italics added).

18. Garrido, Mónica. "La Peña de los Parra según Ángel," http://culto.later cera.com/2017/03/11/la-pena de-los-parra-segun-angel/

19. Parra, *El libro mayor,* 206.

20. Dillon, *Violeta Parra,* 2.

21. Ministerio de las Culturas, "Biografía."

22. Parra, *El libro mayor,* 30.

23. Rodríguez Musso, "La Peña de los Parra," http://www.abacq.net/imag ineria/disc003.htm

24. Ibid.

25. Author's translation of: "La gran casa, que fue creciendo como las legendarias casas de la novela latinoamericana, de haber sido un simple taller de artistas varios, se transformó en verdadera academia de la canción y la artesanía. Comenzó con dos pequeñas salas pero con el tiempo tuvo altillo, comedores, parrón, sala de discos y tienda de tejidos, salas de estudio e información." See Rodríguez Musso, "La Peña de los Parra."

26. Parra, *El libro mayor,* 142.

27. Angel Parra, qtd. in also Parra, *El libro mayor,* 142.

28. In the words of historian Patricia Vilches, "El plebeyo toldo de lona fue el experimento social de Violeta; deseaba reunir a ricos y pobres para enseñarles sobre el auténtico folklore chileno" (The canvas tent was Violeta's social experiment; she wanted to gather the rich and poor in order to teach them about authentic Chilean folklore). Author's translation. Vilches, "Violeta se fue a los cielos de Andrés Wood," 65.

29. Boyle, "Violeta Parra," 174.

30. Author's translation. Subercaseaux and Londoño, *Gracias a la Vida,* 79.

31. Boyle, "Violeta Parra," 180.

32. Author's translation. Parra, *El libro mayor,* 142.

33. Boyle, "Violeta Parra," 178.

34. Boyle, 174.

35. La Peña del Sur was located in the lower Mission District on Twenty-Second Street at Harrison. During its period of operation, the Mission was a vibrant Latino neighborhood with substantial Chicano/Latino communities originating from Mexico, Central America, South America, and the United States. Following the Silicon Valley boom in the mid-1990s, however, white middle-class gentrifica-

tion shifted the district's demographics dramatically. Today, none of the activists or cultural workers discussed in this chapter reside in the Mission area.

36. La Peña Cultural Center, "About La Peña."

37. La Peña Cultural Center.

38. Casasús, "Alejandro Stuart."

39. Alejandro Stuart, email correspondence, June 13, 2012.

40. For an extensive discussion of the politics of new nativism, see Perea, *Immigrants Out!* For a detailed discussion of the increased militarization of the US southern border, see Dunn, *The Militarization of the U.S.-Mexico Border, 1978–1992.* For border-making as a spatial process, see Nevins, *Operation Gatekeeper.* California Proposition 187, which denied "illegal aliens in the United States from receiving benefits or public services in the state of California," was passed by an overwhelming voter majority in November 1994. For a detailed discussion of the ideological and economic rationalization and ramifications of Proposition 187, see Calavita, "The New Politics of Immigration." California Proposition 227, which was legislated four years later, required all public-school instruction in the state of California to be conducted exclusively in English. Proposition 187 was repealed in 2014; Proposition 227 was repealed two years later.

41. Galo Paz, personal interview, June 14, 2014; and Samuel Guía, personal interview, June 12, 2014.

42. "La Peña del Sur," *New Mission News,* 65.

43. Guía, interview; and Stuart, email correspondence.

44. Stuart, email correspondence; and Samuel Guía, email correspondence, June 13, 2012.

45. Paz, interview; and Guía, interview, June 12, 2014.

46. Alejandro Stuart, email correspondence, October 28, 2009.

47. For a more in-depth discussion of these organizational strategies, see Fairley, "La nueva canción"; Tumas-Serna, "The 'Nueva Canción' Movement"; and Reyes Matta, "The New Song."

48. The term *reunion* can connote a meeting or a house party. Here, the concept is invoked in its dual senses, suggesting that leisure and social time might be combined with critical political work.

49. Advertisements for La Peña del Sur's weekly lineup were featured in *Horizontes,* the *Reporter, New Mission News,* and *Cambio.*

50. "La Peña del Sur," 65.

51. La Peña del Sur flyer, created by Alejandro Stuart. Flyer Box M132 (June 1994) Stanford University Special Collections.

52. Alejandro Stuart, email correspondence, October 28, 2009.

53. Casasús, Mario. "Alejandro Stuart: Tengo el archivo mas completo de la nueva canción latinoamericana."

54. Interview with artist, June 12, 2014.

55. Guía, interview.

56. Paz, interview.

57. Here, respatialization refers to the creative reorganization of imposed spatial boundaries.

58. Here I use Siobhan Somerville's method of queer analysis. See Somerville, "Queer."

59. See Cornejo, "Desencuentros."
60. See Pratt, *Imperial Eyes.*
61. Kun, *Audiotopia,* 24.

Works Cited

Bevk, Alex. "'Chilecito,' or San Francisco's Little Chile." *Curbed San Francisco,* October 15, 2012. https://sf.curbed.com/2012/10/15/10317694/chilecito -or-san-franciscos-little-chile
Boyle, Catherine. "Violeta Parra and the Empty Space of La Carpa de la Reina." In *Violeta Parra: Life and Work,* edited by Lorna Dillon, 173–88. New York: Tamesis Books, 2017.
Calavita, Kitty. "The New Politics of Immigration: 'Balanced-Budget Conservatism' and the Symbolism of Proposition 187." *Social Problems* 43, no. 3 (1996): 284–305.
Carrasco Pirard, Eduardo. "The Nueva Canción in Latin America." *International Social Science Journal: Makings of Music* 34, no. 4 (1982): 599–623.
Casasús, Mario. "Alejandro Stuart: 'Tengo el archivo más completo de la nueva canción latinoamericana.'" *El Clarín,* March 26, 2015. https://elclarin.cl/arc hivo/2015/03/26/alejandro-stuart-tengo-el-archivo-mas-completo-de-la-nue va-cancion-latinoamericana/
Cornejo, Giancarlo. "Desencuentros con la identidad en el movimiento LGBT peruano." *Periódicus* 3, no. 1 (2015): 170–82.
Dillon, Lorna. *Violeta Parra: Life and Work.* New York: Tamesis Books, 2017.
Dorr, Kirstie. *On Site, In Sound: Performance Geographies in América Latina.* Durham, NC: Duke University Press, 2018.
Dunn, Timothy J. *The Militarization of the U.S.-Mexico Border, 1978–1992: Low-Intensity Conflict Doctrine Comes Home.* Austin: University of Texas Press, 1996.
Fairley, Jan. "La nueva canción latinoamericana." *Bulletin of Latin American Research* 3, no. 2 (1984): 107–15.
Fischlin, Daniel, Ajay Heble, and George Lipsitz. *The Fierce Urgency of Now: Improvisation, Rights, and the Ethics of Cocreation.* Durham, NC: Duke University Press, 2013.
García, Gabriela. "En busca de la carpa de Violeta Parra." *La Tercera,* August 7, 2011.
Garrido, Mónica. "La Peña de los Parra según Ángel." *Culto,* March 11, 2017. http://culto.latercera.com/2017/03/11/la-pena-de-los-parra-segun-angel/
González, Juan Pablo. "Chile y los festivales de la canción comprometida (1955–1981)." *Boletín Música* 45 (2017): 5–23.
Heble, Ajay, and Rebecca Caines, eds. *The Improvisation Studies Reader: Spontaneous Acts.* London: Routledge, 2014.
Houston, Donna, and Laura Pulido. "The Work of Performativity: Staging Social Justice at the University of Southern California." *Environment and Planning D: Society and Space* 20, no. 4 (2002): 401–24.
Jara, Victor. Liner notes to Victor Jara, *Canto Libre.* Odeon LDC-36726, 1970. LP.
Kun, Josh. *Audiotopia: Music, Race, and America.* Berkeley: University of California Press, 2005.

La Peña Cultural Center. "About La Peña." Accessed June 12, 2014. http://la
    pena.org/about-lapena/

Lewis, George, and Benjamin Piekut, eds. *The Oxford Handbook of Critical Improvi-
    sation Studies*, vol. 1. Oxford: Oxford University Press, 2016.

Ministerio de las Culturas, las Artes y el Patrimonio. "Biografía." Violeta Parra
    100 años (website). Accessed July 2, 2020. https://www.violetaparra100.cl/bi
    ografia/

Moreno, Albrecht. "Violeta Parra and La nueva canción chilena." *Studies in Latin
    American Popular Culture* 5 (1986): 108–26.

Morris, Nancy E. "Canto porque es necesario cantar: The New Song Movement
    in Chile, 1973–1983." *Latin American Studies Association* 21, no. 2 (1984): 117–
    36.

Nasatir, Abraham P. "Chileans in California during the Gold Rush Period and
    the Establishment of the Chilean Consulate." *California Historical Quarterly*
    53, no. 1 (1974): 52–70.

Nash, Catherine. "Performativity in Practice: Some Recent Work in Cultural
    Geography." *Progress in Human Geography* 24, no. 4 (2000): 653–64.

Nevins, Joseph. *Operation Gatekeeper: The Rise of the "Illegal Alien" and the Remaking
    of the US-Mexico Boundary*. London: Routledge, 2001.

New Mission News. "La Peña del Sur, una plataforma para el talento latinoameri-
    cano: Dos años de lucha cultural en el barrio de la Misión." December 1997.

Parra, Isabel. *El libro mayor de Violeta Parra*. Madrid: Ediciones Michay, 1985.

Perea, Juan F. *Immigrants Out! The New Nativism and the Anti-Immigrant Impulse in
    the United States*. New York: New York University Press, 1997.

Pratt, Mary Louise. *Imperial Eyes: Travel Writing and Transculturation*. New York:
    Routledge, 2007.

Reyes Matta, Fernando. "The New Song and Its Confrontation in Latin Amer-
    ica." In *Marxism and the Interpretation of Culture*, edited by Cary Nelson and
    Lawrence Grossberg, 447–60. Champaign: University of Illinois Press, 1988.

Rodríguez Musso, Osvaldo. *La nueva canción chilena: Continuidad y reflejo*. Havana:
    Casa de las Américas, 1988.

Rodríguez Musso, Osvaldo. "La Peña de los Parra." In *Cantores que Reflexionan*,
    Madrid: LAR ediciones, 1984, http://www.abacq.net/imagineria/disc003
    .htm, Accessed July 17, 2019.

Small, Christopher. *Musicking: The Meanings of Performing and Listening*. Middle-
    ton, CT: Wesleyan University Press, 1998.

Somerville, Siobhan. "Queer." In *Keywords for American Cultural Studies*, edited
    by Bruce Burgett and Glenn Hendler, 203–7. New York: New York University
    Press, 2014.

Stanley-Niaah, Sonjah. *Dancehall: From Slave Ship to Ghetto*. Ottawa: University of
    Ottawa Press, 2010.

Subercaseaux, Bernardo, and Jaime Londoño. *Gracias a la vida: Violeta Parra:
    testimonio*. Buenos Aires: Editorial Galerna, 1976.

Thrift, Nigel. "The Still Point: Resistance, Expressive Embodiment and Dance."
    In *Geographies of Resistance*, edited by Michael Keith and Steven Pile, 124–51.
    London: Routledge, 1997.

Tumas-Serna, Jane. "The 'Nueva Canción' Movement and Its Mass-Mediated Performance Context." *Latin American Music Review / Revista de Música Latino-americana* 13, no. 2 (1992): 139–57.

Varas, José Miguel, and Juan Pablo González. *En busca de la música chilena: Crónica y antología de una historia Sonora,* vol. 4. Santiago: Editorial Catalonia, 2005.

Vilches, Patricia. "Violeta Parra: Her Museum and Carpa as Spaces of Nostalgia." In *Mapping Violeta Parra's Cultural Landscapes,* edited by Patricia Vilches, 103–17. Cham, Switzerland: Palgrave Macmillan, 2018.

Vilches, Patricia. "Violeta se fue a los ciclos de Andrés Wood: El naufragio de La Carpa de La Reina." *Revista Internacional d'Humanitats* 29 (September–December 2013): 63–80.

Zolov, Eric. *Refried Elvis: The Rise of the Mexican Counterculture.* Berkeley: University of California Press, 1999.

THREE | "We Are the Ones Who Are Impatient"

Improvising Resistance and Resilience in
Jordanian Hip-Hop and Rap

BEVERLEY MILTON-EDWARDS

Discourse and case studies on sound and conflict emerge from and engage with recent developments in critical studies in improvisation.[1] Critical studies in improvisation also help explain why sound, of various types, is so important in studies of conflict, especially in how it creates alternative ways of knowing and being known through creative risk-taking.

The case study of Jordan that is the focus of this essay forms one fragment of a wider comparative project funded by the UK government under the Arts and Humanities Research Council (AHRC), titled "Sounding Conflict: From Resistance to Reconciliation." This broader comparative project includes the Middle East, Brazil, and Northern Ireland. These sites serve as a basis for evaluating how sound is used to articulate experiences of violence, to support narratives of resistance or resilience, and to promote conflict transformation and reconciliation. The duality of the conceptual framework of improvisation and resistance/resilience highlights specific political conditions through which I analyze the use of sound and music in circumstances where hegemonic authority of the state attempts to silence oppositional voices. This research also addresses a constantly evolving global security environment in which hip-hop and rap music in the Middle East is perceived by political and socioeconomic elites as a threat rather than as a means (particularly for young people) of resistance or an arena for the shared dialogue so necessary to sustaining practices of resilience or reconciliation. This perception that hip-hop and rap are a menace changes their role in sites of exceptional conflict and violence and reduces their usefulness as a vehicle for humanitarian intervention, community building, and conflict transformation within programmatic approaches that seek to build social cohesion among young people by state and nongovernmental organizations alike. I posit, however, that the music of Jordanian hip-hop and rap artists such as The Synaptik offers a powerful vehicle to not only aid young people in such circumstances but also expose the weaknesses of those that claim hegemonic power over them.[2] This music also supports them in making sense of their experiences of conflict and transcends the barriers that are a consequence of forcible displacement and legacies of refugeeism.

In the case of hip-hop and rap in Jordan, this chapter assesses improvisation in terms of community, and social practices as cultural activity.[3] Improvisation here refers to more than a musical performance. It also includes the ways performance contexts are improvised and the ways that knowledge meanings within the wider environment of political and social suppression are subject to ongoing, often fragile moments. I am not so much qualifying the use of the term *improvisation* as I am proposing it as a descriptor of a layered practice engaging with site-specific knowledge production as found in the contested sonic practices associated with hip-hop and rap in the contemporary Middle East.

In this case study, we will see evidence that improvisation is a form of "creative social practice [that] allows for the full spectrum of possibility, including failure . . . that [has] found [its] way into a specific moment" as a means of both resistance and resilience against prevailing social and state norms in the Jordanian context.[4] The performers, performances, and audience experiences I examine deploy forms of risk-taking and encounter that pit participants against state agents as well as private business and social elites. Performance assumes implicit, rather than overt, political signification and consists of strategic messaging in ways that displace state attention from performers articulating alternative or subversive points of view. Yet, when the improvisatory spontaneity of being in the moment or "in the zone" takes over, resistance and resilience, as I shall explain in the following pages, are evident and are released in ways that highlight the political and transformative underpinnings of what are usually highly coded musical practices.

Moreover, in this case study, improvisation assumes new meaning in relation to resilience among refugee and forcibly displaced communities in authoritarian state contexts.[5] Indeed, the majority of the performers discussed here are refugees or their descendants. For example,

Palestinian refugees and their descendants in Jordan account for as much as 70 percent of the population, and more than two million of them still reside in UN-run refugee camps.[6] The experience of enforced displacement is also apparent among more than a million Syrian refugees and tens of thousands of Iraqi, Sudanese, and other refugee populations in Jordan.[7] In this respect, unprecedented levels of displacement as a result of ongoing conflicts in the Middle East inform an "agenda in which arts become part of a larger network tracing the entire human condition" of improvisation and give rise to programmatic and policy alterations among humanitarian and development nongovernmental agencies.[8]

Like Derek Bailey, I think of improvisation(s) in terms of musician and audience response to an event.[9] This frame allows for contextual analysis against the wider socioeconomic and political milieu of a site—specifically the multifaceted, complex dynamic of hip-hop and rap in Jordan in relation to authoritarian, neoliberal, postcolonial, and strategic dependencies of this state and both internal and geopolitical realities. This case study, then, sees improvisation as a sociopolitical, countercultural artifact, a practice that expresses and embodies socioeconomic and political relationships in the Jordanian context. Moreover, improvisation's sonic enactments are analogous to the everyday experiences of youth in Jordan and the power relations that subject young people within that state. In this essay, then, I outline what improvisation means in terms of resistance and resilience in a time of political uncertainty and displacement, as embodied by individual performers. To paraphrase Meki Nzwei, Israel Anyahura, and Tom Ohiaraumunna, what I examine here is how the Jordanian state's "cultural sonic preferences" are at significant odds with the development of hip-hop and rap.[10] The state's configuration of the musical is sympathetic to social preferences for tribally informed and folkloric sounds that align with state self-interest. In this respect hip-hop and rap are countercultural. Ironically the Jordanian state's cultural-sonic preferences are, in many respects, inauthentic—reflecting instead colonial and imperial mimicry, epitomized by the presence of Scottish bagpipes, massed bands, and marching drums in state-managed amphitheaters in towns like Jerash, their performances "marketed" for consumption by tourists rather than citizens. This kind of music is clearly promoted by the state as more constitutively true of Jordan's culture than the creative outputs of its own young citizens in the hip-hop and rap scenes. Site-specific forms of hip-hop and rap in Jordan respond to this milieu, producing unanticipated resonances in the sounds associated with the genre and the performers' improvisatory practices.

The war, conflict, and authoritarian governance that have shaped the Middle East as constitutive of large numbers of forcibly displaced populations should be considered when developing an intimate understanding of how resilience occurs among the current generation of youth, where the majority encounter the everyday on the margins of society rather than at its center. Such resilience is predominantly sourced from peer-based social support networks and can also demonstrate how factors such as hope and steadfastness (*samud*) help youth meet adversity. The majority of youth in Jordan contend with the myriad dimensions and effects of enforced displacement and the dynamic, highly contested spaces of diaspora and refugeeism.[11] What arises from these contexts is a kind of salmagundi improvisation derived in resistance to coercive social, economic, and political contexts enacted against the vast majority of Jordanian youth. Hence its aspirational emancipatory or liberating effects.

Point of Entry

As the taxi speeds from Jordan's main airport into the center of Jordan's capital city, Amman, it takes me on a familiar route. I am on a highway teeming with traffic. As I head toward my destination, familiar sights such as falafel shops and Amman's famous "circle" interchanges reassure me and reinforce a sense of timelessness. If I were to carry on into the city center and terminate in Amman's "real downtown" in front of the small but crowded Husseini mosque plaza, near the markets and ancient Roman amphitheater, that sense of immutability would be reinforced. Five years, a decade, twenty or thirty years or more ago that same journey could have been traced in all-too-familiar detail and completed by a visit to Al Quds Restaurant for a plate of the Jordanian national dish, *mansaf.*

But for once the journey does not finish at this age-old destination. Instead, the taxi enters an area of Amman known as Abdali, or more specifically an area of Abdali designated the "new downtown." It is symbolized in PR and marketing campaigns featuring modern glass and steel high-rises and actualized as a paean to private capital and neoliberal economic visions.[12]

The taxi driver and I are entering unfamiliar territory. We struggle to navigate our way. Both he and I crane our necks and gaze at the carefully planned new buildings and the canyon-like spaces within the Abdali Boulevard and its vast new shopping mall, cafes, restaurants, and high-end hotels. Gated entries and barriers to street openings funnel us around a CCTV-monitored route where we can only be deposited on the outside of the Boulevard complex.

When I leave the taxi, I must pass through a set of security checkpoints that remind me of Northern Ireland and the Troubles, when we lived in a city where the center was typified by security barriers and gates. The vista before me is absent of people. I listen to my own footsteps echo as I move around from one "level" to another, passing empty shop fronts, performance spaces, and cafes. This emptiness strikes me as strange in a city bursting at the seams in terms of demographic density and the mounting pressures on housing, infrastructure, and services from local citizens and refugee populations. I notice that there are more uniformed security officers standing sentinel at all the barricaded entry and exit points than visitors or shoppers.

Sonic Urban Spaces

The soundscape of this "new downtown" stands in quiet distinction to the "real downtown" just some twelve minutes away from me.

The Boulevard has no crowd of busy shoppers thronging the thoroughfare with their clothes rustling, their plastic bags crinkling, their children crying or pleading for juice or candy. No potential buyers stand at shop stalls and carts fingering fruit or feeling the cloth of dresses and jackets for sale and then engaging in vigorous bartering with the shopkeepers or vendors. Nor is anyone there to listen to the competing sonic beats of radios and CD players or the megaphoned repetitive and rhyming exhortations of merchants informing shoppers of the bargain of the day. In the "real downtown," the repetitive footfalls of the thousands of people that occupy the space vie with the call to prayer from the nearby Husseini Mosque, the heavy traffic resonances of motor engines and honking horns made by the drivers of cars, taxis, vans, and buses in the congested streets. Men and women, young and old, employed and unemployed, citizen, migrant, and refugee contribute to the soundscape of the space.

The sonic atmosphere back at the Boulevard does not "welcome" the local but is designed to provide familiarity and comfort for the global-oriented visitor and tourist.[13] Sound in this new urban space also contributes to a global rather than local projection and highlights the disparities and exclusions that stand in contrast to other areas of downtown Amman, which are much more complex, layered, and ambiguous.[14] The global projection is inherent to the project of the Boulevard, financed by foreign capital and marketed as a tourist destination, even including an airport-style duty-free shop where only foreign passport holders can buy alcohol and luxury goods.[15]

Soon, however, the Boulevard's soundscape begins to change. At the amphitheater area young men, and a few women, start to set up for the evening's upcoming events. They set up mixing decks, speakers, and sound systems and lay down cabling. The music technicians engage in a series of sound tests that have the effect of a sonic ricochet bouncing quickly off of the tall buildings around us. These sounds reinforce the constricted feel of the sonic space. Hardly anyone is there, and hardly anyone is paying attention. No one stops in his or her tracks as the assemblage of sound and motion begins to unfold. No one is arrested by the sounds and the samples of music tracks that break the near silence of the afternoon. It is as if a "deaf ear" is being thrown, and the sterile ambient atmosphere is almost impenetrable.

Eventually, people begin to fill the space. From one side of the street, I see one of the Jordanian rappers—The Synaptik—rushing to meet up with some visitors. He has a shopping bag full of mics, headphones, and leads. He has brought this equipment with him to use in an impromptu recording session with some Syrian refugee teenagers. The Synaptik and a small group of French Syrian refugees had worked with these young refugees in a hip-hop and rap workshop earlier in the year.[16] A recording studio will be improvised in a hotel room so that some tracks can be created and laid down for production to take place later. Close by, DJ Sotusura totes a bag of vinyl with him in hopes of getting a chance to play the records on the decks being set up, while MC Satti is using the opportunity of the sound test to hit some beats with the mic and "feel" the sound in the virtually empty amphitheater.

Weaving between tables are the chain-smoking administrators and organizers of the Institut français de Jordanie (IFJ) Amman Hip-Hop Festival. The Franco-Jordanian Chamber of Commerce is a sponsor and exhibitor, and—as Philippe Lane asserts—I am witnessing the IFJ as a "transmitter of culture," promoting a consciously composed and commercial image of France.[17] France was also the proactive element in this 2017 event, interacting with Jordanian governing authorities in ways that the local participants and contributors were unable to do alone. It was clear that IFJ created the festival to achieve a number of institutional aims and objectives reflecting soft diplomacy, French cultural identity, and representations of French state and commerce in Jordan. France's power—as an external, former colonial state—allowed the IFJ to effectively dictate the event presentation, with minimal concern for localized conceptions of culture, music, community and the political. In his public comments at the opening of the event, the French ambassador emphasized the festival as a "celebration of modernity."[18] It was unclear, though, whose modernity he was talking about.

Although the ambassador said that the French ambition was for all events to have free admission and be occasions for access to art and culture for "all without any exception," in reality the strictures concerning access to the Boulevard space would dictate constraint and exclusion. French ambition for the event produced a constitutive tension through its targeted demographic: the young people (including most notably young men) who constitute the majority of Jordan's population. Jordan's neoliberal development project, in contrast, envisions spaces for consumption, entertainment, and shopping that exclude, often deliberately, young men. Their presence is widely considered to be a form of threat and social nuisance. Governing authorities and decision-makers rely on their own narratives about social norms and customs to ban young men from certain spaces—including the Boulevard.[19] Such views also cohere with analyses of the "jihadi" and "home-grown" "terrorist" threat in Jordan, which is perceived as manifest in the milieu of male youth.[20]

The French organizers of the festival were unaware of the ban and the problems this presented in terms of recruiting performers and attracting audience members. Jordanian artists and performers alerted them to this problem, and the organizers then had to make deputations to the local authorities to allow for a temporary lift of the ban. They possessed an agency in relation to power that the excluded youth simply did not have.

As the sun began to set, the experiment in Arab hip-hop and rap unfolded. The small stage area was a slightly raised platform in the basin of the Boulevard's own amphitheater. Black plastic–covered seating cubes mushroomed up. At the edges of the stage area, advertising "cubes" were placed for local mobile photo provider Orange, commercial radio station MoodFM ("Where Music Lives Forever"), and one of the station's local competitors, BeatFM. Yet, around the performance space was an air of unease. One of the French planners admitted to me that they were out of their "comfort zone." While cultural events organized as part of the projection of French presence (and power) in this Amman outpost were not unusual, this event was. "We never tried something like this before, never hip-hop and rap," said the French woman as she puffed away on her cigarette in a state of anxiety. "Usually we have a French pianist or French jazz performance for such a festival. This is the first time we have French and local hip-hop and rap artists and we don't know how it will go. It is a risk."[21]

Spontaneity and Agency in Improvisation

Some dimensions of critical improvisation studies emphasize spontaneity. Rebecca Caines and Ajay Heble alert us to the importance of "spontaneous acts of creativity"—such as the hip-hop performances of Amman— to "offer resources for hope and social transformation," especially in contexts of deeply contested politics.[22] Indeed, the events of the festival were an opportunity for spontaneous performance moments to exert agency, to subvert power, to offer alternative states of being that in turn offered hope and enacted emancipation no matter how short lived.[23] As The Synaptik reflects, "I think improvised rhymes on *the spot* and *in the performance* are more raw, sometimes more melodic, but definitely, they are more emotionally delivered because they are *in the moment* and this is a liberating experience."[24]

It became apparent that for The Synaptik the event was an opportunity to perform at a venue that was usually prohibited not only to him but also to his friends and fans. For him, this concert was a big deal. And access to the venue was an even bigger deal. Under usual circumstances, male youths like The Synaptik, his friends, and his music base were barred from entering. This time was different—kind of. As The Synaptik explains: "at first, there was a group of people who came from [the town of] Irbid to the [security] gate and they [security at the Boulevard] were not going to let them in. So, I got a call and I went and we got them let in . . . they are not normally allowed in on any other night."[25] It is clear that their entry is a form of unprecedented victory.

When his friends and fans begin to arrive, they seek The Synaptik out. They hug, take photos, and phone their mates, thus signaling to a wider cohort the energy and actuality of the event taking place. The spontaneity is thus transmitted to a wider audience, a set of forcibly displaced participants who can't come to the performance because they don't have the money to travel to Amman or they fear that they will make the journey only to be denied admission.

Those actually attending gradually surround the stage and stand along the steps of the amphitheater. They distinguish themselves from the "ordinaries" and "accidental" audience of Others in a variety of ways. First, their dress style and code are visibly different. Many of these guys— there are few young women among them—are dressed in skinny jeans, basketball vests, leather jackets, snapback caps, and high-tops. They have customized their stonewashed denim jackets with embroidered patches and badges and matched the red of their leather bomber jackets with their trainers. Initially, their caps are pulled down low over their foreheads, shadowing their eyes and obscuring their faces. It is as if they want to be an anonymous audience. Second, they are there to dance. But this is not traditional Jordanian *al-dabke* style dancing, which in state-produced cultural narratives is promoted as an authentic "Jordanian" cultural product. In that milieu, traditional Arabic musical tropes such as *zajal* (folk songs), state-manufactured "bedouin," and *al-dabke* performances are firmly tied to normative national identity discourses that are constructed and harnessed by the state to induce societal compliance.[26] Hence, state actors, governing authorities, and societal leaders in Jordan—with few exceptions—tend to look at hip-hop, rap, and the necessary contingencies of improvisation by artists like The Synaptik and hip-hop dancers as a social and political threat. I'm told that rappers are scorned, surveilled, harassed, and threatened by the secret police (*mukhabarat*) and regularly refused spaces to perform or practice. Here at the event, however, through improvised practice, the performance space and audience are transformed, with each instantly and sometimes simultaneously adapting to the opportunities that the event presents. The fans and supporters become performers in their own right: some individually, and some in a series of brief improvised sequences of dance and movement. Street-style dance including breaking, locking, roboting, mirroring, and popping is performed to the sound-check tracks and music excerpts ahead of the main performances by rappers Liqid and The Synaptik.

Music Makes Me Wanna Dance

In a political context of authoritarian rule and conservative social norms, these emergent dance and music practices refuse to engage or even play with "tradition." The dancers are in the zone and appear to exist beyond the dystopian present, where their being is displaced and marginal to power. Down on one side of the performance stage, I watch as a core group of about six young guys break out from among their friends and start dancing. They execute moves for the obvious enjoyment of one another. Often the dance is a duet, an interaction where one guy watches his friend and then replies back with his own steps. They improvise some of the dance to the music. The DJs and MCs who remain above the amphitheater seem to also see the dances unfold before their eyes and spontaneously begin to change the tracks and music that they are playing as if to encourage and ease the opportunity for this improvised performance.

At points, the people on the decks try to ascertain whether the guys below want to dance to specific tracks. Within the improvised dance are sequenced moves. Around the dancers is the rest of the group, who embrace and hug them. They also whoop and chant as the dance progresses. And when the performance is finished, they applaud and call for more. Ciphering here has echoes of Steve Coleman's contention that music and "performance" are "part of a process," with music and dance being "constantly in motion" and sometimes captured as a "snapshot." As Coleman states, "this music is for everyone who can hear it but it is especially for the brothers and sisters in the streets. Hear, Feel, Know."[27]

The dancers are becoming performers. As performers, they nod to one another, and every now and then one or two of the bolder dancers turn to face and interact with the audience of the amphitheater to take his bow, to take either side of the collar of his jacket and turn it up in pride as the audience cheers on. The audience, which by now consists mainly of young men, interacts in moments of intimacy with the dancers. Its members encourage, permit, and amplify the moment that is taking place before their eyes. They do so by moving their own bodies, shouting out to the dancers and applauding them with encouragement; they are also filming, taking pictures, and sharing these shots instantly on social media. Their mobility in relation to the sonic environment is an open form of public defiance that is rarely seen. It has broken free of the strictures of governance. These dances and dancers embody youth resistance in a space that is usually controlled by private business and the state. Through such dancing, youth perform resistance and undertake a "spatial acting-out of place" that, to quote Michel de Certeau, enacts "crossing, drifting away or improvisation . . . [to] transform . . . spatial elements" in urban Amman.[28] This occupation of space playfully mocks the supposed utility of the Boulevard and its projection of ordered forms of consumption and culture, identity and belonging.

The impromptu dancers break back to the front and the first steps of the amphitheater to pause awhile, chat, rest, and even recover before they return to the area they have claimed for themselves. They are projecting fun, positivity, and hope. This is resilience embodied in dance. This is a freestyle moment, "shared and developed," as H. Samy Alim contends, "by a community of interactive" dancers, DJs, MCs, rappers, and the audience.[29] Each time they perform, layers of clothing are peeled off like armor and their baseball caps get pushed back farther from their faces, as they warm to the atmosphere and enjoy the good-will of the growing crowd of spectators. The mask of anonymity is slowly discarded. Ciphering is also a practice in this context and is constitutive of both dancers and performers as they face off and create a communal experience of musical encounter. As The Synaptik states, "I think it's a fun way to practice and enjoy yourself doing what you love doing, which is rapping in my case, also, it turns it into this collective act which helps it become more of a movement than just an art."[30] This communality allows everyone space, and it fosters free-flowing circulation and morphing around the stage, onto the stage, and off again. Small circles of performance are illuminated and made meaningful by other performers, the audience, and the guys in charge of the music decks or the mics.

As the moment extends, something entirely spontaneous and improvised occurs. One group of hip-hop dancers moves, and is not stopped from moving, onto the roped-off area of the stage. It becomes clear that the stage crew and sound mixers in the higher reaches above are assisting, as the sound is turned higher and the audience orients now toward the stage. Sound changes, and so too does the improvisational approach to the music and its audiences. This is a polyvalent, situated set of practices between those mixing and making music. Culture and community are transformed through the interactions among the dancers and the dancer-audience. Sound, and in particular music, changes in this context, with its meaning extended to understandings and practices of being. Familiar beats are mixed to create ownership and empowerment among a contingent group. It is a symbolic challenge to the hegemonic space and bordering of space representing control by the state and neoliberal forces. A local social geography spontaneously produces a polyethnic hybrid of music, generating new sounds. The unexpected contingencies of the hip-hop festival and the encounter between uninvited dancer-performers emerge as an improvisation against that which has come before.

Improvisation and Boundaries

Hip-hop and rap artists like The Synaptik generate forms of rhythm that are dynamic. Such contributions are reinforced among rappers and producers to build a set of counternarratives of resilience to the sonic, musical, and performative environment in which they have grown up.[31] These counternarratives threaten forms of hegemonic ordering that have employed sound and music to build and reinforce the state and control of identity therein.[32]

Enforced dislocation and rupture experienced through direct or descendant histories of refugeeism is also evident in the attempts of such artists to produce and disrupt the protonational cultural arenas in which they reside. In the example of The Synaptik—whose real name is Laith Al Huseini—musical identity and biography are an intimate interweaving of his being both Palestinian/Jordanian and a refugee. His parents are Palestinian refugees living in East Amman, and Laith identifies his musical lineage as rooted in a Palestinian tradition:

> Well, my uncle is a famous Palestinian singer, he is like the biggest in Palestine, like for folk song, *hadday* music.[33] His name is Mousa Hafez. He'd like come here every time one of my cousins had a wedding. He would come and sing and so I like grew up around this kind of folk music. So, my mum's family are like a "*Al Hadday*" family, my grandfather and my uncle's sons they all do this music, *al-dabke* and *al-hadday* and singing at weddings. My mom wanted to be a singer, but she couldn't of course. She had a beautiful voice and she would always tell me stories about how she wanted to go to Egypt to study acting and singing but she could never do that. Yeah, so like singing and this stuff was ok in our house. It was never frowned upon. The voice was in the house . . . my mom would sing . . . not rap though [ha-ha] and I just listened to Eminem and stuff.[34]

Although musicking generally reproduces some sort of power, this hip-hop and rap performance is a momentary act of resistance through a rhythmic form. This act is creative and increasingly accumulative as it transcends national boundaries and speaks to lives lived in almost perpetual dislocation, displacement, and refugeeism. It is deeply indicative of the aesthetic of the improvised. The Synaptik emphasizes how improvisation works for him as the artist, and for his audience.

> It is definitely very different, the dynamic of the scene, yeah our music has changed because the situation [Arab Spring/post-Arab Spring] has gone in different ways. . . . We are no longer explicitly talking about Palestine/Syria because the themes of our dislocation, are the same. The audience is the same, linked directly through displacement, or through a generation of refugeehood. Like, I am a third-generation refugee. So, the audience interprets the songs for themselves in this way. So really the topic and the main theme is about

overcoming. I might actually be wrong about what my audience inter-
prets but for me . . . it's like a message to keep being resilient and to
prevail. Yeah, it's also a bit pessimistic and cynical, but at the same
time it is not nihilistic. It's about how shit the situation is but about
overcoming, yeah, steadfastness [*samud*] this is the mood of [our]
songs.[35]

Here the importance of improvisation is emphasized in relation to how
communities or specifically youth build resilience in the wake of mass
or enforced dispossession and displacement. Furthermore, improvisation is an opportunity for the "third generation" to overcome and resist
physical and geographic barriers enforced by occupying powers and
state actors, barriers that would otherwise separate and fragment shared
identity, community, and belonging. The music—"the songs," as The
Synaptik claims—helps young people feel relevant to themselves in contexts of social and political shunning. Improvisation becomes "a strategy
to circumvent the expected, the constraints of imposed structure, the
monoculture [of state-mediated] histories that forget" this core constituency of the region.[36]

It is evident that a form of community—frequently cooperative but
also competitive—has been established through these improvisational
practices of hip-hop and rap among the current generation. Artists and
audience members apply their own interpretations of American hip-hop
as resistance and conscious rap to their social circumstances to create
an alternative to the dystopian present that surround such youth. This
application and interpretation is not "pure" or complete. It is partial
and in turn reflects the accessibility to the resources of hip-hop and rap
that other, particularly Western, cultures now take for granted. It is about
the everyday experiences and the limits of agency enjoyed or employed
by young people themselves. They are using their music, improvisation,
and forms of performance to expose and find sources of resilience in
their everyday lived experiences of forced displacement, legacies of conflict and the postcolonial state, refugeehood, authoritarian governance
practices, corruption, and endemic and institutionalized practices of
exclusion at the level of society, economy, and politics.[37]

Improvising Daily Life and Identity

Put a bullet in the head of Lawrence then rode on my camel
Till I reached the Jordan river washed my hands in holy water

Shot a hundred fucking ISIS then I started to do the turn-up
Let me finish this falafel then just finish up this warm-up
I'ma about to murder everything, murder everything
I'm doing Dabkeh with the flow, with rows of fucking Bedouins
They say that we the terrorist, well I'ma about to scare you!
Fuck with the middle of the Middle East I double dare you!
  The Synaptik, "Middle of the Middle East"

As refugees or their descendants, hip-hop and rap artists like The Syn-aptik employ music to explore their identity and engage with the politi-cal.[38] This identity, evident from the lyrics of The Synaptik's "Middle of the Middle East," is multilayered, fluid, contentious, and resistant, and it plays with exogenous practices of Orientalist stereotyping.[39] The colonial "Lawrence" (of Arabia) is eradicated through the symbolic act of vio-lence, while the religio-political present is lambasted with the references to the "River Jordan" and ISIS. ISIS, the Islamic State, is rejected and eradicated through the sound of the "bullet" and the "shot" of the gun. Palestinian identity is inherent in the references to falafel (subject to cul-tural appropriation as the national food of Israel) and the now-familiar trope of *al-dabke* dance. The verse is not a paean to culture and identity in Jordan but a rebuke to the ways in which it is imposed, constructed, and reduced. In addition, identity is a fluid mixture of optimism and pes-simism that reflects hope and joy, anger, desperation, depression, and ultimately a desire to overcome adversity. The Synaptik states,

> This is the struggle of daily life and people can relate to that. I don't write about it in this way specifically, but people know it is the same experience for them too. It's the same for everyone and it's the same frustrations too. By the society, injustices, radicalization, lack of educa-tion, the *wasta*,[40] the tyranny, the injustice. Everyone is going through this more or less . . . they are going through it the same. It's not so conscious but yeah, I think at the end also that everything we do is political—even music—even "bragging" music is political because it emphasizes a different kind of context.[41]

Through their encounter with hip-hop and rap such Arab youth use music to provide forms of commentary and narrative that address the realities of displaced (and frequently urban) youth who contend with political, social, and economic inequalities and the psychological scar-ring inherent in experiences of displacement, refugeehood, and identities of not belonging.[42] Yet, because of the authoritarian frame that governs their lives, they are sometimes too scared to blatantly indict the system. Artists like The Synaptik use subversion to begin to resist a system that is predicated on national, ethnic, socioeconomic, and religious hierarchies in communities such as Jordan where identity, nation, and refugeehood are contentious.[43]

In the song "Bedhom," featuring Emsallam and Shouly (and produced by Al Basha), The Synaptik addresses the "struggles of daily life includ[ing] the effect of society and religion on the everyday experience."[44] The Synaptik's sense of futility and the resilience this feeling demands is apparent in the following lines of the song:

> *The movie isn't long,*
> *We are the ones who are impatient,*
> *There is no problem with the sound,*
> *We are the ones with the perforated eardrums,*
> *Our life is flavorless like a boiled chicken,*
> *A crisis after crisis like bazooka shells,*
> *Fatigue fatigue, we're accustomed to it,*
> *They took our shares and did not compensate,*
> *a77a* [Egyptian colloquial for Fuck]

The Synaptik and these other artists know that they must be resilient within a system that barely includes them and that functions through hegemonic practices and "systemic barbarism."[45] They also appreciate the impact of language and the forms of language they employ.

The Language of Resistance and Resilience: Improvising Speech and Lyrics

Traditional practices of improvisation engage with language. Agency and choice of language make "sound change" in the manifestation of realism in Arabic hip-hop and rap because these forms are constantly mediated by language and the debate about the authentic self versus the postcolonial Other. The Other engages (and is often expected to initiate the first encounter) with hip-hop and rap in English or in French. Arab and Arabic-speaking hip-hop artists and rappers like The Synaptik address an experience of tension in terms of the language of expression, representin', and authenticity. The Synaptik understands the role that the English language plays, especially for artists just starting out. His first encounter with the music was with the American and African American rap scene. His encounter narrative is connected with the colonial culture of English in Jordan and its enduring legacies. Sound thus changes in relation to this language, hitched as it is to a colonial legacy of domination, conflict, war, and the dispossession of hundreds of thousands of Palestinians, many of whom are the majority constituent elements of the population in Jordan today. The Synaptik acknowledges his conscious imitation and mimicry as part of this initial encounter. "I originally rapped in English." But he also addresses the uncomfortable feeling it gave him and the pressures that he felt to transition from rap in English to rap in Arabic. "If it's in English then I am contributing in some way to my own inauthentic self."

This experience reflects what Terkourafi refers to as "establishing authenticity of the genre, as well as of oneself as a representative of it." She declares that this, "then amounts to a gesture of emancipation from these multiple lineages, and a declaration of one's own unique identity and right to exist as an independent new identity."[46] For rappers like The Synaptik this "emancipation" struggles to go beyond customs of "gestures" in English but establishes forums of authenticity and relationship in Arabic. Once the audience is local and contained within the realm of Arabic then more meaningful collaboration with fellow travelers takes place. This is limitless in possibility and reinforces the primacy of the audience as local rather than message as global. This localizes culture even when the method of transmissions such as SoundCloud or YouTube is global. It relieves these artists of a tension frequently apparent in postcolonial discourses of language and identity. As Williams contends, "through localization of hip-hop culture, the artists are re-defining what it means to be . . . in terms of language choice and self-expression" and political form too.[47]

As The Synaptik explains of his song "Thalathat Wujouh" ثلاثة وجوه—إنتاج يدخن (produced by Smokable), "this track is about wanting to leave the Middle East, and about the refugees' journey in those boats to Europe. And about the longing afterward for the lost countries and how it is a void that you can never fill."[48]

> I've been pushed from one shoulder to another, stepped on, stood up, alienated, from all this world
> Leave the ظ Letter for Arabs I'm leaving for the ZAZA land, where the propaganda is fresh, and freedom is a new catch,
> It's okay I'd sleep in the cold, as long as my neighbors don't care what I do in my bedroom, Forget the "he said she said," forget the prison sentence, and the "supreme leader," and shit on radio in the morning, in the Arab land where we only rest after we die.

I've reserved a spot at the checkpoint, was in a hurry so I had to park in the
  handicapped area, write "Arabeezi," on my passport forget about the classic
  font,
Leaving the land to laugh, and drink bitter estrangement, it's better than
  drinking air strikes, in a curfew neighborhood,
And now we sing for the motherland from afar, "oh your soil, your sun, your
  land. . . ." Nostalgia, brings us near, like a feeling of hope after the storm
  zoloft, we have fallen into the trap. . . .
. . . And the sea, let you waves hug our kids because the land has betrayed
  us, the land has betrayed us

These lyrics (translated by The Synaptik for the author) exhibit localized themes, but they are not rooted in patriotic or nationalist brands; they address wider political exigencies of status—marginalized, excluded, displaced, and stateless—and global themes of migration, conflict, and security.[49] Such a product encapsulates both a desire to be and a desire to depart.

At work in the act of cultural transmission here are appropriations of transcultural practices that can commence as mimetic Americana but that become, through processes of improvisation, a fusion of Arabic rhyme, poetry, oral traditions, and beats. Take for example the hip-hop and rap festival organized in Amman. In representin' and presentin' themselves, the youth who perform, attend, and dance look to all intents and purposes like proponents of contemporary, American hip-hop and rap culture. By using their bodies to display what are recognized as American-inspired "authentic" hip-hop and rap clothing brands such as OBEY and PYREX, these young Jordanians transmit signals of both inward belonging and outward difference in the site-specific context. It is only perhaps in the intimation of army green camouflage jackets, the wristbands in the red, black, green, and white of the Palestinian flag, and the "peace" T-shirts that local preoccupations may be detected.

The personal becomes political as rappers like The Synaptik fashion words and catchphrases to transmit messages of resistance, resilience, overcoming, banality, fun, and ambition. Witness the lyrics of The Synaptik's "Different Times" (produced by Al Basha):

Man, I love Rap,
But the odds are depressing,
Why do I have to dream big then wake up in the desert?
Why do you need a message just to listen to my record?

I swear to god this shit is hard and I'm so close to saying fuck,
But I know that I can't escape it,
Get back to writing rhymes when the walls start caving

This song reveals a need to nuance and speak in codes and metaphors in order to share with the audience a joint experience and endurance of oppression. Here, a complex transmutation of cultures is at work in the improvisational possibility of hip-hop and rap, which promise resistance but speak to the reality of contemporary being in a Middle Eastern state where the majority of the population is young but is marginalized and excluded from socioeconomic and political power.[50]

This opportunity for performing, creating, and improvising music is grounded in a site-specific and mediated environment where the interconnected meanings of sound and hip-hop and rap are mimetic but distinct. The practices at work here are creatively coproduced but also reveal tensions among musicians and their surrounding contexts. Here class, national background, and freedoms come into play within the stratified social milieu of Jordan, with its "East Bankers," tribes, "bedouin lore," Palestinians, and refugee populations of Iraq and Syria. This context creates a rich site of situated improvisatory practices that are evident in hip-hop and rap. Identities of resistance and resilience flow within and across these groupings to establish very different performance situations even as autonomy is difficult to claim. This is an event horizon that is created and determined by others but in which opportunities for cocreativity, resistance, and mutation become apparent.

Rap *Rihla*

The Synaptik's *rihla* (journey) in improvisation is still underway. He has something to say about where and how improvisation is situated within his realm of musicking.

> For me, improvisation is coming up with the content on the spot, either the words, the melodies, or the whole thing together. It [improvisation] is definitely present in my process of making music, I improvise the initial melody of how I want the song to sound like on the beat. Lyrically, it is also present, sometimes I come up with whole lines on the spot, sometimes I come up with a great analogy or an idea for a line that I can work on later and turn into a final line. I think it can be a way to communicate the culture of confrontation to the masses.[51]

Within his performances, The Synaptik experiments and engages in improvisatory processes, contemporaneous coproduction, and collaborations with other rappers, DJs, and producers. Rap battles, for example, provide a vibrant and energetic forum to present that which is composed and prepared beforehand while embracing the moment onstage when improvisation becomes necessary to score a point against the opponent.[52] For him, hip-hop and rap are a continuous and (often exhausting) journey of improvisation. Whether he is writing lyrics and rhymes above a chicken shed on the outskirts of Amman, performing at the French cultural extravaganza in the "new downtown" of the city, making beats in a studio on Rainbow Street, or performing onstage at the Palestine Music Expo (PMX) in Ramallah, he is creating and cocreating in his artistry.

For The Synaptik, as for so many other Arab youth, hip-hop and rap music, performance, production, and interaction are forms of resistance that make their own point of entry. Nevertheless, these young people and artists are constantly challenged by a lack of access to resources, sociability, and spaces where they are welcomed. Hence, they demonstrate their resilience by creating and honing their cultural product, overcoming these obstacles and the dire circumstances of war, conflict, enforced displacement, dislocation, and the authoritarian state that are the everyday experience. For the most part, such artists have little by way of musical training. Instead, they have an improvised route into the realm of music itself. This is a territory where they find a way to make a two-bar loop, create beats, and draw sounds and samples together. "It was the beat of the computer game machines that I heard as a high school student and, of course, Eminem himself that first spoke rap to me," says The Synaptik. "Then I started myself. I started singing and making M-beats with a cheap pair of headphones and some crappy software on my computer." From this kernel of artistry and improvisation came a voyage into performance. The act of putting it out in public was an encounter with fear—not so much fear born of the audience of peers but rather fear bred by life in a tightly controlled surveillance state. "The first time was really scary. I was shaking, literally shaking," says The Synaptik.[53]

The process of explication is just that—a process. Positions and political resistances are undertaken. Opposition to authority grows through performance and through the subsequent responses of society and governing authorities to this performance. Through their music, these artists take up an argumentative position, reconnaissance into the contentions of politics such as endemic corruption and unemployment in Jordan. The axioms of power and resistance, however, largely remain intact.

Enemy State Subordination

Here in Amman, and through hip-hop and rap, Arab artists are creating spaces within a dominant cultural frame for something that is far more improvised, fluid, and transcendent of their geopolitical reality. They have attempted to walk under the cover or shade of relations with state-mediated forms of culture but have run afoul of political, social, and cultural norms that fail to truly include or accommodate them. Their sense of outsider status leaves such performers and artists disconnected.

They want full inclusion but know the price they will have to pay, so they reject it at the same time. They are in a state of constant evolution and improvisation as they use their hip-hop and rap statements, beats, and rhythms to both reflect the activist messages of African American hip-hop and rap and voice their own defiance, framing, signification, and liminal occupation of the temporal space and oppressive state. Henry A. Giroux describes such contexts as "hollowed out," as the state "shifts its emphasis away from providing for people's welfare, protecting the environment, and expanding the realm of public good, it relies more heavily on its militarizing functions and the criminal justice system as a model for how to manage and contain populations with a wide range of public spheres."[54]

Youth in Jordan, as with other states in the Middle East and North Africa, live in authoritarian contexts. Their cultural products, particularly music, are contained and regulated.[55] The popular culture universe is populated by artists that the hip-hop artists and rappers reject as nothing more than saccharine for consumption. For them, mainstream music does not reflect their daily struggles or those of their parents and grandparents before them. Indeed, cultural artifacts of Arabic poetry and literary traditions are also absented from this popular form of saccharine pop music of the *habibi* (my love) type.

Yet, increasingly, historical iterations of Arabic poetry and literature are sampled into some Arabic hip-hop and rap. This is music for the masses but not for mass consumption, as the state ensures that it continues to be seen as nonrepresentative and marginal. The social commentary embedded into the Jordanian hip-hop and rap scene implicitly critiques the authoritarian state, or occupation, for the violence and the enforced displacement of populations. This critique is not something that the state will embrace and explains why governing authorities are so hostile to this music. As The Synaptik observes, "we have grown up watching the struggles of our parents, of our families who are distanced from us by war and conflict and we know we are a lost generation. We know what has been denied us by the governing authorities in terms of rights, opportunities, and a future. I am not talking about one, two, or three young people but thousands and millions of us."[56] This generation of Arab youth sits on the margins of their own society.

So, it may be contended that within some iterations of Arabic hip-hop and rap a generation of youth inhabit a cosmos where they can articulate their experiences and sense of community in a medium that they enjoy some autonomy and power over. This music is identity formation by and for youth. It is a new form of resistance, with which the state and governing authorities must contend. These forces have variously attempted to co-opt it and subvert it, but usually they just work to prevent it. Such music forms repertoires of resistance for a generation of young people who have come of age amid a region in turmoil and a time in which the largest instances of forced displacement in the last century have taken place. It is in the lyrics, performance, and production of such music that acts of resistance are occurring.

Improvisation as enacted by Jordanian hip-hop artists and rappers is an opportunity for insight into youth in this context and the creative dimensions of risk-taking that are foundational to their milieu. These dimensions of risk-taking are evident in case studies that emphasize critical improvisation as part of a global practice of cultural, socioeconomic, and political (non)dialogue. Yet sound changes and accrues a meaning in the Jordanian context that is unique. As we have also discovered on the "Sounding Conflict" project, most contemporary studies on conflict and the arts emerge from arts-based disciplines. The research for this case study, in contrast, starts in the social sciences and seeks to construct a bridge to the humanities through critical studies in improvisation, in order to understand the integration of sociopolitical and emotional dynamics and effects that are produced by music-making, sound art, and the performance of narratives of conflict. Such socially engaged and site-specific practices offer a key mechanism for investigating relationships between the political, socioeconomic, and aesthetic dimensions of conflict experiences, rooted in forms of political activism, civic engagement, and community building. Improvisation allows us to be alert, in this case study, to the powerful intersections of hip-hop and rap music, conflict, and political dynamics.

* * *

The Jordanian rappers explored in this case study use their music to speak to and connect with the daily forms of resistance and resilience building that shape their identities and the music they make. Navigating upheaval, protest, disruption, dislocation, and uncertainty, these artists use hip-hop and rap not only as a vehicle of resistant expression but also as a transcultural practice of diasporic identity that encompasses resilience. These insurgent musical practices form telling sites of dissonance at odds with the localized state power and more global authorities seeking to contain them. Among those engaged in hip-hop and rap, improvisation is a vital way of being and affirming their identities, but also a tactic for testing agency, action, and resilience in the shadow of an authoritarian state working to limit liberty and emancipatory expression for the majority of its youth.

Notes to Chapter 3

1. A professor of politics at Queen's University Belfast, Northern Ireland, the author is also a co-investigator in "Sounding Conflict: Resistance to Reconciliation," a multi-year project funded by the UK Arts and Humanities Research Council (AHRC). The author expresses her thanks to Arab hip-hop artists and rappers, producers, managers, and their community of fans and supporters. Without them this research would not have been possible.
2. Fanon, *The Wretched of the Earth.*
3. Said, *Culture and Imperialism.*
4. Fischlin and Porter, "Improvisation and Global Sites of Difference," 16.
5. Atallah et al., "Decolonizing Qualitative Research."
6. UNRWA, "Where We Work."
7. UNHCR, "Jordan Fact Sheet."
8. Fischlin and Porter, "Improvisation and Global Sites of Difference," 2.
9. Bailey, *Improvisation.*
10. Nzewi, Anyahura, and Ohiaraumunna, *Musical Sense and Musical Meaning,* 6.
11. Dal Pra, "A Refuge for Refugees."
12. Parker, "Tunnel-Bypasses and Minarets of Capitalism," 116.
13. Daher, "Neoliberal Urban Transformations in the Arab City."
14. Ababsa, "Social Disparities and Public Policies in Amman."
15. Al Rabady and Abu-Khafajah, "Send in the Clown."
16. Dahi, "Wameed."
17. Lane, *French Scientific and Cultural Diplomacy,* 35.
18. "French Week Brings Paris to Amman," *Jordan Times.*
19. Milton-Edwards, *Marginalized Youth.*
20. Yom and Sammour, "Counterterrorism and Youth Radicalization in Jordan."
21. Neyrat Manyon, IFJ administrator, Amman, Jordan, personal interview, October 18, 2017.
22. Caines and Heble, *The Improvisation Studies Reader,* 2.
23. Fischlin, Heble, and Lipsitz, *The Fierce Urgency of Now.*

24. The Synaptik (Laith Al Huseini), Amman, Jordan, personal interview, August 3, 2018.

25. The Synaptik (Laith Al Huseini), Amman, Jordan, personal interview, October 18, 2017.

26. Massad, *Colonial Effects*.

27. Coleman, liner notes to *The Way of the Cipher*.

28. Certeau, *The Practice of Everyday Life*, 98.

29. Alim, *Roc the Mic Rights*, 93.

30. The Synaptik, interview, August 3, 2018.

31. McDonald, *My Voice Is My Weapon*.

32. Shalhoub-Kevorkian, *Militarization and Violence against Women*.

33. The *hadday* sing *hadadi* and far'dwi songs at Palestinian weddings, reinforcing culture and traditions from past celebrations.

34. The Synaptik, interview, October 18, 2017.

35. The Synaptik.

36. Fischlin and Porter, "Improvisation and Global Sites of Difference," 3.

37. Massad, *Colonial Effects*.

38. Maira, "We Ain't Missing."

39. Milton-Edwards, *Contemporary Politics in the Middle East*.

40. *Wasta* is broadly defined as being reliant on networks of influence of family, friends, and other social groups to access power.

41. The Synaptik, interview, October 18, 2017.

42. Gana, "Rap and Revolt in the Arab World," 32.

43. Milton-Edwards and Hinchcliffe, *Jordan*.

44. The Synaptik, interview, October 18, 2017.

45. Evans and Giroux, *Disposable Futures*, 126.

46. Terkourafi, *Languages of Global Hip-Hop*, 7.

47. Williams, "We Ain't Terrorists but We Droppin' Bombs," 68.

48. The Synaptik, interview, March 23, 2018.

49. Milton-Edwards, *Marginalized Youth*.

50. Milton-Edwards.

51. The Synaptik, interview, August 3, 2018.

52. Talty, "Meet the Middle East's Battle Rap Gods."

53. The Synaptik, interview, October 18, 2017.

54. Giroux, "Zero Tolerance," 59.

55. LeVine, "Music and the Aura of the Revolution."

56. The Synaptik, interview, October 18, 2017.

Works Cited

Ababsa, Myriam. "Social Disparities and Public Policies in Amman." In *Villes, pratiques urbaines et construction nationale en Jordanie*, edited by Myriam Ababsa and Rami Daher, 205–31. Beyrouth, Lebanon: Presses de l'IFPO (Cahiers de l'Ifpo), 2011.

Alim, H. Samy. *Roc the Mic Rights: The Language of Hip-Hop Culture*. New York: Routledge, 2006.

Al Rabady, Rama, and Shatha Abu-Khafajah. "'Send in the Clown': Re-Inventing Jordan's Downtowns in Space and Time, Case of Amman." *Urban Design International* 20, no. 1 (2015): 1–11.

Atallah, Devin G., Ester R. Shapiro, Nidal Al-Azraq, Yaser Qaisi, and Karen L. Suyemoto. "Decolonizing Qualitative Research through Transformative Community Engagement: Critical Investigation of Resilience with Palestinian Refugees in the West Bank." *Qualitative Research in Psychology* 15, no. 4 (2018): 489–519.

Bailey, Derek. *Improvisation: Its Nature and Practice in Music.* New York: Da Capo Press, 1992.

Caines, Rebecca, and Ajay Heble, eds. *The Improvisation Studies Reader: Spontaneous Acts.* Abingdon: Routledge, 2015.

Certeau, Michel de. *The Practice of Everyday Life.* Berkeley: University of California Press, 1984.

Coleman, Steve. Liner Notes to Steve Coleman and the Metrics, *The Way of the Cipher*, BMG 74321316932, 1995. M-Base. Accessed July 5, 2020. https://m-base.com/recordings/the-way-of-the-cipher/

Daher, Rami. "Neoliberal Urban Transformations in the Arab City: Meta-Narratives, Urban Disparities and the Emergence of Consumerist Utopias and Geographies of Inequalities in Amman." *Environnement urbain/Urban Environment* 7 (2013): 99–115.

Dahi, Rémy. "Wameed, a Project That Gives Voice to Those Who Are Reduced to the Word 'Refugee.'" *Takam Tikou*, 2017. http://takamtikou.bnf.fr/vie_du_livre/2017-07-20/wameed-un-projet-qui-donne-une-voix-ceux-que-l-on-r-du it-au-mot-de-r-fugi-s

Dal Pra, Amelia Marie. "A Refuge for Refugees: The Historical Context and Socioeconomic Impact of Palestinian Refugees in Jordan." *Global Tides* 11, no. 1 (2017). https://digitalcommons.pepperdine.edu/globaltides/vol11/iss1/4

Evans, Brad, and Henry A. Giroux. *Disposable Futures: The Seduction of Violence in the Age of Spectacle.* San Francisco: City Light Books, 2015.

Fanon, Frantz. *The Wretched of the Earth.* Translated by Constance Farrington. New York: Grove, 1963.

Fischlin, Daniel, Ajay Heble, and George Lipsitz. *The Fierce Urgency of Now: Improvisation, Rights and the Ethics of Cocreation.* Durham, NC: Duke University Press, 2013.

Fischlin, Daniel, and Eric Porter. "Improvisation and Global Sites of Difference: Ten Parables Verging on a Theory." *Critical Studies in Improvisation* 11, no.1–2 (2016). https://www.criticalimprov.com/index.php/csieci/article/view /3949

Gana, Nouri. "Rap and Revolt in the Arab World." *Social Text* 30, no. 4 (2012): 25–53.

Giroux, Henry A. "Zero Tolerance, Domestic Militarization, and the War against Youth." *Social Justice* 30, no. 2 (2003): 59–65.

Jordan Times. "French Week Brings Paris to Amman." October 17, 2017. http://vista.sahafi.jo/art.php?id=968b5d537ec1fef6c7ec935dedad4157fefe7903

Lane, Philippe. *French Scientific and Cultural Diplomacy.* Oxford: Oxford University Press, 2013.

LeVine, Mark. "Music and the Aura of the Revolution." *International Journal of Middle East Studies* 44, no. 4 (2012): 794–97.

Maira, Sunaina. "We Ain't Missing": Palestinian Hip Hop—A Transnational Youth Movement." *CR: The New Centennial Review* 8, no. 2 (2008): 161–92.

Massad, Joseph. *Colonial Effects: The Making of National Identity in Jordan.* New York: Columbia University Press, 2001.

McDonald, David A. *My Voice Is My Weapon: Music, Nationalism and the Poetics of Palestinian Resistance.* Durham, NC: Duke University Press, 2013.

Milton-Edwards, Beverley. *Contemporary Politics in the Middle East.* 4th ed. Cambridge: Polity Press, 2018.

Milton-Edwards, Beverley. *Marginalized Youth: Toward an Inclusive Jordan.* Policy Report. Doha, Qatar: Brookings Doha Center, 2018. https://www.brookings.edu/research/marginalized-youth-toward-an-inclusive-jordan/

Milton-Edwards, Beverley, and Peter Hinchcliffe. *Jordan: A Hashemite Legacy.* Abingdon: Routledge, 2009.

Nzewi, Meki, Israel Anyahura, and Tom Ohiaraumunna. *Musical Sense and Musical Meaning: An Indigenous African Perception.* Amsterdam: Rozenberg, 2009.

Parker, Christopher. "Tunnel-Bypasses and Minarets of Capitalism: Amman as Neoliberal Assemblage." *Political Geography* 28, no. 2 (2009): 110–20.

Said, Edward. *Culture and Imperialism.* New York: Vintage Books, 1994.

Shalhoub-Kevorkian, Nadera. *Militarization and Violence against Women in Conflict Zones in the Middle East: A Palestinian Case-Study.* Cambridge: Cambridge University Press, 2009.

Talty, Alexandra. "Meet the Middle East's Battle Rap Gods." *Roads and Kingdoms,* April 11, 2018. https://roadsandkingdoms.com/2018/arab-rap-battle/

Terkourafi, Marina, ed. *Languages of Global Hip-Hop.* London: Continuum International, 2010.

UN Human Rights Council (UNHCR). "Jordan Fact Sheet." February 2018. https://reliefweb.int/sites/reliefweb.int/files/resources/FactSheetJordanFebruary2018-FINAL_0.pdf

UN Relief and Works Agency (UNRWA). "Where We Work." Updated December 1, 2016. https://www.unrwa.org/where-we-work/jordan

Williams, Angela. "'We Ain't Terrorists but We Droppin' Bombs': Language Use and Localizations in Egyptian Hip Hop." In *The Languages of Global Hip Hop,* edited by Marina Terkourafi, 67–95. London: Continuum, 2010.

Yom, Sean, and Katrina Sammour. "Counterterrorism and Youth Radicalization in Jordan: Social and Political Dimensions." *CTC Sentinel* 10, no. 4 (2017): 25–30.

FOUR | Nomadic Improvising and Sites of Difference

SALLY MACARTHUR AND WALDO GARRIDO

Improvisation is made possible through movement. We extend to improvisation what the philosopher Gilles Deleuze says about music, that it "is lodged on the lines of flight that pass through bodies."[1] Improvisation is the movement of the body joining with the movement of the sonorous material that intensifies it. It is an interchange of vibratory movements, spontaneously unfolding music in the moment of its creation, passing through time, moving in time. As with the performance of all music, improvisation is caught up in the intensity of musical sound, the changes of energy that give rise to its expressive and affective qualities. Improvisation is driven by bodies interacting with one another. Chris Stover astutely observes that improvising bodies are not only performers but also "musical-objects-as-bodies," always in a state of transition, encountering one another "in affective exchanges of intensities."[2] The self, as much as the music, lives in transition, taking on the character of the nomad: the itinerancy of the improvising nomad means that it inhabits an identity but never makes identity permanent. This formulation is analogous to Rosi Braidotti's idea that the nomad "never takes on fully the limits of one national fixed identity. The nomad has no passport—or has too many of them."[3] Eugene Holland characterizes improvisational jazz as nomadic in the way that it "foregrounds processes of 'itinerative following' rather than 'iterative reproducing.'"[4] Following Deleuze and Félix Guattari,[5] Eva Aldea says that for nomadic people, "land is not distributed to the people . . . rather, they are distributed on

101

the land," whereas in a static, sedentary space "a piece of land belongs to the people."[6] Put differently by Claire Colebrook, sedentary space "remains what it is and is then divided and distributed. Nomadic space, however, is produced through its distribution."[7] For Vida L. Midgelow, who is focused on dance improvisation practices, nomad dancers are comfortable with transition and change, and they resist clinging to illusions of permanence and stability.[8] In the popular imagination, regardless of the genre in which it takes place, improvisation is nomadic: it invents musical material on the spot and, in so doing, constitutes itself as continuously emergent in each moment of its production.

Since 2007, the Improvisation, Community and Social Practice (ICASP) research project, now morphed into the International Institute for Critical Studies in Improvisation (IICSI) at the University of Guelph, has focused attention on the idea that improvisation is a site for the analysis of social practice. Research under ICASP and IICSI auspices aims "to promote a dynamic exchange of cultural forms and to encourage new, socially responsive forms of community building across national, cultural, and artistic boundaries."[9] The broad idea is that improvisation can serve as a model for the ways in which communities negotiate differences, learn how to accept risk and contingency, and engage in respectful dialogue across cultural divides in a world in which such differences are so often marginalized or subordinated to a dominant group.

Some research published in the peer-reviewed journal *Critical Studies in Improvisation / Études critiques en improvisation* and on the ICASP and IICSI websites, and also language used in the marketing materials for the Guelph Jazz Festival, has fetched scathing criticism. Scott Currie claims that in these sites an "ideal-type" of improvisation is privileged and serves as a standard against which other forms of improvisation are measured and then, by implication, deemed to be inferior.[10] Currie says that the persistent unmarked use of the term *improvisation* effaces the wide-ranging differences and culturally specific meanings found in improvisational practices worldwide. For Currie, universalistic characterizations that envision its "core qualities" as "democratic, humane, and emancipatory" are troubling, for such notions do not apply to all improvising practices. In his view, minority improvising groups are disempowered, subsumed under what he identifies as the dominant form of Western improvisation, namely, transatlantic "free improvisation." Accordingly, producers and curators of cross-cultural collaborative free improvisation events are likely to produce cultural power asymmetries.

In a recent Bourdieusian sociological study of the Indigenous/non-

Indigenous distinction in Australia, the editors give a nuanced reading of how power asymmetries are produced, focusing on the cultural and social inequalities that emerge in capitalist and settler-colonial societies.[11] In their view, what is and is not valued is arbitrated, reproduced, and reinforced according to a system of widely shared ideas. In Deleuzian thought, this system of ideas is conceptualized as the collective assemblage of enunciation. Typically, there is a link between cultural value and the dominant white settler-colonial class, showing that the latter has more pedigree that emerges from its association with economic and political power. Yet, as these writers also point out, it is not simply a matter that the colonized will have more or less of the cultural capital that is valued by the colonizing culture. The colonized will also maintain and reproduce their own ideas about what is to be valued,[12] and, indeed, they will engage in their own "community-based and family-based storytelling."[13] This means, for example, that the colonized Indigenous Australian has never ceased to produce various versions of their identity, an idea that could be applied to any subordinated identity group living in a capitalist-colonized culture. In Australia, which includes a colonial-settler order with an increasing salience of the Indigenous/non-Indigenous binary, a growing anxiety exists among the dominant white Australian class that a nonwhite Australian (multicultural) class could threaten its dominance.[14]

If we take this broader view and map it onto improvising contexts, it is equally possible, then, to conceive of situations in which subordinated cultures will tip the balance of power. Stover makes the point that each improviser inevitably brings their own histories, inclinations, desires, and wills to an improvising context and, in so doing, affects what happens as an improvisation begins to unfold.[15] In this scenario, an improviser who is situated outside of the dominant culture can bring their music and lineage to the space and, in turn, mark the space in new ways. From a Deleuzian perspective, we suggest that improvising musicians will always be engaging in acts of territorialization and deterritorialization. As Kylie Message observes, however, these acts will not reinforce the dichotomous relationship between the territory and its deterritorialization but will always be "a malleable site of passage . . . in a state of process whereby it continually passes into something else."[16] While improvising will establish connections with representation, it will not project a fixed image of itself. In this way, connected with nomadic space, improvisation will continuously engage movement as a force of territorialization, deterritorialization, and reterritorialization.

Such a reading allows us to shift from identity thinking, in which the identity category is polarized, to an idea of identity as a becoming, constantly being constituted (and reconstituted) through its rich entanglement of heterogeneous groupings and intersectional differences. The critique offered by Currie, with its emphasis on identity thinking, represents improvisers as occupants of sedentary space. We are making the case that nomadic thought exists in a place of potentiality, thereby enabling improvisation to always occupy that potentiality, to open onto something that exceeds the bodies that create it.

In *A Thousand Plateaus*, Deleuze and Guattari view the concepts of nomadic and sedentary space as analogs of smooth and striated space.[17] Tom Conly explains that a "'smooth space' is one that is boundless and possibly oceanic, a space that is without border or distinction that would privilege one site or place over another," whereas striated space is "drawn and riddled with lines of divide and demarcations that name, measure, appropriate and distribute space according to inherited political designs, history or economic conflict."[18] Composer Pierre Boulez, as cited by Deleuze and Guattari, contends that in a smooth space-time "one occupies without counting," while in a striated space-time "one counts in order to occupy."[19] But, as Deleuze and Guattari point out, space will always vary according to its degrees of smoothness and striation. They write: "The two spaces exist only in mixture: smooth space is constantly being translated, transversed into striated space; striated space is constantly being reversed, returned to a smooth space. In the first case, one organizes, even the desert; in the second, the desert gains and grows; and the two can happen simultaneously."[20]

In this essay, we explore the interactions between smooth/nomadic and striated/sedentary space in the specific sites in which improvisation takes place. We foreground the cultural and social allegiances of musicians and musical genres in two case studies, focusing on the markers of ethnicity and gender. In their treatise on nomadology, Deleuze and Guattari posit the concept of the war machine, which is constituted as part of the assemblage of nomad thought.[21] They use this concept to disrupt the fixed categories of identity. Indeed, Colebrook stresses that the war machine is not a metaphor for stable and "proper beings, each with their identity, that must be distributed according to their essence and definition. . . . It is not, for example, that there are masters who then dominate and govern the slaves."[22] Rather, for Deleuze and Guattari, the master becomes a master "through an exercise of force."[23] To put this point slightly differently, it is through the process of exercising force that the master is produced. The master-slave relation is thus shaped, changing the distribution of power and the distinct hierarchies and identities that are affected by it.

As a model of the master-slave relation, then, improvisation functions as a war machine, constantly shifting the dynamics of the master musician–slave musician relationship, opening up possibilities for individuals to assume a dominant role within a single improvising group or—using improvisation as an engaged political practice—to articulate a nonviolent collective action to advance a political cause. As a collective activity, the improvising war machine is driven by a collection of desiring machines. The improvising war machine is carved out of its creative, musical processes, taking up nomadic forms of group belonging and creating distinctive minority identity positions, yet refusing permanent identification with one minority group or another. We regard this image of thought as positive and productive. It "thinks" difference without, as Yolanda Spangenberg writes, "reducing it to a *pre*supposed, *pre*determined and ultimately restrictive identity."[24] According to Deleuzian philosophy, "dogmatic images of thought," such as those anchored in identity, proceed "by objectifying and comparing the new with the known or what has already been experienced,"[25] thereby excluding what may exist but, as a virtual quality of pure difference, may not yet be actualised. As Spangenberg explains, representational images of thought perpetuate "a reductive and damaging illusion that hides reality seen in terms of pure difference or difference 'in itself.'"[26] For her, pure difference is "the virtual condition for (the possibility of) all actual identities," experienced as intensities or forces.[27] In this view, representation locks improvisation into a rigid set of boundaries, setting one musician or identity group or musical genre against another.

We attend to some of the ways in which the literature on gender, music, and ethnicity in diasporic communities in capitalist-settler societies engages, or not, with the concept of the war machine and nomadic thought. We follow this discussion with an analysis of two case studies, captured as interview data that has been mined from improvising identities in the very local site of Sydney, yet not necessarily bound by the limits of that city. From the findings of our interview data, we then make a case for a nomadic improvising practice that is driven by the forces of the war machine, even as it arises from the connections it makes in the various temporary circumstances in which it finds itself.

The interviewees' valuation of cultural identity suggests that improvising or making music as a cocreative activity in a given moment gives rise to its transformative potential.

Three voices—one author, one improviser, and one author-improviser—speak to questions that arise from sedentary identity thinking and the ways in which such thinking can be transformed by improvisation as a practice of nomadic thought (the war machine), giving rise to the concept of difference in itself. The lead author, Sally Macarthur, acts as facilitator in these quasi ethnographic/autoethnographic conversations, inserting a Deleuzian thinking process into the writing of this essay, and undertaking interviews with Jessica Arlo Irish and Waldo Garrido. As coauthor, Garrido provides insights that inform the ethnographic and autoethnographic material as it speaks to the Deleuzian framing of the essay. In addition to the interview material, he contributes specific information about his experience of migrating and of being a Chilean musician working in Australia. With Garrido, Macarthur thematizes the data into qualitative categories that enable the ensuing nomadic analysis to probe between the gaps and across the lines that divide one music and one cultural identity from another. Instead of focusing on the meanings that may emerge from the interview data, this chapter explores improvising's effects on the identities or selves or bodies who improvise.

Nomadic and Sedentary Sites of Difference in Music

Sedentary approaches used to study feminist work in music tend to turn women and their music, through the processes of capture, into conditions of subordination. Statistics are often used in feminist music research to demonstrate the need for change.[28] In relying on stable categories, such as male/female, statistics mostly end up supporting a narrative of victimhood, reinforcing the negative conception of women. Statistical work also tends to validate what is already known, that women's music is significantly underrepresented. Statistics are stratifying acts that capture the numerical information from the multiplicity, fixing this data as numerical entities in grid-like categories that do not account for the complexity of information that they represent. Statistics normalize the status quo and are then ripe for repeated use.

An overview of the literature that has for several decades examined women's marginalization in music, using both statistical information and a variety of qualitative methods, indicates that a correlation between the amount of research conducted and the performance of women's music in the concert hall.[29] It argues that when the research tapers off and feminist issues take a back seat, the amount of women's music performed in the concert hall also decreases. In the sedentary space of their analysis, the authors argue that if the issues continue the pattern of decreasing and increasing, feminist work will continue to perpetuate a circular model of argument about identity politics such that "what goes around keeps coming around." Similar styles of analysis have been conducted about gender and sexuality in improvising contexts, notably by Lucy Green, Sherrie Tucker, and Ellen Waterman.[30] The binary thinking in these studies frames identity as grievance and/or victimhood and metaphorically posits identity groups as warring tribes.

Similar stratifying methods concerned with the disadvantage of non-white social groups have characterized the work on ethnicity in music. Some of this work, however, tends to avoid the question of disadvantages of minority, multicultural groups, presenting, instead, a heroic, celebratory discourse that extols the benefits of having a culturally plural nation. A comprehensive review of the work that pays attention to diasporic communities asks how ethnic identities and cultures are maintained and transformed through music in their new surroundings.[31] The conclusion suggests that music is important for immigrants and refugees to develop their identities in their new situations.

Other issues are at play, as Laurie Bamblett, Fred Myers, and Tim Rowse point out about the broader research in Australia, notably that the social imaginary has a tendency to conceive of the nation as fundamentally unitary. Accordingly, through the process of assimilation, all Australians become indistinguishable from one another.[32] Furthermore, these authors suggest that two idioms of representation have emerged, one that addresses the critique of inequality and the other that is a positive or celebratory evocation of the richness of Indigenous (to which we would add multicultural) heritage. The simultaneous projection of "the population" and "the people" gives rise, says Bamblett, Myers, and Rowse, to an unstable contradiction in which difference is understood as both inequality and plurality.[33] In the discourse about "the population," Indigenous Australians (and other disadvantaged cultural groups) are perceived to have a deficit. In the discourse about "the people," they are affirmed for their plurality of ideas.[34] In this view, diversity is a valued trait. These narratives of representation, exemplifying sedentary thought in action, produce a concept of difference that highlights the structural problems associated with identity: that power and gender, and power and race, produce structural relationships that are seemingly immutable. In agreement with Daniel Fischlin and Eric Porter, however, we acknowledge that the structure of power in improvisation can be *both* simultaneously. It can be "riven by gendered, racial, ethnic, and class-based exclusions, conflicts, and symbolic (and occasionally real) violence" and yet also serve as a model for how alternatives to such asymmetrical power relations may be explored.[35]

Indeed, in an earlier article, without explicitly framing their ideas in Deleuzian philosophy, these authors offer some compelling examples of nomadic thought (the war machine) in action, conceiving it as a progression toward the disintegration of the self. Beginning with a series of aphorisms that are woven into their entire article, they map improvisation as a global phenomenon with multiple sites of difference: as a continuous stream with no beginning or end;[36] as a "system of difference, a blend of contextual specificities, an experience of disparate possibilities";[37] as the source of sound that traverses a waterfall in which the listener will hear the singer and "the ghost of the cascade and the flow of which it is a part";[38] as regenerative potential, thriving in opportunity, turning dissolution and degeneration into creative refiguration;[39] as something that occurs in beaches, streets and squares; and as "the readiness to remake things out of crisis."[40] These, among many others, imply the presence of a self but without specification. The implication is that improvising employs the power of its machinic assemblage to open up the multiplicity and, in so doing, to exercise its capacities to affect and to be affected, forging an identity as an exercise of political force, tapping into an infinite source of new material,[41] and engaging in the notion of *wu-wei*, which is to say, the notion of "effortless non-doing."[42] In our reading of this article, improvising is Deleuzian. It is a war machine par excellence.

Such a reading, then, illuminates the ways in which improvisation connects with its surroundings rather than dwelling on its meaning in its surroundings (as in a sedentary reading). According to Tamsin Lorraine, three lines compose the assemblages or multiplicities, themselves always in a state of flux as they continuously make (and remake) themselves in the moments of their cocreation. The molar line "forms a binary, arborescent system of segments,"[43] interacting with the world as a closed, deterministic system, similar, in this respect, to sedentary thought. The molecular line is more fluid and elastic but not entirely free, characterized by both sedentary and nomadic thought. The molecular line may undertake deterritorializations, but these may also return to the sedentary operations of the molar line. The line of flight is a path of pure mutation, a transformation "that can evolve into creative meta-morphoses of the assemblage and the assemblages it affects."[44] In the reading of improvisation above by Fischlin and Porter, the line of flight emerges through the connections made between disparate animate and inanimate objects, such as between the sound, the waterfall, the listener, and the singer. In so doing, it gives rise to improvisatory becomings as dynamic transformations.

Oscillations between Nomadic and Sedentary Thought in Two Local Case Studies

The binary logic underpinning sedentary research, as we have seen, structurally locks it into resemblances of itself with no apparent lines of escape. And yet, sedentary research has, significantly, drawn attention to the structural inequalities to which we have been referring, as well as the contradictions that emerge when two ideas, such as "the population" and "the people," are represented in terms of inequality and plurality. To follow the line of thought offered by Anna Hickey-Moody and Peta Malins, we suggest that when improvising identities and genres are subjected to preexisting, ready-made identity categories and their corresponding modes of musical enunciation, they are limited in what they are able to reveal about a given genre or identity and likewise may "conceal as much as they express."[45] As these authors continue, while categories create a stable sense of self and can be useful for political purposes—such as mobilizing gender and race issues and their relationships with specific improvising genres—they are also limiting, "reducing the body to particular modes of being and interacting; affecting not only how the body is understood but its potentiality; its future capacity to affect and be affected."[46] Deleuzian thought enables us to deploy conceptual tools that potentially transform the rules and structures that organize thought and liberate the social bodies that are constrained by them.

In this vein, we will now undertake a mapping, through the machinery of the interview, of the local practices of two (Australian) Sydney-based improvisers, Jessica Irish and Waldo Garrido. The overarching question for these two case studies is whether improvisation means the same thing in all circumstances or whether it is a master trope that erases difference. The interviews, consisting of open-ended questions, were designed to elicit data about the following themes, understanding that these themes inevitably push the data into sedentary space: cultural identity, including ethnicity and gender; the influence of musical genre on improvising;

appropriation and power relations in improvising collaborations; and definitions of improvisation.

Interviewee Jessica Irish (Jess) highlights the multiple musical sites and improvisational practices that an early-career musician inhabits. She moves across collaborative spaces of various configurations that involve teaming up with artists in the Irish Celtic tradition, popular song writing, film/video music, and intercultural, experimental "free improvisation." She is a doctoral student, moving toward the completion of her degree at Western Sydney University, and she teaches music performance and song writing as a casual lecturer at that institution. Interviewee Waldo Garrido (Waldo) is a seasoned, internationally renowned bass player and improviser, and also the coauthor of this essay. He is a Chilean-born musician, residing in the Blue Mountains, west of Sydney, and he lectures in music at Western Sydney University. His work spans genres in mainstream and Latin jazz, world music, and other popular music traditions, such as funk and rock.

Unfolding the Findings

As a microcosm of a global practice, Western Sydney University and its extended improvising communities have become a battleground between musical genres: "free," modernist, Western classical music improvisation accrues more symbolic value than other forms, such as traditional jazz and popular music. For the modernist aficionado, the practice of playing instruments in an unusual manner (including in ways that resemble those of the 1950s and 1960s), and of incorporating live sound processing onstage, is perceived to be complex and clever, which, in turn, aligns it with musical excellence. Such improvisation is often nothing more than a reinvention of the wheel, with the music displaying minimal musical technical proficiency as it sets in motion slow-moving canvasses of sound that drift aimlessly across the sonic space with minimal interaction between the collaborators and minimal engagement between the performers and their audience. Such music is frequently derivative while, paradoxically, making itself inaccessible to listeners. This music takes us back to 1958, when Milton Babbitt published his manifesto "Who Cares If You Listen?"[47]: the listener is cast in this scenario as the least important part of the improvising equation. Closer inspection of the music will also show that it adds nothing particularly new, lacks a coherent structure, and seems devoid of purpose, cohesion, and musicality. This kind of improvising, within the context of the Western art music progress narrative, creates an inferior replica of the original and is driven more out of ego than out of musicality.

In counterpoint to this characterization, Waldo (bass guitar and band leader) and his six-piece jazz ensemble improvise music that belongs not in a privileged, linear, classical music tradition, but in systems of music-making that have several intercultural lineages. Some of these lineages trace back to Africa through the enslaved who were taken and transported to the Americas, and to the Chilean music that was already there and that continues to be played and performed in the present day. Since Waldo migrated to Australia in 1976, his bands have been variously labeled Latin, Latin jazz, world music, and funk. His music is linked to multiple roots and occupies multiple sites of difference. Traces of many kinds of music move about, interacting with one another, in the spaces of Waldo's improvising bands. The performers, who all exhibit high levels of technical expertise, always seem to be in the moment, enjoying the moment, as they perform and improvise, incorporating movement of bodies and conversational banter as part of the act, drawing on high-level listening skills, and "wowing" the audience, which is always invited to participate actively.

Waldo's story is unlike that of the many Chileans who migrated because of the political situation in Chile. He writes:

> Contrary to what might be perceived as a uniform migration experience to Australia—as a reaction to the post-Pinochet regime in Chile—my circumstances were different. We did not come to Australia for either economic or political reasons. My father was a well-known musician in Chile, and my mother was a schoolteacher who was part of an upper-middle-class family. Our move to Australia had to do with resolving family issues. In fact, my parents decided to migrate in order to save their marriage. My father was involved in the music industry which tends to encourage and promote certain problems in behaviour, such as drinking, womanising, and drugs. It took me many years to find my place in Australia.

Waldo recognizes three distinctive waves of Chilean migration to Australia during the latter half of the twentieth century. A small group arrived as a result of the economic crisis during the presidency of Eduardo Frei (1968–70); others, worried about the economic and political future in Chile under the subsequent presidency of Dr. Salvador Allende, arrived between 1970 and 1973; the last group, by far the largest, immigrated as a result of the coup d'état led by General Augusto Pinochet on September 11, 1973. The first groups to arrive in Australia tended to belong to a wealthy, upper-class Chilean oligarchy. Those that migrated when Pinochet was in power, however, consisted mostly of Chileans of working-class and lower-middle-class backgrounds. They were a largely homogenous population of skilled workers.

In Waldo's experience, integration in the new country was difficult, and like many others, he experienced racism and discrimination, not just from the dominant white Australians but also from those Chilean refugees, mostly from the lower middle classes, who had migrated in the 1970s. He explains that he was frequently called a "wog," and he often experienced discrimination by his teachers. Music was his refuge, making life bearable. Like many of his compatriots, however, he had very little contact with mainstream Australians, living in a ghetto with high concentrations of South Americans, and maintaining a strong attachment to his traditions and customs, among them music, food, dance, language, and poetry. According to Waldo, culture and memory are important to Chileans, and music serves as a social glue, linking him and his compatriots to the home country. For Waldo, music is a powerful marker of his homeland, one that helps him maintain a strong connection with Chile.

Jess's experience is entirely different from that of Waldo. She was born into a privileged, white, middle-class family, and like many in her situation, she experienced a life of relative comfort and opportunity. While it is the case, as demonstrated in the literature, that women are inclined to be sidelined as creators/composers, often experiencing discrimination, in Jess's case as a relatively young musician at the beginning of her career, she has managed to escape such discrimination. Like Waldo's music, Jess's improvising is marked by high levels of energy, especially in her work as an Irish Celtic fiddler in Damien Leith's Irish Celtic band and in her cross-cultural collaborations with the internationally acclaimed Korean *taegum* improviser Hyelim Kim. With a focus on intercultural and cross-genre improvisation, Jess stretches her Irish Celtic–influenced vocals and violin/viola improvisations to intersect with multiple influences, specifically, those with East Asian sensibilities. As a practice-led researcher, she looks for opportunities to fracture her improvisational stylistic boundaries. In her collaborative work, Jess uses the concept of *clash-collaboration*, which she herself coined, to bring together seemingly disparate musical elements or genres or musicians in such a way that they will fracture each other and create new sonic territories.

In a Deleuzian sense, then, these two musicians—one a female musician who inhabits a minority social position while also belonging to a dominant white Australian class, and the other a Chilean improviser who is marginalized by the dominant white postcolonial Western culture in Australia—counter the above characterization of the "modernist," technically stagnant musician. Jess and Waldo are both exemplary improvisers who are at the top of their game.

To make their musicianship visible, however, they must engage in a form of nomadic violence (war machine) against the sedentary structures of the norm, which, in this case, is imagined as a "free" modernist improvisation practice that has dominance. The sedentary improvisatory structures of modernist free improvisation in this local site obscure the open space of the nomad improviser in other forms of improvisation. Nomads can be the objects of violence as enacted by the sedentary modernist free improvisers. To change the dynamics of the fixed master-slave relations, nomads must become war machines, shifting the power relations between themselves and the oppressor modernist improvising machinic assemblage, acting against its oppression, and expressing themselves joyfully, in the face of sedentary violence, as musicians of distinction. As nomads, Jess and Waldo take up temporary occupancies of their marginalized improvising practices, some of which involve cross-cultural collaboration, and, in so doing, open a space of limitless energy and potentiality that is guided by the war machine.

The findings reveal that Jess and Waldo consider their cultural identities to be important in shaping who they are as people and as improvisers. We also discover that they have a propensity to oscillate between nomadic and sedentary space.

Cultural Background: Ethnicity and Gender

Waldo states that his Chilean background is a crucial part of his identity:

> My cultural background is very important to everything I do. It informs my musical direction, and it is essential to my creative process. The decisions I make when I am playing music have a lot to do with the ideas that I have collected throughout my career as a musician and as a person: they have been critical to the formation of my identity. Improvisation is for me a practice that relies on my ever-expanding toolbox of musical motifs that I have collected over time. I use structures in my music that are known to be culturally common to many musicians of Latin origin.

Jess also acknowledges the importance of her white Australian cultural background, but she explains how encountering different cultural traditions of music, such as Irish Celtic, rock, and film music, changes the way she improvises, stating that:

> My cultural background . . . has had a massive impact on who I am as an artist . . . it can be disrupted and pushed into new territories when you deliberately engage with people of a different cultural standing. So, whilst it's still got its history and roots in the cultures you have established yourself from, it has formed a new meaning . . . it forms like this amalgamation of all of them, which in a sense is new.

Jess was asked whether her gender played any part in constructing her identity as an improviser and whether it had a negative effect in terms of the power relationships in the improvising space. While acknowledging that inequality still exists, she says that she had the good fortune to be born into a time in which sexual equality has been more broadly addressed. In terms of her own experience, she proffered that she has been well respected as an artist when working in male bands, continuing that:

> It becomes more about my craft and being respected for my craft than it does about gender, which is what I would hope because I wouldn't want my gender to come into it. I'm in that environment because of what I have to offer and because of my skills and what I have learnt and that's not going to be different for a male or a female. It should come down to that. It shouldn't be about gender. . . . I don't struggle with confidence issues when I'm improvising. I don't struggle with feeling able to express myself in those environments and push my agenda if I need to. . . . I wouldn't say I'm 100 percent feminine and I wouldn't say I'm 100 percent masculine. I'm in the middle of those two stereotypes.

In this account, improvising is less about gender and more about the craft of improvising, which, for Jess, is conceived as gender neutral. However, as Macarthur has argued elsewhere, gender codes are always embedded in music, oscillating between the actual and the virtual.[48] If the dominant code is actualized as masculine, then the transgression of that code (regardless of the gender of the transgressor), will be feminine, which is extracted from the virtual. In this scenario, the masculine code of music would undergo a "becoming-woman," opening up the new as a "becoming-other" of music. We might surmise that Jess, as an improviser, is too close to the action to be fully cognizant of this possibility. However, the Deleuzian-nomadic, analytic intervention that we are making allows us to entertain the thought that the deterritorialization of the masculine code would give rise to a productive potentiality for the improvising space.

The Influence of Musical Genre on Improvising

Given that genres are always in process, never settling into fixed, stable categories, especially in terms of their hybridizations, border crossings, and intercultural collisions, Jess was asked whether genre boundaries are constraining. Regardless of genre, Jess views improvising as a cocreation of music on the spot, generating a new piece of music in which each of the collaborators has an equal part to play. She discusses her work with the Irish Celtic musician Damien Leith and his band, as well as the free cross-cultural improvisation she undertakes with Hyelim Kim and Yantra de Vilder, stating:

> With Damien Leith's music—he's the front man—I am improvising to add to the whole and not to be the star, not to give it too much glamour. I'm trying to just raise the track itself. The cultural background comes into it because I'm aware that I want it to have an Irish flair, but I want it to be contemporary. I don't want to dominate. I'm trying to hear the parts where it needs a lift, the parts where it just needs a melodic undertone, the parts where it needs a solo, so I'm constantly listening. It's probably more fatiguing doing that kind of improvising, whereas working with Hyelim Kim and Yantra it's a combined project, fifty-fifty. I have more creative power in that moment. . . . I'm less familiar with Asian cultures and their traditional music. . . . I'm probably pushed further out of my comfort zone because I do understand Celtic music a lot more than I do East Asian music. I'm feeling my way through it rather than analysing my way through the improvisation.

Waldo proffers the insight that genre feeds into his ethnicity and class identity, suggesting that, in Australia, Latin musicians are stereotyped as sex merchants ("playing to get laid") in contrast to the more subdued, restrained performances of white postcolonial musicians. A white postcolonial formulation of Australian music, according to Waldo, effectively disempowers people of other ethnic backgrounds by making them objects of musical knowledge over which white postcolonial Australians have control. This idea is based in Edward Said's anti-imperialist agenda.[49] In this reading, Latino music performed by Latin musicians is viewed as kitsch, but Latin music performed by an Anglo jazz ensemble is seen as "cool." According to Waldo, Latin American ensembles are viewed as primitive. Waldo says that in his time in Australia, his music has been regarded variously as not Latin enough for the Latinos, too Latin for the Anglo audiences, and not jazzy enough for the jazz musicians.

In different ways, Jess and Waldo are aware that their improvising is continuously under construction, forming different kinds of genre assemblages that interact and connect with different bodies in different contexts. The assemblage of the improvising machine, then, cuts across the categorical divisions between genre and musician such that the classical fiddler moves in and out of the foreground and background, and the Latino improviser tests the boundaries of jazz, opening up the possibilities for transformations of Western jazz by Latin jazz, and vice vera.

Appropriation and Power Relations in Improvising Collaborations

Waldo and Jess were asked whether they were sensitive to the power relations that can occur between musicians of different cultural backgrounds. In relation to her collaborative work with Hyelim Kim, Jess underlines that:

> I don't think engaging with other cultures within a culture means that you're erasing the culture you're engaging with. I think it forms the basis of the improvisation, and it is important in the end product because it's still there, and the end product couldn't have resulted without that initial culture that you've engaged with and the new one that you're currently working within as well. If I'm not fully listening to her, I'll miss the point. It doesn't mean that because I'm listening to her that my culture is being erased [or vice versa]. . . . If one was eradicating the other it wouldn't actually work. It would just die . . . the whole point . . . is that the cultures do survive but they just form a new meaning together. You can't stop that from happening.

She further added,

> if Western musicians do not engage with non-Western musicians, the music of non-Western cultures could run the risk of being unknown

and unheard by future generations outside the non-Western tradition. By engaging with older, non-Western music traditions, we bring them with us into modernity whilst simultaneously promoting the culture and the history of the tradition. . . . As long as we're respectfully engaging with them, and they with us, then I think it's completely appropriate to engage with them.

For Waldo, there are instances in which appropriation and power imbalances can emerge. As he comments:

You need a good basis from which to proceed in working with another culture. You can't just go in there and be superficial. You need to understand the cultural values before you begin working with musicians in different cultural groups. I've also found that in some instances it might be "cool" to have a Latin or ethnic musician, and this can have a favourable impact on their careers. I've also found that jazz musicians are eclectic, adopting or using musical elements from other cultures to generate more interest in their music. But I've also noticed that these collaborations between musicians of different cultures can be one-sided in that the Western musicians will often have agenda of advancing their careers at the expense of the ethnic minority groups with whom they're working.

The line governing these responses to the power relations question is characterized, on the one hand, by sedentary thought, and on the other hand, by nomadic thought. The idea in Waldo's response that ethnic minorities are "used" to advance the careers of a dominant culture is locked in a sedentary mode of thinking, while, as he also indicates, nomadic thought is likely to emerge when musicians focus on what an intercultural collaboration would enable. Jess similarly discusses power relations as a sedentary concept within a binary construct (us/them) while simultaneously pointing to the importance of listening as a way to move into nomadic thought.

Definitions of Improvisation

We then explored whether our interviewees think that improvisation is a universalizing term that covers over difference. In her search for an adequate definition, Jess speaks about the familiar and preestablished templates that improvisers use compared with the more unfamiliar forms, such as those in free improvisational cross-cultural collaborations. According to Jess, cross-cultural free improvisation pushes her into uncomfortable territory. She deploys the term *clash collaboration* to suggest the idea of music in one culture clashing with another and explains the necessity for finding common ground. As Jess explains:

> I think improvising is so hard to define because there's improvising within a pre-established structure and improvising within familiar structures [such as] Irish music. I've got a pretty good idea of where it's going. . . . The same thing with pop music. Pop music is quite formulaic. . . . Then there's true improvisation, which is improvising in situations that are uncomfortable, which is where I come into clash collaboration—a term I've coined—which is just improvising in situations with people and with genres and traditions that are unknown and probably uncomfortable. So, they actually clash with your aesthetics. . . . I have found that that is really the only way you're ever going to experience yourself doing anything new. If you try and stick to your original structures that you would have normally used it just won't work. . . . You need to try and understand each other in order to move forward, or you just get stuck at this point with no push and pull. It's just like a battle. I've found that that's probably been the thing that's pushed me the most. . . . There are different types of improvisation, and it really depends on its purpose. . . . Is it for someone else? Is it for yourself, just for enjoyment? Is it for a situation that you're familiar with? Or, is it in a situation with which you're unfamiliar?

For Waldo, improvising is tied very strongly to his Chilean background, which he perceives to be a minority group in Australia. When he began working as a musician and composing—suggesting that his compositions could be regarded as improvisations—he was always coming up with new musical ideas. He established himself as a highly regarded improviser, and he believes that this focus gave him a sense of power and self-worth because others began to recognize him as a creative musician. Waldo says that improvising is:

> the idea that you as a musician can express musical ideas freely, to some point. I also believe that great improvisation comes from having a substantial amount of experience, training, and maturity. It involves collecting motifs, working on your theory, expression, and values, and expressing your personality.

For Deleuze, Jess's "uncomfortable territory" would move her improvisation beyond the sedentary operations of the molar line to open a path of pure mutation or a line of flight. In Waldo's case, the contested notion (in elitist music circles) of improvisation as equivalent to Western composition prepares the ground for two disparate music traditions— Chilean music and Western jazz—to transform each other through the acts of bodies connecting with these two sonorous systems.

Discussion: The Data and the War Machine

Following Elizabeth Gould,[50] we argue that this interview data is produced by the war machine. The female improviser who traverses multiple sites of difference and the Latino jazz improviser who is aligned with an ethnic minority group are, in their very presence, objects of institutional violence because they carry the mark of difference: the first is not a man and can never become a man; the second is not a white Australian and can never become a white Australian. As Gould says, the goal of nomadic violence is to "liberate difference," in this case, from the grip of the academic music machine and its dominant "free" improvisation, which can also be considered as an act of resistance (nomadic violence) as it undermines "the foundations on which the profession is enacted and understood."[51] Following Gould, we suggest that for these to be effective sites of resistance, they must make connections and these nomadic improvisers must be seen (and heard). In the academic music setting dominated by white masculinity, the success of the two improvisers from minority groups depends on their ability to use their difference as a source of value. They must embody their improvising as consummate artists in a way that shifts the power dynamics from the idea of a preestablished master improviser that dominates over a fixed composition of subordinated musicians, to the idea of an ever-changing, mobile power relationship of all musicians in a collaborative, improvising context, moving in and out of the master-slave relationship while simultaneously constructing it.

This idea emerges in the interview data when Jess talks about herself as being between the idea of maleness and femaleness. She also believes that an improvising space is a collaboration of improvisers who work with one another on an equal footing, with the dynamics constantly shifting from one improviser to another. In the Irish Celtic context, which requires significant concentration and listening ability, Jess is constantly moving in and out of the foreground and background.

In Waldo's interview data, a striking image emerges in his character-ization of his music as not being Latin enough or being too Latin for Anglo audiences or not being jazzy enough. The implication of the last is that the Latin rhythms underpinning the music are toned down for the Australian context, but they are not toned down enough or they are not "white" enough for white "man's" jazz. In our reading, however, Waldo's minoritarian status can be likened to Deleuze and Guattari's reading of the writer Franz Kafka.[52] As Colebrook puts it, Kafka's literature belongs in a minor tradition, and it responds "to the problem of writing in German as a Czech national."[53] Kafka did not occupy a language "that he could consider his own or identical with his being."[54] His work was the vehicle for the creation of identity rather than the expression of identity. When a term is expressive, in this sense, it is majoritarian. Conversely, when it is creative, it is minoritarian, implying an identity to come, or a becoming.[55] Kafka is regarded as great because he wrote "not as a being with an identity, but as a voice of what is not given, a people to come."[56] Colebrook explains that "great" literature is not necessarily the litera-ture of minorities, although this can be the case. A great writer like Kafka writes without a standard notion of "the people."

Following this Deleuzian reading of Kafka by Colebrook, we can con-ceive of the nomadic improvising of Waldo as Kafkaesque: his music cre-ation is a response to his positioning as a Chilean national in Australia. Waldo's interview data reveals that his musical language operates outside of the conventions of the insider "white" jazz traditions in Australia. His performances can be understood as not beginning and ending with his identity but as inserting a voice of what is not given, presaging, in the Deleuzian sense, a people to come.

Conclusion

Nomadic moments (the war machine) can be read in the interview data as acts of resistance, articulating, in Stover's analysis, a tension inher-ent in the territorializing networks that seek to define the improvisa-tional plane in terms of its boundaries while simultaneously conceiving it as "always in process of being defined, immanent to itself, unfolding a double action of territorialization and deterritorialization through which the emergent identity of the context is inscribed."[57] For Stover, the constant flux of movement of improvising bodies produces forces in which "affect is always already in a doubled state of transition or pas-sage," as the bodies transition "from one affective state to another."[58] In improvising "there are no states other than transitional states; there is only, always, passage."[59]

Stover posits improvisation as an event, a happening, an in-between, a transition, and a passage, all of which work in tandem to produce the affective space.[60] In his reading, improvisation constitutes the nomadic space that we have been discussing. It is created by the capacity of the body to be affected, and by the body's positioning as always in the middle, or in-between, an idea that Jess and Waldo affirm. In this way, affective forces cut across the improvising assemblage with their loci residing in the body. Accordingly, improvisation constantly shifts between smooth/nomad and striated/sedentary space: the affective actions or encounters of an improvising event leave their effects as a trace on the bodies that inhabit this transitional space. Bodies are constituted by these actions and encounters while simultaneously constituting them.

Notes to Chapter 4

1. Deleuze, *Francis Bacon*, 47.
2. Stover, "Affect and Improvising Bodies," 5.
3. Braidotti, *Nomadic Subjects*, 33.
4. Holland, "Studies in Applied Nomadology," 25.
5. Deleuze and Guattari, *A Thousand Plateaus*. In particular, Aldea refers to chapter 12, "Treatise on Nomadology," 351–423.
6. Aldea, "Nomads and Migrants."
7. Colebrook, "Nomadicism," 187.
8. Midgelow, "Nomadism and Ethics," 2.
9. Heble, "About ICASP."
10. Currie, "The Other Side of Here and Now."
11. Bamblett, Myers, and Rowse, introduction.
12. Bamblett, Myers, and Rowse, 7.
13. Bamblett, Myers, and Rowse, 8.
14. Bamblett, Myers, and Rowse, 8.
15. Stover, "Affect and Improvising Bodies," 11.
16. Message, "Territory," 281.
17. Deleuze and Guattari, *A Thousand Plateaus*, 474–500.
18. Conly, "Space," 261.
19. Quoted in Deleuze and Guattari, *A Thousand Plateaus*, 477.
20. Deleuze and Guattari, 474.
21. Deleuze and Guattari, 351–473.
22. Colebrook, "Nomadicism," 187.
23. Colebrook, 187.
24. Spangenberg, "Thought without an Image," 89 (italics in the original).
25. Spangenberg, 92.
26. Spangenberg, 92.

27. Spangenberg, 92.
28. See, for example, Adkins Chiti, "Secret Agendas in Orchestral Programming"; Brown, "Female Composers Largely Ignored"; Hirsch, "Lend Me a Pick Ax"; and Hope, "All Music For Everyone."
29. Macarthur et al., "The Rise and Fall."
30. Green, *Music, Gender, Education*; Tucker, "When Did Jazz Go Straight?"; and Waterman, "Naked Intimacy."
31. Lidskog, "The Role of Music in Ethnic Identity Formation in Diaspora."
32. Bamblett, Myers, and Rowse, introduction, 12–13.
33. Bamblett, Myers, and Rowse, 18.
34. Bamblett, Myers, and Rowse, 17.
35. Fischlin and Porter, *Playing for Keeps*, 4.
36. Fischlin and Porter, "Improvisation and Global Sites of Difference," 1.
37. Fischlin and Porter, 1.
38. Fischlin and Porter, 2.
39. Fischlin and Porter, 5.
40. Fischlin and Porter, 5.
41. Fischlin and Porter, 10.
42. Fischlin and Porter, 10.
43. Lorraine, "Lines of Flight," 147.
44. Lorraine, 147.
45. Hickey-Moody and Malins, *Deleuzian Encounters*, 5.
46. Hickey-Moody and Malins, 5.
47. Babbitt, "Who Cares If You Listen?"
48. Macarthur, *Towards a Twenty-First-Century Feminist Politics of Music*, 109–71.
49. Said. *Orientalism: Western Conceptions of the Orient.*
50. Gould, "Nomadic Turns."
51. Gould, 155.
52. Deleuze and Guattari, *Kafka.*
53. Colebrook, *Understanding Deleuze*, xxxiv.
54. Colebrook, *Gilles Deleuze*, 103.
55. Colebrook, 104.
56. Colebrook, 104.
57. Stover, "Affect and Improvising Bodies," 6.
58. Stover, 8.
59. Stover, 8.
60. Stover, 8.

Works Cited

Adkins Chiti, Patricia. "Secret Agendas in Orchestral Programming." In *Culture-Gates: Exposing Professional Gate-Keeping Processes in Music and New Media Arts*, by ERICarts, 325–60. Bonn: ARCult Media, 2003.
Aldea, Eva. "Nomads and Migrants: Deleuze, Braidotti and the European Union in 2014." *Open Democracy*, September 10, 2014. https://www.opendemocracy.net/en/can-europe-make-it/nomads-and-migrants-deleuze-braidotti-and-european-union-in-2014/

Babbitt, Milton. "Who Cares If You Listen?" *High Fidelity Magazine* 8, no. 2 (1958): 38–40.

Bamblett, Laurie, Fred Myers, and Tim Rowse. Introduction to *The Difference Identity Makes: Indigenous Cultural Capital in Australian Cultural Fields*, edited by Laurie Bamblett, Fred Myers, and Tim Rowse, 1–37. Canberra: Aboriginal Studies Press, 2019.

Braidotti, Rosi. *Nomadic Subjects: Embodiment and Sexual Difference in Contemporary Feminist Theory*. New York: Columbia University Press, 1994.

Brown, Mark. "Female Composers Largely Ignored by Concert Line-Ups." *Guardian*, June 14 2018. https://www.theguardian.com/music/2018/jun/13/female-composers-largely-ignored-by-concert-line-ups

Colebrook, Claire. *Gilles Deleuze*. London: Routledge, 2002.

Colebrook, Claire. "Nomadicism." In *The Deleuze Dictionary*, rev. ed., edited by Adrian Parr, 185–88. Edinburgh: Edinburgh University Press, 2010.

Colebrook, Claire. *Understanding Deleuze*. Crows Nest, Australia: Allen and Unwin, 2002.

Conly, Tom. "Space." In *The Deleuze Dictionary*, rev. ed., edited by Adrian Parr, 260–62. Edinburgh: Edinburgh University Press, 2010.

Currie, Scott. "The Other Side of Here and Now: Cross-Cultural Reflections on the Politics of Improvisation Studies." *Critical Studies in Improvisation / Études critiques en improvisation* 11, nos. 1–2 (2016): 1–10.

Deleuze, Gilles. *Francis Bacon: The Logic of Sensation*. Translated by Daniel W. Smith. Minneapolis: University of Minnesota Press, 2003.

Deleuze, Gilles, and Félix Guattari. *Kafka: Toward a Minor Literature*. Translated by Dana Polan. Minneapolis: University of Minnesota Press, 1986.

Deleuze, Gilles, and Félix Guattari. *A Thousand Plateaus: Capitalism and Schizophrenia*. Translated by Brian Massumi. Minneapolis: University of Minnesota Press, 1997.

Fischlin, Daniel, and Eric Porter. "Improvisation and Global Sites of Difference: Ten Parables Verging on a Theory." *Critical Studies in Improvisation / Études critiques en improvisation* 11, nos. 1–2 (2016): 1–19.

Fischlin, Daniel, and Eric Porter. *Playing for Keeps: Improvisation in the Aftermath*. Durham, NC: Duke University Press, 2020.

Gould, Elizabeth. "Nomadic Turns: Epistemology, Experience, and Woman University Band Directors." *Philosophy of Music Education Review* 13, no. 2 (2005): 147–99.

Green, Lucy. *Music, Gender, Education*. Cambridge: Cambridge University Press, 1997.

Heble, Ajay. "About ICASP." Improvisation, Community, and Social Practice (ICASP). Social Sciences and Humanities Research Council of Canada. Accessed June 28, 2019. http://www.improvcommunity.ca/about

Hickey-Moody, Anna, and Peta Malins, eds. *Deleuzian Encounters: Studies in Contemporary Social Issues*. Houndmills: Palgrave Macmillan, 2007.

Hirsch, Lisa. "Lend Me a Pick Ax: The Slow Dismantling of the Compositional Gender." *New Musicbox*, May 14, 2008. http://www.newmusicbox.org/article.nmbx?id=5576

Holland, Eugene. "Studies in Applied Nomadology: Jazz Improvisation and Post-Capitalist Markets." In *Deleuze and Music*, edited by Ian Buchanan and Marcel Swiboda. Edinburgh: Edinburgh University Press, 2004, 20–35.

Hope, Cat. "All Music for Everyone: Working Towards Gender Equality and Empowerment in Australian Music Culture." *Limelight*, December 5, 2018. https://www.limelightmagazine.com.au/features/limelight-in-depth-cat-ho pe-all-music-for-everyone/

Lidskog, Rolf. "The Role of Music in Ethnic Identity Formation in Diaspora: A Research Review." *Authors International Social Sciences Journal* 66, no. 219–220 (2017): 23–38.

Lorraine, Tamsin. "Lines of Flight." In *The Deleuze Dictionary*, rev. ed., edited by Adrian Parr, 147–48. Edinburgh: Edinburgh University Press, 2010.

Macarthur, Sally. *Towards a Twenty-First-Century Feminist Politics of Music.* Farnham, England: Ashgate Press, 2010.

Macarthur, Sally, Dawn Bennett, Talisha Goh, Sophie Hennekam, and Cat Hope. "The Rise and Fall, and the Rise (Again) of Feminist Research in Music: 'What Goes Around Comes Around.'" *Musicology Australia* 39, no. 2 (2017): 73–95.

Message, Kylie. "Territory." In *The Deleuze Dictionary*, rev. ed., edited by Adrian Parr, 274–76. Edinburgh: Edinburgh University Press, 2010.

Midgelow, Vida L. "Nomadism and Ethics in/as Improvised Movement Practices." *Critical Studies in Improvisation* 8, no. 1 (2012): 1–12.

Said, Edward. *Orientalism: Western Conceptions of the Orient.* London: Penguin Books, 1978.

Spangenberg, Yolanda. "'Thought without an Image': Deleuzian Philosophy as an Ethics of the Event." *Phronimon* 10, no. 1 (2009): 89–100.

Stover, Chris. "Affect and Improvising Bodies." *Perspectives of New Music* 55, no. 2 (2017): 5–66.

Tucker, Sherrie. "When Did Jazz Go Straight? A Queer Question for Jazz Studies." *Critical Studies in Improvisation / Études critiques en improvisation* 4, no. 2 (2008): 1–16.

Waterman, Ellen. "Naked Intimacy: Eroticism, Improvisation, and Gender." *Critical Studies in Improvisation / Études critiques en improvisation* 4, no. 2 (2008): 1–20.

FIVE | "That Which Exceeds Recognition"

Sound and Gesture in Hassan Khan's Dom Tak *and* Jewel

JEMMA DECRISTO

You are standing in two different rooms: one flushed with bright light that flickers against bare white walls while anthropomorphic speakers stand stolid in the distance; the other almost entirely dark, but partially blue lit by the moving images on the screen. Both rooms, in radically different ways, are awash in Egyptian Shaa'bi music produced by Egyptian artist Hassan Khan. These are two different times, two different moments, at the same time: *Dom Tak Tak Dom Tak* (2005) and *Jewel* (*Jawhara*, 2010).[1] Though *Dom Tak* and *Jewel* appear quite distinct and were composed differently, both installations unfold from their engagement with Egyptian Shaa'bi music, and they oscillate between automation and improvisation.

These installations are playing you back to yourself in the isolation of the gallery space, and the process may be revealing nothing more than what you have always felt and always lived, but have rarely been taught to know. None of this you is fully settled; it moves in a kind of perpetually migratory musical process. Yet, the formal constitution of a self, as one of Khan's oft-cited intellectual influences R. D. Laing argues, always requires the regulation and disavowal of the massive realities of these experiences and processes.[2] Laing's writing, which Khan has explicitly engaged in his art, analyzes the psychic paradox of the self as the container and mediator of experiences.[3] As the self becomes the dominant conceptual arbiter of experiences, it also always destroys the complexity of such experiences by conceptually reducing them to the analytical container of experience. For Laing, it was as much the analyst as the patient who was frozen into a denial of experiences as the formal rigidification of a self qua experience.[4] Khan's work formally posits that the artist (as commodity producer of experience) and the audience (as consumer of experience) rely on a similarly rigid framework in the self. Through the enactment of distinct forms of automation and improvisation, Khan's work critiques this preponderance of the self, opposing the massively overrepresentative function of the self to the formal nuances, references, memories, and experiences that the self so often attempts to swallow whole.

The resonance between Shaa'bi music and Khan's work dwells somewhere in the automated and improvisatory movements, the flourishes and gestures, that disrupt the axiomatic function of sound to reflect the singularity of the self. The improvisational traditions of Arabic music-making—especially as they have been standardized within Western models of musical conservatories as the dominant (though by no means only) institutional mode of musical education—have, perhaps increasingly, relied on a formal context wherein improvisation is the affirmation of a self, of the individual musician's virtuoso interpretation in relation to the longer musical-social tradition.[5] Not entirely unlike the kind of restrictive models of improvisation that recording foisted on jazz into the 1960s, many Arabic art musics over the twentieth century increasingly framed improvisation as an assertion of the individual's performance in relation to the ensemble and in opposition to the collective.[6]

Present in Khan's work is the historical, cultural, empirical, and technological image of the self as an audible, psychic, and discursive embodiment. Khan, however, treats this self as a material—one among many—that can be sonically sculpted and played through its very structures of recognition. Thus in Khan's work the self can just as easily be a visible figure on-screen, as we see more explicitly in *Jewel* (a character, a body, a language), as it can be the invisible structure of interpretation, what Khan has called the "invisible audience" that recognizes a sign's capacity to speak.[7] The pertinent strand in Khan's work, then, as it pertains to this essay, is the question that it poses to improvisation, a question that reverberates in the aesthetics of the Black radical tradition: what would it mean to improvise something beyond and before the self?[8] The poetics of Khan's work emerge from his deeply held suspicion as to the "purity" or singularity of a self as that which is opposed to a collectivity.[9] Khan's distrust is not articulated through an idealistic self-assertion disguised as self-negation, an approach common to certain modernist practices of sonic experimentation.[10] This kind of "modernist fantasy," as Khan has called it, rests on its disavowal of the artistic and social collectivity that brought it to fruition.[11] Shaa'bi (lit. "of the people") music, on the other hand, is a "collectively produced genre" with its own complex forms of self-possession and class consciousness that are formally invested in "recognizing the position through which one speaks."[12]

Khan is not a Shaa'bi musician but an artist who works primarily in well-funded international art spaces. Therefore it is not only or perhaps even primarily the automated modes of sound making in Arabic musics that Khan wishes to unsettle; rather, in parallel, Khan seeks to disquiet the drives of "engineered cultural spaces" in Cairo and abroad: museums, galleries, and art institutions. These spaces produce a codified consumable image of Cairo; they cohere and succeed by "promoting the experiences of the 'free' and 'informed' museum visitor, art history student or seeker of knowledge."[13] It is these genres of the self, the consumer, and the listener that Khan's work aims to complicate and disturb through sound. Through his intricate methods of composition and sonic experimentation, Khan wishes to coax the listener to improvise something beyond their own listening.

In *Dom Tak Tak Dom Tak* (2005), a programmed visual and sonic environment, and *Jewel* (2010), a choreographed sound and video installation, Khan quite profoundly and subtly undoes the standpoints, the gestures, and the forms against which a self is often recognized and measured as a listener and a viewer in culture.[14] Khan discusses the self in his work and in culture as a kind of automated and automatic process, a series of programmed rules and functions prescribed by culture. He also conjectures that not just reception but also production unfolds in this automatic loop. Many modes of improvisation conform to this kind of automation, wherein improvisation is itself a kind of rule-governed automated process that does not disrupt but perhaps reifies hegemonic conceptions of self that arise in genre, form, and the ever-present social ascriptions of race, class, ethnicity, language, and voice. Thus Khan's sonic installations *Dom Tak* and *Jewel* theorize that improvisation in its most radical instantiations can interrupt, unsettle, and re-create the most immediate and immanent moments of the social, moments that are too often regulated and subsumed by the self. In this regard, Khan theorizes something that we can only grasp at with improvisation and automation, but which more pointedly revolves around the actively charged and spontaneous (though always culturally rooted) reimaging of sound by shifting the context and meaning of its social referents.

The sound track to *Dom Tak* and the visual-choreographic language of *Jewel* are both composed of intricate methods of improvisation derived from the Shaa'bi genre of music commonly heard at street festivals, weddings, and *moulids* throughout Cairo, Egypt.[15] *Dom Tak* was produced and composed by Khan through a highly regimented process in which Khan hired six Egyptian Shaa'bi studio musicians: an accordionist, a *kawala* (reed instrument) player, a backing keyboardist, a solo keyboardist, a trumpeter, and a violinist. Khan then isolated each musician from the others, gave them a conventional key and mode in which to play, and provided them with a generic Shaa'bi beat that he had composed; he gave them no melody. The musicians were then sonically blindfolded from hearing what the others had played. This process of recording broke down the common conventions of performing and recording Egyptian Shaa'bi music and encouraged each musician to imagine a set of projected others with whom they were playing. The recorded product of this experiment was then rematerialized as a highly "programed environment," wherein a computer's metronomic clock initiates a series of thirty-second lighting and sound changes that operate indifferently in relation to the audience's presence in the space.

In *Jewel*, a choreographed video installation, Khan took an equally unique, yet subtler and perhaps even more complex, approach to improvisation. *Jewel* began as an "unconscious fantasy," a kind of daydream one day while he was cabbing home in Cairo. As Khan peered out the window of the car, he saw two young men dancing to Egyptian Shaa'bi music amid the refracted lights of the city streets. This distinct yet commonplace sight triggered in Khan a rich and profound scene of music, sound, body, image, and interaction, which eventually led him to hire two actors with varying levels of training to engage and realize the conscious dimensions of this scene. Khan worked with the actors in isolation from each other and provided them with only a bombastic Egyptian Shaa'bi beat that would become part of the video's sound track. This reverberating Shaa'bi beat also provided a context against which these two performers could develop, along with Khan, an improvised language of gestural and choreographic communication to eventually be "spoken" at, to, and with each other. The resultant interaction became the primary sonic and visual imagery of *Jewel*. While the context and especially the mode of exhibition of *Dom Tak* and *Jewel* differ markedly, the two works share an obvious common referent in their engagement with Egyptian Shaa'bi music, a music traditionally produced with improvisational practices. Hence each work quite subtly emerges from a highly specific, and at times even personal, language of improvisation.

Hassan Khan is no improviser-technician. He is not formally trained in any one instrument or discipline, but his work and his practice have materialized from a critical and promiscuous relationship with forms, gestures, and references. Khan notes that as a teenager in Cairo, "I came at art through noise . . . feed-backing TVs and guitars at peoples' homes. This was basically the beginning of my practice."[16] Khan and his friends Mahmoud Refat and Amr Hosni, among others, were as youths part of the burgeoning 1990s noise scene in Cairo, which eventually led to Refat founding the first experimental record label in Cairo, 100 Copies Music.[17] Khan's practice, however, has radically shifted over the course of his twenty-year career, from his early video and sound works in the mid-1990s, to his more recent sound/visual/textual installations. Yet his work has persistently reflected a profound engagement with the excess of technical, functional, and technological structures of recognition through which something like a self is thought to emerge. Specifically, Khan's work reveals a protracted fascination with automation as a site through which to think and rethink the terms of the self. While Khan frequently deploys images and figures of the technical, the functional, the technological, the automated, and the conditioned in his work, these images are also decoys, partial objects through which the self might desire recognition.[18] I suggest then that Khan's engagements with improvisation in *Dom Tak Tak Dom Tak* and *Jewel* deploy the self as a technical and technological image, a decoy, a material through and against which new materials, forms, and languages can be realized.

Dom Tak Tak Dom Tak and the Embodied Automatism of Shaa'biyat

In a pithy 2006 article for the art publication *Bidoun*, Khan ruminated on the emergent forms of Shaa'bi music (what Khan then called New Wave Shaa'bi, but what has more recently been dubbed *Mahraganat*), which had been colliding with and shifting his thoughts over the preceding five years. While the potency of electronic sounds as a medium for understanding and critiquing the production of a self was a dominant theme in much of Khan's early video work, Shaa'bi music had not arrived as a prominent epistemic through which to approach this endeavor. Video works such as *Lungfan* (*Nafs*, 1995) and *Do You Want to Fight?* (*Anta Awaz Tatakaaneq*, 1997) engaged the notion of *a-nafs el-mashruta*.[19] This notion, "the conditioned self," was a term invoked by Khan in some of his earlier work to reflect the way in which a self is conditioned and composed by a prescribed set of social rules or formal patterns that allow it and coerce it to function. In these video works, Khan was invested in the immediacy of sounds, gestures, and forms that could disrupt the audience, as a way of perhaps calling attention to the contours of this conditioned self. While Khan's early work explored the dimensions of the self as a determinant object, a skepticism materialized as to the self's finite singularity in representation.[20] At this point in Khan's practice, Shaa'bi became more important and resonant.

In Khan's 2006 article for *Bidoun*, he writes, "Shaa'biyat [Shaa'bi forms of music] is a genre that can potentially evacuate itself to present us with a form that is open enough for an engagement that is not merely based on interpretation. This is a genre that refuses to be ruled by the logic of any of the master signifiers or tropes of Egyptian popular culture. Class, although implicit, has been abandoned as a subject; eroticism is practiced rather than represented; and narratives to draw lessons from have disappeared. We're left with a charged object to be encountered, loud, dumb, and present."[21] Khan's investment in Shaa'bi music emerges from an organic resonance between the genre and many of his own practices, forms, and investments. By avoiding novel symbolic references to and reifications of prescribed social orders such as class, Shaa'biyat produces operational practices and vocabularies through which class is lived and realized. The context for improvisation in Shaa'bi, then, arises not so much out of the discrete sounds or their formal-technical production, but from the sounds' facilitation of a formalization of the everyday. What is improvised is what has always been lived in its immanence, and the sound becomes the material language for the realization and production of experiences and selves that are not reducible to any simple master trope.

The speedy, bass-heavy rhythms and wailing, animated vocal lines inherent to the forms of Shaa'biyat to which Khan is referring were birthed within the drug-laden carnivalesque context of Egypt's *moulids*.[22] *Moulids* are large public festivals: feasts, tradeshows, revivals, and musical gatherings that draw hundreds of thousands (perhaps even millions) of people to Egypt's urban centers, most notably Cairo. The *moulid* is both the tropological referent of many Shaa'bi tracks and the social milieu in which Shaa'bi formally evolved, perhaps most fittingly because *moulids* have often been a dynamic and grotesque meeting point between the sacred and the profane, the religious and the secular.[23] Fueled by a mixture of aggressive amphetamine consumption (Cairo's *silaba* pills) and the residual transcendentalism of Sufi *Zikr/Dhikr* music, sophisticated practices of life and music materialized. In the *moulid,* and eventually in the recording studio, pathologies of working-class life and pathologies of musical form, motivic or otherwise, were bypassed and undone.

Zikr music, much like its (somewhat more secular) cousin *Tarab*—and, indeed, something like the social ideal of the *moulid* that hosts it—has historically privileged a kind of transcendental escapism. The self-conscious formalism and virtuoso ideal at the center of classical Arabic musical forms such as *Zikr* and *Tarab* have, especially in the context of the *moulid,* come to function as vehicles for working-class fantasies of escape and *tarab* (ecstasy).[24] In *Tarab,* soloistic instrumental virtuosity within the context of the larger ensemble is highly prized. This instrumental virtuosity is put to the use of producing *tarab* for the listener as well as the practitioner. Prior forms of Egyptian Shaa'bi music, however, at least as far back as the 1970s, centralized notions of class and discussed the material and discursive obstacles of working-class life. The notion of "the political" in prior forms of Shaa'bi often congealed through the lyrical form of a message or statement about working-class conditions. The Shaa'biyat forms that Khan draws from and that he identifies with the moniker New Wave Shaa'bi complicate several of these dominant musical conventions. Shaa'biyat forms—or New Wave Shaa'bi, or *Mahraganat*—have increasingly shirked the virtuoso musicianship and instrumental specialization characteristic of earlier, more classical forms of Arabic music. Instead, Shaa'bi musicians have increasingly adopted electronic instrumentation, not just the ubiquitous Korg Triton, which has been backing a wide variety of Arabic musics since the early 2000s, but also drum machines, various synthesizers, digital samplers, and computer-based virtual instruments. In fact, the materials of musical production bear more resemblance to hip-hop and contemporary electronic musics than to prior forms of Arabic music. Similarly, the vocal instrumentation, how singers craft and sculpt their voices, has balked at and nearly parodied the improvised virtuoso melisma and textual stretching of classical Arabic forms.

Shaa'bi singers like Abdel El-Rewash ("Cool Abdel"), Nasser El-Sukran (Nasser the Drunkard), and Ashraf El-Brins (Prince Ashraf)—all of whom Khan cites as innovators at that time—stretch their voices into various shouts and shrieks, engaging in such dramatic and excessive pitch-shifting even on single tones and syllables that one would think it is mere digital affect. And sometimes it is. The digital affects in New Wave Shaa'bi secure the intricate otherworldly narratives of class and the political, which are rendered contextually rather than semantically or symbolically. Even as recently as the early 2000s the popular forms of Shaa'bi that dominated the mainstream imaginary were tracks by artists like Abdel Basset Hamouda, whose vocal style, *fasaaha* (clarity of enunciation), and phrasing bore a more striking resemblance to classical forms and techniques of vocalization. Hamouda's lyrical aesthetic often revolved around a statist and internationalist politic of appeal, a sentimental plea, albeit one tinged with cynical humor and melancholic resignation. At that juncture Shaa'bi lyrics often formalized the political into the functionalism of appeal, a convention that has undoubtedly, to varying degrees, come to define a broader postcolonial/neocolonial, post-*nahda* (post-renaissance: the period after the 19th century cultural rebirth that took place across much of the Arab world) aesthetic in Arabic musics. In New Wave Shaa'bi, this self-conscious politic is jettisoned for the materiality of the aesthetic that carried it. One can still detect an air of Hamouda's broken-down hoarseness, his visual and musical aesthetic of absolute depletion in the face of social and sonic digital perfection. Hamouda's straining vocals point to the tonal limitations of conventional Shaa'bi's improvisatory vocal modulation; Hamouda's voice, although perhaps dismissed as popular or paltry, actually improvises as the formal materiality and immediacy of the voice. The "grain" of Hamouda's voice that strains against the image of the form—the genre in which his voice is contained and in which it (mostly) contains itself—becomes the sculptural clay of New Wave Shaa'bi or Shaa'biyat forms.[25] In New Wave Shaa'bi lyricism, such depletion is the ground floor, the baseline materiality through which lyrical fantasies and perverse doubles of Cairo's urban life are imagined and materialized.

But what materiality is this? What forms of life, subjects, modes of subjection and selves, can be found in this move? In *Dom Tak* and *Jewel,* Khan seems to be thinking through these questions rather than trying to define Shaa'bi as a kind of exotic reference. Khan adds: "I am not interested in the Shaa'bi reference as some kind of validation, or street cred or some kind of funkiness. That's fusion. I am not trying to just export some hip sounds or some exotic sounds; that's not the interest."[26]

What then is Khan's investment in Shaa'bi? For that matter, what is Shaa'bi as it is evoked in and through Khan's work? Khan's eloquence in describing his interests and motivations is illustrative here:

> I am interested in automation. This word is important for me in general not just for music. It is part of what I am most profoundly interested in as an artist in general, which is the thin line between our sense of self as a result of a set of gestures that are inherited and programmed and our ability to counter that, it sounds really trite like free will versus determination, but that's not what I mean. What I

mean is that there is a sense in which culture is a set of automated rules in a way; more than that, not just rules, but a set of gestures and thought patterns etc. And at the same time there is a space where your sense of self is distinct from that and part of that. I think this is operational in all contexts, not [just] speaking about traditional and non-[traditional]; I am speaking in the widest possible sense. Therefore, that's why for example in *Dom Tak Tak* I am working with a musical culture and presenting that musical culture through its own sense of automatedness. So the musicians play without listening to each other, they are recorded without listening to each other, so that means that they revert to the basic, let's say DNA, of the form or the basic code of the form. Because they are imagining the other musicians, they're not just playing a scale, but because they are not playing with someone they need to imagine their musical culture to perform it. There is a higher level of conscious fantasizing involved, and by doing this the musical product that is coming out in a nonscientific fashion is the result of that automatedness. It's not the genre itself, because the genre itself has that automatedness—but it is also played—what is played is its ghost or twisted twin or something like that, because its rules are being performed.[27]

Khan's investment in automation and his investment in Shaa'bi converge around the operations through which a self is simultaneously recognized and undone. This context, in which a self is produced and recognized, is something like what we often call culture, and this automation that Khan speaks of is something like what we might identify as the *recognition* of culture. More precisely, Khan is using the Shaa'bi genre to think about the documentation and recognition of culture as automation or as something automated.

Khan's formulation of culture as "a set of automated rules . . . a set of gestures and thought patterns," which the self is both part of and distinct from, recalls the late cultural theorist Stuart Hall's distinction between *encoding* and *decoding*.[28] In his now classic media theory and cultural studies essay, Hall argues that the hegemonic structures of meaning that are produced by (mass) culture and encoded by the larger economic enterprises of capitalism are not the only "networks of production" at work. While the messages encoded in mass cultural formations are prescribed by the dominant order, the "relative autonomy" of the messages within this system allows for different interpretations and interventions in decoding these presumably dominant meanings. Hall's use of *auton-*

omy instead of automation is significant here. Autonomy grants fluidity to the signs of communication, but only as they manifest in recognition (of the gestures, words, and names that form a self) and eventually settle into meaning and culture. A self, then, is cast as a kind of singularity, a determined yet still autonomous object of the sign's interpellation. In his characteristically generous brilliance, Hall notes that this dynamic between encoding and decoding is asymmetrical and riddled with mis-recognitions within and beyond the structures of recognition. Because of this asymmetry, the calculus of signs and the calculus of selves—for they must surely be selves now—become charged and unwieldy; they exceed the presumed singularity of meaning and culture as they exceed the container of experience. *Dom Tak* is thus distinguished from the (hegemonic) culture or experience of Shaa'bi because the piece divests from the prescribed will of the performer or the consumer that consti-tutes the formal culture or genre—a distinction Khan makes explicit in the above passage. Through the specific practices of automation and improvisation at work in *Dom Tak*, Khan muddies the waters of Shaa'bi's prescribed modalities of subjection and recognition.

The synonymy of automation and musical genre is one of the chief conceits of *Dom Tak*, and this synonymy is what allows Khan to estab-lish the terms of recognition both for the participating Shaa'bi artists and for the viewing/listening audience that encounters *Dom Tak* in the fine art gallery. For the production of *Dom Tak*, as noted, Khan invited six Egyptian Shaa'bi studio musicians—an accordionist, a *kawala* (reed instrument) player, a backing keyboardist, a solo keyboardist, a trum-peter, and a violinist—to record separately in individual studio sessions. These musicians were given the same backing Shaa'bi beat produced by Khan and a musical mode in which to play, but they were not given a mel-ody or a theme, and they did not hear or see what their fellow musicians had played. Crucially, these musicians were all session musicians rather than bandmates in an already formed group or ensemble, although they may have, at some point in their careers, worked together.

Some of the musicians who showed up to the recording sessions with Khan recognized one another socially or informally, but none of them were privy to the sounds the others would produce. So while these musi-cians were likely at least partially familiar with the others' respective sounds and some of their tendencies, they had not formally practiced together in any single coherent group context. Moreover, (and much like Khan himself) they had no exact idea of the larger sonic output to which they were contributing. Thus, while each musician, as in any genre or form, had their own musical tendencies, they could not base their tendencies on the playing of their fellow musicians. This lack of a leading voice is an especially important in the face of Shaa'bi's typical modes of play and performance.

The formal conventions for playing and performing Shaa'bi music have become sedimented through the studio context. Not unlike some classical forms of Arabic music such as *Mawaal* or *Tarab*, with which Shaa'bi shares some formal roots, Shaa'bi music's instrumental composition revolves around the configuring of and improvisation on Arabic musical scales or *Maqaamaat*.[29] While long-form improvisation tends to dominate the various live performance contexts in which musical forms related to Shaa'bi are performed, Shaa'bi music has curtailed the broader spirit of improvisation in the recording studio, largely limiting it to shorter tracks that are dominated by vocal leading. Within either a live performance or a studio recording session, Shaa'bi musicians conventionally play off of the sonic and visual presence of their fellow musicians, most especially the vocalist, and they use such a presence to develop a point of reference from which to improvise and solo.

Individuality or autonomy for Shaa'bi musicians emerged through the contrasting modalities of "live" and "recorded" recognition within the structure of the ensemble. Increasingly, in the studio context, Shaa'bi has tended to lean toward popular forms of Arabic music that produce shorter-length lyrical tracks. This inclination in the Shaa'bi form has been nurtured through its rigidification into a genre replete with an established discursive context and a set of standardized operations, gestures, sounds, and signs. These operations have become established terms of recognition against which a self or other supposedly identifies in and as the music.[30]

The studio musicians in *Dom Tak* are not encouraged to break with these terms of recognition, this automatic gesture, or this genre. Khan does not offer these musicians "freedom" or "agency" either within or without the genre in which they play and make their livings. As George E. Lewis has pointed out in his writing on Black experimental music and the European avant-garde, art musicians, in service of their own fantasies of artistic freedom, have often produced works that presumptuously appropriate the labor and condescendingly admonish the practices of genre-based musicians.[31]

Dom Tak implicitly acknowledges (on the part of Khan and the Shaa'bi musicians) that genre indeed represents the terms of recognition against which they must define themselves, not merely a kind of aesthetic or political limitation. Their identity and their sense of self is produced through the absented/projected other: the other musician whom they imagine to be playing the genre of the production, and the genre of the self that is accompanying, accenting, leading, or improvising with that projected musician. The musicians' performances become uncanny doubles of themselves; they hear themselves playing their tendencies, playing the genre, engaging in the kind of self-analysis of which Cecil Taylor so eloquently speaks.[32] They must reckon with that sonic self, with their instrumental individuality, precisely as they sonically name these terms of recognition within the larger event of the sound track of *Dom Tak*.

When you walk into *Dom Tak* you are faced with a profound presence that refuses to recognize you. Off in the distance a set of anthropomorphic speakers of varying heights both suggest and negate a corporeal presence; in the corner of the room lies a visible yet visually subdued computer running a program that synchronizes the lights to the music; every musical track corresponds to a different light setting. Abruptly, the timer ticks audibly, ominously, for exactly thirty ticks, leading into thirty seconds of white light, after which a sudden explosion of Khan's Shaa'bi composition blares forth. *Dom Tak* presents you with violent indifference; it refuses to recognize you even as it (re)presents the common terms of recognition you require.

What is being automatically sounded in *Dom Tak* is not Shaa'bi music; as the earlier quote from Khan suggests, it is genre: "what is played is its ghost or twisted twin or something like that, because its rules are being performed." The split that occurs in *Dom Tak* is something like the rupture between genre and idiom. Or, to put this more sharply in terms of Nathaniel Mackey's formulation of the improvisational ruptures of Black music, *Dom Tak* partially initiates a "movement from noun to verb," which the Shaa'bi music enacts through and against its categorization and commodification.[33] Not unlike that profound movement from jazz to improvisatory free forms of something else, which Mackey engages in his work, Khan's piece engages the Shaa'bi form, displacing the expectations of its practitioners and most especially its audience that it must function as an "autonomous" object for their interpretation and consumption. Khan elaborates on this effect: "While we were installing [*Dom Tak*], I had a sensation when I was adjusting the volume, I suddenly had a sensation that listening, it was as if Shaa'bi music has gone to a psychoanalytical session and I was witnessing all of its neurosis; a little nervous breakdown, what it wants, what it hates and what it loves and what it's afraid of was kind of speaking to me. . . . The moment you come in the

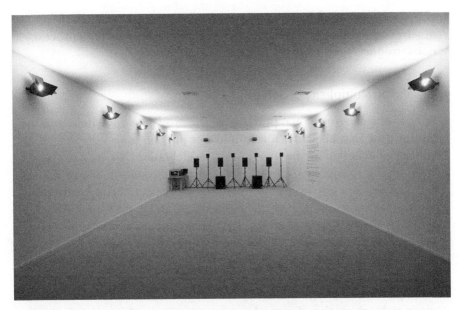

Fig. 5.1. Hassan Khan's *Dom Tak Tak Dom Tak* (2005), displayed in SALT Gallery, Istanbul, Turkey, 2012. (Image courtesy of the artist and Galerie Chantal Crousel.)

room and the lights go on and [the music ends] then the lights go off. That's actually also the moment when the audience feels the rupture in their experience of the piece as something they're consuming and their experience of the piece outside that."[34] Somewhere between the neurotic excess of Shaa'bi's automation and the indifferent automation that unfolds in front of and over the audience, *Dom Tak* emerges as a liminal space. Autonomy is foreclosed when Khan asks the musicians to adhere to the sonic output of their genre, but only under constraints that disrupt Shaa'bi's conventional performance dynamic. Neither, equally profoundly, does Khan allow the listener/viewer of *Dom Tak* to adopt a kind of autonomous consumer/viewer relationship to the form. Khan "is playing the musical culture itself rather than just the music."[35] This is a moment and a space of mutual misrecognition among musicians and audience that thwarts the apperceptive recognition of the studio and the gallery. The selves and their respective others are rendered as images in a mirror, sounds in a speaker, notes in a score, and elements in a work that, though it has been materially inscribed, has yet to be performatively realized. As Lewis notes of improvisation, "the listener also improvises."[36] The shattering of the self's fantastic singularity in recognition opens up a vocabulary through which we can start to think in terms of selves as points and sounds wherein meaning is perpetually a process, not a product. *Jewel* invites us to go there, too.

Jewel: The Multiplicity of Selves

By 2010 the congregational practices of the *moulid* had overflowed into the form of Shaa'bi, as the music, and not just the now somewhat distant religious ceremony, became cause for celebration. Not only did New Wave Shaa'bi conjure images of working-class life, much like its antecedent forms, but the music and the form also began to cohere around spectacular and fantastic movements, gestures, and ways of operating by working-class musicians, dancers, DJs, MCs, and various practitioners. New Wave Shaa'bi morphed into a more self-consciously sound system–driven culture, a "bass culture" of sorts.[37] New Wave Shaa'bi ascended to a larger organized public presence through sound system parties organized primarily through Shaa'bi producers, MCs, and dancers. At these street or block parties, dancers became a significant draw as their fluid and jagged movements developed a nuanced formal language to speak in and along the booming bass and the rapidly rolling tabla strikes—*dom tak tak, dom tak, dom dom tak tak.* Yet the compositional contexts of New Wave Shaa'bi began to shift to radically informal spaces of practice as well.

The music's relative ubiquity throughout Cairo's working-class neighborhoods led to organized and spontaneous scenes of dancing right within the packed density of Cairo's crowded streets and squares. Shaa'bi thus became a kind of quotidian "spatial practice," in which street dancers have produced their own vocabularies, syntaxes, and grammars of movement that occupy social class not as a point of symbolic reference, but as a milieu from which to speak. How these vocabularies emerge is irreducibly connected to Cairo and its manifestation in these contemporary Shaa'bi practices as an improvisatory "way of operating"; that is what Michel de Certeau once called "a space of enunciation," a context to be practiced and performed.[38] The complex gestures, gesticulations, and movements that characterize Shaa'bi's culture of improvised street dancing compose subjects whose trajectories and projections of selves cut across both the "vertical" narratives of the city and the horizontal narratives of Shaa'bi's marginality, which would reify those vertical narratives.

Attempts to nominalize Shaa'bi and package it for mainstream Egyptian society as *the* authentically marginal form of culture emanating from Cairo's vibrant slums have been relatively successful both nationally and internationally, as with, for example, Hind Meddeb's 2013 film *Electro Chaabi*. The commercialization of Shaa'bi also corresponds to a longer history of the novelization and authentication of urban and folk Egyptian cultural forms within fine art and mainstream commercial contexts. Both state-funded and private, often Western, nonprofit art contexts have played host to works that idealize and profit from what Khan succinctly calls "the Shaa'bi reference."[39] As Omnia El Shakry and Jessica Winegar point out in their respective works, Cairo's contemporary neoliberal art landscape of private and state-funded art often privileges works that represent a perceived authentic (*Asili*) Egyptian aesthetic or, conversely, a global artistic modernist "contemporary" aesthetic (Mu'asiri) that presumably appeals to a Western global art world.[40]

Both discursive art contexts—which still dominate many of Egypt's fine art institutions—have sought to produce a consumable "experience" of Cairo, whether that is the exoticized experience of the Western art "outsider" or the state-sanctioned experience of the putative national subject who frequents the official spaces of display. Khan's work with Shaa'bi in *Jewel* enters the fray precisely at this nexus.

In the dark expanse of a room, only a single bulb illuminated in the back, the wall across from the entrance becomes a screen: the text/image *Jewel/Jawhara* appears, while a slow-winding *kawala* whispers. The text/image disappears, and—just as an accordion joins the *kawala*, and a suggestive galloping tabla beat is heard, replete with rhythmic *riqq* (tambourine) accents—the screen-wall is ornamented in blue-lit flickers. A bejeweled anglerfish swims across the screen amid the blue speckles of light, and the introductory passage of the Shaa'bi track ruminates. As the track hovers in place, a chorus of *mizmar* (shawms or reed instruments) sharply cuts through; the anglerfish freezes and is transubstantiated into a series of abstract lights that line the surfaces of a rotating speaker. When the camera pans out, the audience is faced with two men: one clearly younger, the other clearly older, dancing on either side of the speaker and facing each other. Their movements, a series of gyrations, undulating pops and locks, and sweeping hand gestures, partially resemble the dance repertoire of Shaa'bi street dancers, yet these moves have an uncanny, wayward quality that veers from the expected conventions of that form. Shaa'bi street dancing often adheres to a battle style, wherein dancers deploy their bodies in the most spectacular and undulant of positions in an attempt to trump their opponent, who usually dances a mere foot in front of them.

In forms like *Tarab* and *Zikr*, dancing often achieves self-possession

and ecstasy and affirms the body's function in securing the transcendental potentialities of the self.[41] These classical forms emphasize that the
machinations of the body are teleologically *for* or *about* the spiritual ends
that the self can attain. In Shaa'bi, however, the dancing body becomes a
material site through which the formal experiences of a self are config-
ured and realized at every instance; through gesture and movement they
become ends in themselves. *Jewel* uncannily references the formal constraints of the Shaa'bi cipher in the dancers' distance from each other,
the presence of the (fish-adorned) speaker, and of course the booming
sound track. *Jewel* does not regressively freeze the Shaa'bi form into a
semantic rendering of the self in language. The performers are speaking their own secret language, and they are part of a more complex fantasy of their own invention that frolics in the face of externally imposed
forms of class overdetermination and meaning.

   Jewel evolved from a reverie that Khan had while cabbing home
through Cairo one night, when he saw two men dancing in the glimmer
of the streetlights; this scene triggered an elaborate fantasy for Khan.
The video installation that is *Jewel*, Khan admits, is amazingly similar to
that fantastical scene that he concocted. In fact, he had such a sharp
image of the two men dancing in his dream that Khan chose the two performers in *Jewel*—Ahmed Mohamed Abdel El Rahman and Shehta Abdel
El Aziz—based in large part on their resemblance to those fantasized figures. Yet, the sublimity of *Jewel* perhaps belies the complex and organic
methods of improvisation and practice that brought the work into being.
In *Jewel*, much like in *Dom Tak*, Khan engages the Shaa'bi reference, and
yet again in *Jewel* Khan is not interested in the reification or romantic
celebration of that reference.

   In some consonance with how Shaa'bi street dancers enact the materiality of their bodies, Khan engages Shaa'bi as a referent and a context
from which a language and the inherent excess of a self can emerge.
That emergence is not detached or naively decontextualized, but rooted
within a stark and perhaps oblique juxtaposition to that figure of the
anglerfish that begins *Jewel*. On the one hand, the anglerfish ushers in
the specter of an "instrumental rationality" of evolutionary and social
theory. The anglerfish is aesthetically cloaked in the shadow of the inhu-
man and the inscrutably monstrous, even as the categorical nature of
evolutionary thinking justifies its appearance under the designation of
the fish's rationalized functionalism. Khan adds:

   Another reason the fish interests me so much is that it is formed by its
   context, it looks the way it does, because it lives in that place, where

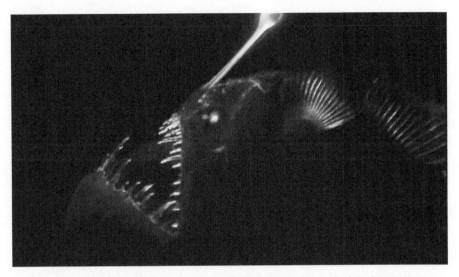

Fig. 5.2. Hassan Khan's *Jewel* (2010), displayed in SALT Gallery, Istanbul, Turkey, 2012. (Image courtesy of the artist and Galerie Chantal Crousel.)

> there is no light. How it looks is also how it survives, it's an anglerfish, it uses that light to attract prey. That kind of basic situation is translated into a cultural format with the two men with their language. I don't know if it's about reducing things, but about really connecting basic conditions with complex conditions. . . . So in a way I had an interest in bringing these two things together in a smooth way, not in a way where there is conflict. It's almost as if your deepest core is also your farthest point, something like that, but it's also the farthest thing from the self.[42]

Not unlike the improvised language of the dancers Abdel El Rahman and Abdel El Aziz, the anglerfish is conditioned by a context that is perceived as natural and that, tautologically, determines its perceived nature and ultimately its projected abjection, its monstrous appearance. Yet, on the other hand, all the paradigms that render the fish monstrously intelligible also always facilitate ways in which its forms of being are otherwise. The specific movements and decisions it makes as an image, an object, and a figure in *Jewel* are facilitated, for example, by it appearance even though they remain opaque to our prescribed terms of recognition. Something like its self remains remote and unintelligible to us precisely at its greatest point of (monstrous) intelligibility.

The choreographic language that Abdel El Rahman and Abdel El

Aziz are "speaking" appears opaque to the audience. The music frames
their movements as seemingly within the Shaa'bi genre, yet their interaction is not quite a rehearsal: there is no agreed upon genre or form,
no codified set of conventions and determinations, even though this
is the context in which their movements become visible and partially
intelligible. Khan in his collaboration with Abdel El Rahman and Abdel
El Aziz enacts something like what Fred Moten identifies as the phonochoreography invoked by Blackness.[43] In analyzing radical Black aesthetics, Moten asserts the language of phonochoreography as a way to
understand Blackness in apposition to language: Blackness exists and
is made by making meaning in the world through, yet also against, the
pathological determinations of language, genre, sound, and the ontol-
ogy of the self. In thinking of phonochoreography as an interruption
to "ontological explanation," Moten posits Blackness not strictly as an
identitarian possession of individual selves; rather, Blackness operates as
a radical, formal disruption of the very structure of the self in sound and
movement. Khan's description of the process of producing *Jewel*, which
he was gracious enough to share with me, speaks to the way in which he
was attempting to produce a language of form that does not reify the
determinations—musical, political, racial—of pathology and genre:

> So in working with each of them [the performers] separately I devel-
> oped a physical gestural language where they could talk, threaten,
> and express love, or respect, or hesitation. Of course it is not a totally
> refined language; it's gestural, there's no words. I connected it to
> each of them personally to what they knew personally. I would then
> start to connect it to the music. I would then play them bits of the
> music, they would get to listen to some of the music, I'd bring my
> laptop with my multi-track and I'd play some of the beat only, and
> then while they're working with that add another instrument in. So I
> made them very familiar with the music with this process of playing
> different parts of the music to them in different ways and connecting
> their movements to it. Then I brought them together. I wanted them
> to meet each other when they both had a language so that they could
> talk to each other through that language. So then the conversation
> begins; that's kind of how it was built.[44]

The improvisatory process that Khan developed with Abdel El Rahman
and Abdel El Aziz reveals some of the resonance between *Dom Tak* and
Jewel, or perhaps the endless revision of the one by the other. A pho-

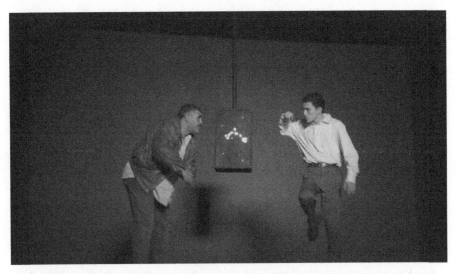

Fig. 5.3. Hassan Khan's *Jewel* (2010), displayed in SALT Gallery in Istanbul, Turkey, 2012. (Image courtesy of the artist and Galerie Chantal Crousel.)

nochoreographic space is opened up in *Dom Tak*, in *Jewel*, somewhere between and beyond the interstices of genre and form. The Shaa'bi genre provides a kind of familiar referential context for Abdel El Rahman and Abdel El Aziz, but it is also merely one material with which they work and through which they improvise; versions and even languages of selves emerge.

The process by which Khan, Abdel El Rahman, and Abdel El Aziz produce a grammar, a vocabulary, a language through *Jewel* complicates both the pathology of genre and the pathology of a self through improvisation. In their collaborative development of a vocabulary of movement, Khan prompted the performers with a generic set of moves and gestures that he had imagined and composed. This vocabulary was nonetheless subjected rigorously to the irreducibly complex set of memories, references, and figures that each performer brought to each session. So while Shaa'bi might have ostensibly provided the overarching musical context for their movements, the syntax, diction, and indeed the whole repertoire of movements that Abdel El Rahman and Abdel El Aziz imagined came from the divergent and at times contradictory indexes that had marked them and that they had marked. Yet the artists did not engage these references with the intention of representing their sources. These moves had been composed with an indexical web of meanings; Khan invoked mass cultural references, presumably shared sensations, and experiences as points of orientation with Abdel El Rahman and Abdel El Aziz.

Khan is not trying to affirm an indexical relationship to these references wherein they could be reified as such. The dancers' improvisatory language possesses an idiomatic quality that grades against the standardized conventions of genre, language, and self-expression. There is a distinct yet irreducible sense that Abdel El Rahman and Abdel El Aziz are having a sonic, visual, and gestural conversation through their movements, but not a conversation based on the functional nature of communication. Rather, their conversation is entrenched in the density of poetic gestures, as if a conversation in verse, where the weight of meaning is tethered to the discursivity of a form, of their histories and their bodies, but not reducible to any of these.[45] Quite explicitly, *Jewel* reproduces a kind of self/other relation between the two performers, but Khan works with the inherent excess of that relation, of the charged others and selves that are always already there.

A modernist impulse toward the simultaneous recognition and fugitivity—the otherwiseness—of the self through gestures, words, and forms permeates Hassan Khan's work. Khan's work evinces a suspicion of the apparatuses of representation through which this self is asserted and against which its fugitivity is defined and recognized in so many modernist artistic and musical practices. While Khan's work primarily circulates and participates within fine art contexts in Cairo and abroad, his creations also disturb the normative valuations of those spaces' exceptionality and consumptive drives. At the level of the material, both *Dom Tak* and *Jewel* unsettle the way in which that otherwiseness characteristic of the modernist impulse must hinge on the commodified autonomy of the artist through and against the commodified autonomy of the consumer. The automated nature of this exchange is the material basis from which Khan's work pushes forms to improvise beyond these designations.

If *Dom Tak* partially alienates the audience from the experience of consumption of an art object by drawing the viewers' attention to that commodified, mirror-like structure through which they constitute their notions of self as consumer/listener/patron, then *Jewel* delves further into how this mirror is thinking, speaking, sounding, and moving.[46] *Jewel* basks playfully in that space of negated assumptions, just beyond the pale of recognition, because it is interested not in creating intelligible, communicative, and consumable signs, but in producing an active immersive reality, a process where context is perpetually formed and refashioned.[47]

The underinterrogated ethos of freedom that underwrites improvisation, and against which genre is pitched as its opposite, presumes the singularly of a self, or perhaps more subtly the standpoint from which a self is wholly produced and identified. *Dom Tak* and *Jewel*, in powerful yet distinct ways, depart from that formal opposition between genre and improvisation, automation and improvisation. Yet by exploring and disturbing the terms of recognition and meaning through which a self is recognized, Khan's oeuvre veers toward the realization of a new context, time, and reality not reducible to the self's interpellative function as the experience of the work. In that improvisatory moment, that set of decisions that are perpetually decisions, that phonochoreography of sounds, images, words, and materials, somewhere amid the elusive infinity of selves that are conjured and denied in language, *Dom Tak* and *Jewel* speak, and move, and sound there.

Notes to Chapter 5

1. I encountered both works at SALT Gallery in Istanbul, Turkey, which hosted a retrospective of Hassan Khan's work in 2012.

2. See Laing, *The Voice of Experience*. Additional works by Laing that resonate with Khan's thinking are *The Divided Self* and *Self and Others*.

3. See, for example, Khan's crystalline sculpture *The Knot* (2012), which references Laing's text *Knots*.

4. Laing, *The Voice of Experience*, 19.

5. A. J. Racy, in *Making Music in the Arab World*, discusses the institutionalization of Arabic musics specifically in terms of two critical shifts that emerged from the 1932 Cairo Congress of Arab Music: a push to standardize the notational conventions of Arabic music into an even-tempered system, and a call to integrate more Western instruments into Arabic ensembles. Beyond these thrusts, however, and important in light of my discussion of Khan's work, the Cairo Congress also led to the standardization of the actual structures and modes of improvisation.

6. For a discussion of this development in relation to improvisation studies, see Lewis, *A Power Stronger Than Itself*.

7. Khan, *Nine Lessons*.

8. See Fred Moten's *In the Break* and Cecil Taylor's famous equation of improvisation as "self-analysis (improvisation)," which is cited in the liner notes to *Unit Structures*. I would extend Taylor's formulation into a critique and analysis of *the self* (not just a self) in Western civilization.

9. See, for example, Khan's radio drama *Purity* (2012).

10. John Cage's approaches to composition, especially as he describes them as incommensurate with improvisation, tend to revolve around self-assertion disguised as self-negation. See Cage, "Composition as Process." Also see an oft-cited quote from Cage: "People frequently ask me if I'm faithful to the answers,

or if I change them because I want to. I don't change them because I want to. When I find myself at that point, in the position of someone who *would* change something—at that point I don't change it, I change myself. It's for that reason that I have said that instead of self-expression, I'm involved in self-alteration." Quoted in Larson, *Where the Heart Beats*, 179. My critique of Cage here has been shaped by conversations with Hassan Khan, as well as by Lewis, *A Power Stronger Than Itself*; and Braxton, *Tri-Axium Writings*, vol. 1.

11. Khan, "The Big One: Performance Program" Queens Museum, Hassan Khan, May 2011. In reference to what Khan would characterize as this canonical "modernist fantasy," see *Electronic and Experimental Music*, in which Thom Holmes argues in rather minimal terms that the Euro-American avant-garde of the twentieth century was constituted by a practical collectivity of artists and musicians. Holmes's points about collectivity are rather myopic in the context of the larger work, in which he disavows the centrality of improvisation and its extensive emergence within Black music. Holmes approaches the topic of turntablism exclusively through the work of Christian Marclay, a white art-music turntablist. This treatment is an egregious disavowal of the work of Grand Wizard Theodore, Grandmaster Flash, DJ Jazzy Jeff, Rob Swift (and the X-Ecutioners/X-Men), DJ Qbert (and the Invisibl Skratch Piklz), DJ Mutamassik, DJ Craze, and many, many others who have experimented with the turntable. Holmes excludes the impact of postcolonial experimentalists such as Afro-jazz-funk musicians Fela Kuti and King Sunny Ade and dub musicians King Tubby and Lee "Scratch" Perry, and he offers a condescendingly nominal inclusion of Halim El-Dabh— whom some have called "the father of African electronic music"—under the moniker "international artists," revealing the provincial Euro-American supremacy that pervades the electronic-experimental avant-garde. For a more useful perspective here, see Schütz, "Making Music Together."

12. Hassan Khan, Cairo, Egypt, personal interview, August 28, 2010.

13. Khan, "In Defense of the Corrupt Intellectual," 5.

14. Khan's thought and work resonate with what Fred Moten, in various incarnations, has outlined as the irruptive force of Blackness, which troubles the equation of personhood as selfhood and by extension the tenets that supposedly make the self possible. Undoubtedly, some of this resonance between Khan and Moten emanates from a shared Fanonian reservoir that differently shapes their work. See Khan's ongoing performance work entitled *READFANONYOUFUCKINGBASTARD* (1997–); and see Moten, *In the Break*; and Moten, "Blackness and Nothingness."

15. Anna Madoeuf offers a broader treatment of *moulid* festivals and feasts in Cairo, including more information on their religious contexts, as events that emerged historically from Sufi gatherings, among other traditions. See Madoeuf, "Feasts."

16. Khan, interview, August 28, 2010.

17. See 100 Copies Music: 100copies.com. Accessed August 24, 2010.

18. See Kuo, "Trusted Sources."

19. Hassan Khan, Istanbul, Turkey, personal interview, September 24, 2012.

20. One can start to sense this shift—though it was also always there all along— most prominently in a short video by Khan titled *Sometime/Somewhere Else* (2001) and in one of Khan's most expansive video works, *The Hidden Location* (2004).

21. Khan, "Loud, Insistent and Dumb," 82–83.

22. Khan, 82–83.

23. Madoeuf, "Feasts."

24. For a historical and formal distinction between *Zikr* and *Tarab*, see two key texts on Arabic music: Al Ghazali, *Ihya 'Ulum al-Din*; and Racy, *Making Music in the Arab World*. Eleventh-century Al Ghazali is generally considered to be the most influential writer on Arabic music in the classical period. His perspectives on music, specifically in relation to *Tarab*, are further explicated by Racy.

25. Roland Barthes's formulation of the "grain" harmonizes with Khan's space for working with Shaa'bi, especially in terms of how the grain—as "the materiality of the body speaking its mother tongue; perhaps the letter, almost certainly *signifiance*"—operates through yet strains against the signification, the communicability or even functional recognition of the form (Barthes, "The Grain of the Voice," 182, 186–87).

26. Khan, interview, August 28, 2010.

27. Khan, interview, September 24, 2012.

28. Hall, "Encoding/Decoding."

29. For more on the formal influences of Shaa'bi music, such as Islamic *Mawaal* and *Muwashshah*, and on the legacy of instrumentation between these musics and Shaa'bi, see Touma, *The Music of the Arabs*; and Shawqi, *Ibn Al-Munajim's Essay on Music*.

30. See Meintjes, *Sound of Africa!*

31. See Lewis, *A Power Stronger Than Itself*; Lewis, afterword; and Braxton, *Tri-Axium Writings*.

32. Here I am referring again to Cecil Taylor's instantiation, "self-analysis (improvisation)."

33. Mackey, "Other: From Noun to Verb." *Representations*, Summer, 1992, No. 39 (Summer, 1992), 51–70.

34. Khan, interview, September 24, 2012.

35. Khan, interview, August 28, 2010.

36. Lewis, "Improvising" 14.

37. See Bradley, *Bass Culture*; and Brewster and Broughton, *Last Night a DJ Saved My Life*.

38. Certeau, *The Practice of Everyday Life*, 98.

39. Khan, interview, August 28, 2010.

40. See El Shakry, "The Hidden Location." For a treatment of Egypt's art scene, see El Shakry, "Artistic Sovereignty in the Shadow of Post-Socialism"; and Winegar, *Creative Reckonings*.

41. See Racy, *Making Music in the Arab World*.

42. Khan, interview, September 24, 2012.

43. Moten, "The Case of Blackness," 180.

44. Khan, interview, September 24, 2012.

45. This centering of form may partially explain why every time *Jewel* has been exhibited, it has conjured an asymmetrical response from young men, who frequently gather in the piece and dance in partial imitation of the performers on the screen. Khan attested to this phenomenon in a conversation that I had with him via Skype, June 23, 2014. I also witnessed this phenomenon at SALT Gallery in Istanbul, Turkey, in September 2012.

46. See Marriott, *Haunted Life*.

47. In examining the status of the graphical sign in southern Cameroon under colonialism, Achille Mbembe writes: "In these conditions, the great epistemological—and therefore social—break was not between what was seen and what was read, but between what was seen (*the visible*) and what was not seen (*the occult*), between what was heard, spoken, and memorized and what was concealed (*the secret*). To the extent that reality had each time to be transformed into a sign and the sign constantly filled with reality, the problem for those whose main activity was publicly to decipher the world was to interpret simultaneously both its obverse and what might be called its negation, its reverse." Mbembe, "The Thing and Its Double," 144. In *Jewel*, Khan seeks to disrupt the simulacrum of language (words whether spoken or written) as representation of a reality.

Works Cited

Al Ghazali, Abu Hamid. *Ihya 'Ulum al-Din*, vol. 2. Damascus: Maktabat 'Abd al-Wakil al-Durubi, 1976.

Barthes, Roland. "The Grain of the Voice." In *Image-Music-Text*, translated by Stephen Heath, 179–89. New York: Hill and Wang, 1977.

Bradley, Lloyd. *Bass Culture: When Reggae Was King*. New York: Viking, 2000.

Braxton, Anthony. *Tri-Axium Writings*, vol. 1. San Francisco: Synthesis Music, 1985.

Brewster, Bill, and Frank Broughton. *Last Night a DJ Saved My Life: The History of the Disc Jockey*. New York: Grove Press, 2000.

Cage, John. "Composition as Process: 1. Changes (1958)." In *Silence: Lectures and Writings by John Cage*, 18–55. Middletown, CT: Wesleyan University Press, 1973.

Certeau, Michel de. *The Practice of Everyday Life*. Berkeley: University of California Press, 1984.

El Shakry, Omnia. "Artistic Sovereignty in the Shadow of Post-Socialism: Egypt's 20th Annual Youth Salon." *e-flux journal* 7 (June 2009). https://www.e-flux .com/journal/07/61388/artistic-sovereignty-in-the-shadow-of-post-socialism -egypt-s-20th-annual-youth-salon/

El Shakry, Omnia. "The Hidden Location: Art and Politics in the Work of Hassan Khan." *Third Text Asia* 1, no. 2 (Spring 2009): 71–85.

Hall, Stuart. "Encoding/Decoding." In *Culture, Media, Language: Working Papers in Cultural Studies, 1972–79*, edited by Stuart Hall, Dorothy Hobson, Andrew Lowe, and Paul Willis, 128–38. London: Center for Contemporary Cultural Studies, University of Birmingham, 1980.

Holmes, Thom. *Electronic and Experimental Music*. New York: Routledge, 2002.

Khan, Hassan. "In Defense of the Corrupt Intellectual." *e-flux Journal* 18 (September 2010). https://www.e-flux.com/journal/18/67447/in-defense-of-the-cor rupt-intellectual/

Khan, Hassan. "Loud, Insistent and Dumb: Shaabiyat and the Return of the Moulid as Charged Referent." *Bidoun* 11 (Summer 2007). https://www.bido un.org/issues/11-failure

Khan, Hassan. *Nine Lessons Learned from Sherif El-Azma / 9 Durus Mustaqa min Sharif El-Azma*. Cairo: Contemporary Image Collective, 2009.

Kuo, Michelle. "Trusted Sources." *Artforum International* 52, no. 2 (October 2013). https://www.artforum.com/print/201308/trusted-sources-43120

Laing, R. D. *The Divided Self.* New York: Penguin Books, 1969.

Laing, R. D. *Knots.* New York: Vintage Books, 1972.

Laing, R. D. *Self and Others.* New York: Penguin Books, 1971.

Laing, R. D. *The Voice of Experience.* New York: Pantheon Books, 1982.

Larson, Kay. *Where the Heart Beats: John Cage, Zen Buddhism, and the Inner Life of Artists.* New York: Penguin, 2013.

Lewis, George E. "Afterword to 'Improvised Music After 1950' The Changing Same." In *The Other Side of Nowhere: Jazz, Improvisation and Communities in Dialogue,* edited by Daniel Fischlin and Ajay Heble, 163–72. Middleton, CT: Wesleyan University Press, 2004.

Lewis, George E. *A Power Stronger Than Itself: The AACM and American Experimental Music.* Chicago: University of Chicago Press, 2009.

Lewis, George E. "Improvising Tomorrow's Bodies: The Politics of Transduction." *E-misferica,* vol. 4.2, November 2007, pp. 1–15.

Mackey, Nathaniel. "Other: From Noun to Verb." *Representations,* No. 39 (Summer, 1992), pp. 51–70

Madoeuf, Anna. "Feasts: Panoramas in Town—The Spaces and Times of the *Moulids* of Cairo." In *Urban Africa: Changing Contours of Survival in the City,* edited by AbdouMaliq Simone and Abdelghani Abouhani, 68–95. New York: Zed Books, 2005.

Marriott, David. *Haunted Life: Visual Culture and Black Modernity.* New Brunswick, NJ: Rutgers University Press, 2006.

Mbembe, Achille. "The Thing and Its Double." In *On the Postcolony.* Berkeley: University of California Press, 2001.

Meintjes, Louise. *Sound of Africa! Making Music Zulu in a South African Studio.* Durham, NC: Duke University Press, 2003.

Moten, Fred. "Blackness and Nothingness (Mysticism in the Flesh)." *South Atlantic Quarterly* 112, no. 4 (2013): 737–80.

Moten, Fred. "The Case of Blackness." *Criticism* 50, no. 2 (2008): 177–218.

Moten, Fred. *In the Break: The Aesthetics of the Black Radical Tradition.* Durham, NC: Duke University Press, 2003.

Racy, A. J. *Making Music in the Arab World: The Culture and Artistry of Tarab.* New York: Cambridge University Press, 2003.

Schütz, Alfred. "Making Music Together: A Study in Social Relationship." In *Collected Papers II: Studies in Social Theory,* edited by Arvid Brodersen, 159–78. The Hague: Martinus Nijhoff, 1964.

Shawqi, Yusuf. *Ibn Al-Munajim's Essay on Music and the Melodic Ciphers of Kitaab Al-Aghani / Risala Ibn Munajim fi Kashaf Rumuz Kitab Al-Aghani.* Cairo: Ministry of Culture Centre for Editing and Publishing Arabic Manuscripts, 1976.

Taylor, Cecil. Liner notes to Cecil Taylor, *Unit Structures.* Blue Note 784237-2, 1987 (1966). Compact disc.

Touma, Habib Hassan. *The Music of the Arabs.* Translated by Lauri Schwartz. Portland, OR: Amadeus Press, 1996.

Winegar, Jessica. *Creative Reckonings: The Politics of Art and Culture in Contemporary Egypt.* Palo Alto, CA: Stanford University Press, 2006.

SIX | Improvising Mythoi and Difference in the Asian/Woman More-Than-Tinge

MIKE HEFFLEY

Referring to a Cuban rhythm, Jelly Roll Morton named "the Spanish tinge" as a key ingredient in the creole music called jazz that he helped concoct in New Orleans. Morton's notion is at odds with the fact that the rhythm in question was more accurately sourced to Africa than to Spain, and was arguably more a core than a "tinge" component in the bigger history of the music. Since such blithe confusion of genealogies and their significance is what this collection illuminates, I will take up and modify Morton's well-established "tinge" trope accordingly. I suggest a similar infusion—of an Asian more-than-tinge, through four women's voices— to the current profusion of improvised music first spawned, through African/European/American music hybrids, in the Atlantic triangle of the slave trade. The Atlantic region's history has dominated the narratives about power, race, and gender in modernist and postmodernist accounts of such music; the Pacific Rim's equally colonialist-imperialist past, though less about African enslavement and more about Asian struggles of a different order, deals with similar racial and gender dynamics. The tales told in the music of these four women engage that past, mainly by bespeaking much more a present and potential future well beyond its disparities of power. The difference they infuse in the music of the Atlantic emerges not from *changing* their traditional Asian aesthetics and techniques, or even their gender identities, so much as from *resetting* them all in the West's different contexts, and that to change the latter.[1]

These four expatriates living in North America—Jin Hi Kim from

Korea; and Han Mei, Wu Man, and Min Xiao-Fen from China—have labored long and extensively in Canada, the United States, and Europe to establish themselves within those originally Atlantic-world contexts of musical improvisation grown from jazz, free jazz, aleatoric and maverick composition, "noise," and other such experimental music scenes born and grown over the last century. They have done so by bringing their variously different and similar Asian-traditional instruments, sounds, techniques, and aesthetics, first as newcomers (as "hosted guests") to such improvisational practices and their larger discourse. I trace the arcs from their original styles and contexts to their various situations as budding improvisers, then as greater adepts in their cross-cultural, transcultural, and transhistorical (distinctions between the three ahead) collaborations and contexts. Those arcs (from nonimprovising roots) culminate in their flowerings in the different voices and statements they have brought to the Western improvisatory *milieux*, statements recently sounding in Asia as well.

I view those arcs through the bifocal lenses of *logos* and *mythos* to frame key features of their processes. The Greek terms are more conventionally used to denote the hierarchy of the rational over the mythical in intellectual history.[2] Here, instead, *logoi* refer to the techniques employed (mostly left- and right-hand mechanics of plucking and bending notes, since all are string players), and *mythoi* refer to the original (Asian-traditional) and different (Western, more-than-tinged) contexts in which the music is performed. Mythoi encompass, for example, conventional renditions of traditional folk or composed material as they are, as cross- or transcultural collaborations, as experimentally spontaneous and unscripted improvisations, or as newly conceived transhistorical formations for composition and improvisation.

All four musicians share similar logoi and mythoi in their overlapping career paths, and the complementary Greek terms serve to catch them all well. That said, I discuss Kim and Han more in terms of their logoi, and Wu and Min more in terms of their mythoi for two reasons: first, the technical details that "change" the sound by changing only its context will reach from Kim and Han to cover Wu and Min; and second, Wu and Min share a point of origin as pipa interpreters of the same notated classical repertoire but have taken divergent though overlapping lines into the Western contexts of improvised music, showing how the same original sound can change to any number of new mythoi (an insight that will then reach back to cover Kim and Han).

The woman part of the "more-than-tinge" can be seen in three ways:

all four women left their cultures of origin to seek wider musical horizons in the West in part because they felt their gender limited them where they were; all worked their way into roles as novice improvisers (first in the Western contexts of the practice, later in contexts of their own design) and relatively quickly established themselves as leaders in those roles more usually played by men; and all worked in ways that are as reflective of their gender as of their Asian identities, as they drew on their histories to "difference" the post-jazz Western improvised-music scene. I conclude the chapter with a meditation on hybridized notions of improvisatory discourse that produce sound changes.

Korean composer and *komungo*[3] master Jin Hi Kim comes from a country with strong, living roots in a woman-centered, improvisation-rich shamanism, which shares cultural space with other, more patriarchal traditions—Buddhism, Confucianism, Western classical music, jazz—that are variously improvisatory and scripted, transmitted through literary and oral/aural means. From China, *zheng* master Han Mei mines her traditional instrument and its ancient Taoist contexts—some in the instrument's traditional repertoire, much more in the West's new-and-improvised music scenes and various world-music genres—for how they might speak in and to that West about the more global creative-music terrain. And Min Xiao-Fen and Wu Man, both conservatory-trained *pipa* masters, have similarly turned from their original backgrounds in the Chinese classical repertoire to their respective improvisation-charted paths. The three Chinese musicians, unlike Kim, come from a musical milieu and practice devoid of improvisation, which they encountered only after moving to North America. They have each since made excursions into Chinese music history to rediscover and revive improvisational aspects of that tradition. The different mythoi couching the rubric of improvisation in both Korean and Chinese traditions will be distinguished from Western ones in the details ahead.

Jin Hi Kim (Composition and *Komungo*)

To summarize Kim's telling of Korean history,[4] it began some three thousand years ago when Tungusic tribal nomads from Mongolia settled in the region, building an agricultural state. Their Siberian shamanism was central in the state until, around the seventh century CE, Buddhism took shamanism's place in the courts. Confucianism supplanted Buddhism in the fourteenth century, and later periods, through the twentieth century, were marked by Japanese occupation and then Western cultural domination. While the ancient shamanism, Buddhism, and Confucianism have endured in the folk culture, by Kim's time the Western influence was at its height.[5]

Kim's interest in musical aspects of this history manifests directly in her contemporary offerings as a composer, improviser, and theorist. She was born in Incheon to devout Catholic parents, and her first exposures to music in school and church were Western, both religious and classical. When she was a musically precocious thirteen-year-old, her father enrolled her in the new national high school devoted to Korean traditional music (part of a traditionalist revival to elevate the social status of shamanism).[6]

Masters of the folk music styles *minyo* and *pansori*, mostly sung by ordinary people and rooted in shamanic traditions, taught Kim's favorite classes. *Sanjo*, a related genre developed in nineteenth-century shamanist practice, centralizes a rhythmic cycle (*jangdan*, similar to an Indian *tala*) under a master melody, generating both improvisation and trance. Unlike formal court styles, it is for both singers and players a vehicle for individual creativity and emotional expression. Kim writes, "Playing sanjo was difficult for me. Other students from the Southern province, where sanjo was created, already knew the melody at a young age, and they had already picked up the phrases very fast and created their own tone gestures within the phrases. . . . In order to play good sanjo, one should be gifted with a 'folk soul.'"

Yielding to that block of birth and nurture, she challenged another one. "I chose to major in the komungo—a fretted board zither with six strings, and a traditionally male instrument—over *gayageum*, the 12-stringed 'female' zither. I was attracted to komungo because it was known as the Confucian scholar's instrument. I questioned why a woman shouldn't play it; I liked the challenge. I was told that to play komungo one must be intellectual like a scholar, and that it was a difficult instrument to learn." Her training on this instrument in both full court orchestra and (especially) the smaller ensemble for the vocal genre *kagok* (or *gagok*, literally "lyric song," in which it is the more active lead instrument) brought her through its challenges to its full potential on foreground display.

Kim enrolled in 1976 at Seoul National University to major in traditional music, while auditing as many Western-music courses as she could. Her goal was to be a composer, and she had some initial public success with pieces she created for Korean and Western instruments, unusual at that time. Having thus found her tastes and niche in Korean classical styles, aesthetics, and instruments, she conceived her mission as a composer to fuse these elements with the Western classical tradition in which she had been brought up, to make her case for both traditions as equals. To immerse herself in that previously "occupying" music on its home turf, she thought it best to move to the West (specifically to the United States, as the Western society more multicultural than Europe) for her graduate studies. Her decision was also driven by the lack of opportunity and respect both for women and for folk music that she saw blocking her potential to be recognized as either composer or *komungo* master in Korea. "The society was still under the shadow of Confucianism. The male is better and the older is better. I was hopeless as a young female there."

Starting with her move to San Francisco in 1980, she studied composition and electronic music with composers John Adams, David Rosenboom, Lou Harrison, Larry Polansky, Terry Riley and others at both the San Francisco Conservatory of Music and Mills College, where Kim earned an MFA in electronic music and composition. A big part of her education was her work as a correspondent for a Korean magazine, writing columns about and interviews with composers at the yearly New Music America Festival. The experience exploded and exposed as too quaint her initial vision of joining East and West. "I was surprised to see how people respected all different kinds of music styles, including improvisation. . . . In fact, American composers are more focused on world music, while not looking at European classical music as much. From this, I witnessed the future of traditional music, and an infinite possibility to become successful as a musician."

Full of and liberated by this anything-and-everything-goes spirit, she developed a concept of composing that incorporated systematic improvisation on the level of a single note. Her signature "Living Tones" concept was developed to use in both scored pieces and collaborations with improvisers. It was inspired by the Korean element of *sigimse* (intonation). This Korean word suggests more than the Western concept of intonation, which, since the Baroque period, has meant rigid conformity to the equal-tempered scale. *Sigimse*, rather, conceives of each tone as having its own unique character and identity to be brought out and expressed in performance; what is expressed is a signature voice, similar to the "personal sound" of a jazz musician. In 1986, Kim composed the string quartet *Linking* for the Kronos Quartet, developing a special notation system for performance articulations and gestures, that extended traditional Korean techniques into her Living Tones: written directives and oral directions general enough to allow for the personal inflections of an outsider to the tradition.

Here is a good point to begin considering what is tinge, and what is more-than-tinge, and why. To my hearing, and from my reading of Kim's memoir, her Living Tones is far more than a "tinge," which would be something like writing a piece for a Western string quartet that adhered to fundamentally Western compositional and improvisational conventions, but with a garnish of Korean sounds and inflections sprinkled across its surface. Both Kim's words and the sound of the piece define it as more-than-tinge, a meeting of Korea and West as equals. The piece sees—and then actualizes—the de facto Western improvised/experimental music's intrinsic potential to *be* as Korean as Western, and raises it from that *potentia* to her agency's *actu.*

Kim's work as a composer since then has drawn similarly from various elements of Korean music, including shamanism's rural, agricultural, and folk practices; female fertility, based on Confucian principles of *yin* and *yang* in the cosmological forces that social and musical order were thought to reflect; and Buddhist rituals and chants. Her work and identity as a free improviser with other free improvisers began around this time too. Guitarist Henry Kaiser invited her to play freely improvised duets on *komungo*; similar collaborations with other leading guitarists and instrumentalists on the transatlantic scene followed, leading her to electrify the *komungo* (the first such instance worldwide) to bring its volume up to their usually greater levels. She attributes to her grounding in Korean traditional music—even the elitist introverted court styles—an unintended training for unscripted improvisation, as this traditional music was collective and leaderless, fostering vigilant and sensitive interactive listening to others while playing one's own part.

Kim, arguably, most fully solidified her approach to improvisation in the West when she was able to tap into the more extroverted folk-cultural aspects of the shamanist styles from which she first felt alienated. This development occurred when she discovered Ornette Coleman, Cecil Taylor, the Association for the Advancement of Creative Musicians (AACM), and African American music generally. "New Orleans reminded me of the Southern Jolla province in Korea, where improvisational music like pansori, *sinawi*, and sanjo were born. . . . If New Orleans is the birthplace of recent hybrid musical products, then Southern Jolla is an ancient such hybrid, with Siberian Shamanism, centuries ago. Both places made a similar mark as cradle of improvisational spirits and atmosphere."

The comparison is apt. Her improvisational style, Kim says, focuses more on texture than on melody. *Pansori* is a vocal style marked by rough texture to express raw, powerful emotion, in dialogue with percussion; speaking about similarly textured and percussive African American music, Amiri Baraka (when he was still going by his birth name LeRoi Jones) has said that "the whole concept of Afro-American music is hinged on vocal references."[7]

A more destructive clash of cultures led to an improvisatory performance context stemming from America's racially fraught history. The 1992 riots following the acquittal of four Los Angeles police offers charged with beating Rodney King included conflicts between Koreans and African Americans in Los Angeles's Korea Town. They prompted the Korea Society to commission Kim to stage a "concert to heal the wounds" at the Los Angeles County Museum of Art. She put together a trio with saxophonist Oliver Lake and bassist William Parker that she called Quagmire, "which meant in our context that 'difficulty and beauty are coexistent.' . . . *In this context, recognition of Korean and American culture/tradition was not so important.* We as human beings were bonded and moving together toward one destiny. Each individual sound of the trio melted well into one voice . . . I cannot avoid the feeling of insecurity when I mingle with a different race/culture, but at the same time I gain strength that I alone could not generate . . . The important part is not to try and avoid uneasiness but to deal with it." One might justifiably read the same attitude toward racial and cultural tension in the woman leaving her comfort zone to negotiate a violent male world. Further, the free-improvisation method itself trumps the idea that one culture or another dominates the dialogue. It is a *trans*cultural *statement* more than a hierarchical or clearly bordered *cross*-cultural *dialogue*.

In 1989, Kim and fellow musician and partner reed player Joseph Celli drew on their multicultural New York pool of peers to form the No World Improvisation ensemble, featuring acoustic and electronic instruments and players from Korea, India, Australia, and Senegal. "The name [No World Improvisation] signals the message that all music, regardless of nation and economic differences (the First World or the Third World/rich or poor), is equal. . . . I also experienced that when I do free improvisation with non-Western traditional musicians there is a common old-time sense among us, which is grounded, that the outcome is not so urgent and chaotic. . . . At the end it shapes its own organic form. Let it be." Kim has brought her Living Tones concept to her work as a free improviser as well as a composer. It "is based on not only unique tonality," she writes, "but also a time sense that is different from Western music. The Living Tones function best in a slow tempo where enough space is available to shape notes, which does not work well in a strict time frame. . . . The ensemble sound flows horizontally within a heterophonic melody in which each individual instrument creates its own nuances and specific articulation. All this is happening slowly and within a calm space."

That slow time first piqued my interest when Kim explained it in a workshop at Wesleyan University. What struck me as mysteriously regular yet unmetered was in fact something that she could count off for students, vocalizing what she was doing silently, to demonstrate the rhythm internalized. It immediately struck me as like what has been racially stereotyped by White people as Black people's "natural rhythm" (Anthony Braxton calls it "existential" to distinguish it from metered rhythm),[8] with the same affect of open cooperation with, rather than controlled manipulation of, one's/nature's rhythms and cycles—the difference being that Kim's slow time was a comfort and familiarity with the slow and serene rather than the fast and excited end of the spectrum.

Han Mei (*Zheng*)

Like Kim, Han Mei has produced a tome (in this case, her 2013 dissertation) covering all aspects of her work in music, including much autobiography and a chapter on the role of improvisation at issue here: "Improvisation as a Tool for Zheng Performance and Composition," with a subsection titled "Discovering an Individual Voice through Free Improvisation." Improvisation for her, too, was not a part of her early musical training or knowledge; it became so only after she came to the West as an adult professional musician who was accomplished on her instrument in both traditional and contemporary styles and repertoire. It drew her in then as a vehicle for personal expression and actualization of creative potential, and as a means of developing her own fresh and vital reprise of traditional Chinese music and theory.

Like Kim, Han came of age at a time when official repression of her natal culture's music was lifting, and she benefited from some of its brightest surviving torchbearers. At age eleven, in 1971, she began her *zheng* studies with the celebrated Shandong master Gao Zichen. The instrument itself—a plucked, horizontal zither born to Han China around the first century CE, grown since from as few as five to as many as fifty strings—embodies in its design a set of fundamental aesthetics

reflecting Confucianism and Taoism. "While these ancient Chinese philosophical principles delineated ideal standards of sound, meaning, and
performance, they also fostered spontaneity and extemporization," Han
writes.[9] More specifically, the "ideal standards" are conceived in the balance between Taoism's *yin* and *yang*, and Confucianism's *sheng* (sound)
and *yin* (music). Yang comprises everything fixed, finite, concrete—the
right hand's generation of the sound itself by plucking the string, a composition fixed in notation, mechanical or rote performance of same; yin
is the metadescriptor of what the left hand does with the raw sound and
patterns to turn them into personally and culturally expressive music,
through improvised bends of pitches, timbral/textural effects, dynamics, and so forth. Such processes are described in more nuanced terms
such as *jiahu* (ornamentation, "adding the flower" to the "bone tune"),
yi (intent), and *yun* (sophistication, refinement, and beauty). While conventional (and conventionally extolled) technical virtuosity is a mostly
yang display, Han borrows from music and education scholar Jane
O'Dea the concept of *craft skills* to apply to the subtler, deeper deployment of *yun* in *zheng* playing. "When I asked composers what attracted
them to write for the zheng, their answers often included 'bending,'
'portamento,' 'inflection,' or 'timbre,' effects primarily achieved with
nuanced use of left-hand bending techniques and right-hand plucking
techniques. These techniques would fall within the craft skills, which
'have to do with discerning and utilizing the interpretive potential of
subtle tonal colours.'"[10]

The *zheng*'s original, richly improvisatory and oral-traditional practice
spanned the male (intellectual, official) and female (sensual, emotional,
informal) poles of the culture, much like the piano in the equally patriarchal West. That practice has waned over the last couple of centuries,
giving way to a traditional canon fixed in notation, largely conscripted
for nationalistic propaganda as Han came of age. Even so, she took to
the instrument's sound as a gentler counter to the martial music heard
in her military family. When she was sixteen, in 1975, the army recruited
her into the Qianjin Song and Dance Troupe in Shenyang; in 1980 she
auditioned for and won the coveted position of solo *zheng* player in the
nationally prestigious People's Liberation Army Zhanyou Song and
Dance Ensemble. As Han told me in June of 2007, "The troupe began in
the 1940s. It had several hundred artists when I was there (dancers, singers, and musicians). It is very much like the army troupes in the Soviet
Union. . . . Many nationally famous artists were at Zhanyou (the Army
had the privilege and advantage to recruit top artists)." Throughout the

1980s, as China opened up to outside influences, pop music (electric) instruments and sounds began taking over, including in that ensemble. The *zheng* and other traditional instruments receded, and she lost interest and left.

A confluence of events—historical, emotional, intellectual—triggered a desire in Han to leave China for Canada, which she did in 1996. She sought a master's degree in ethnomusicology at the University of British Columbia in Vancouver, and she embarked on a range of performance events including Western chamber music, new music, free improvisation, electroacoustic, and world music genres in collaboration with musicians and composers from different cultural backgrounds.

Han's first exposure to free improvisation came through meeting Vancouver musician Randy Raine-Reusch. His specialty is collecting Asian traditional instruments, *zheng* among them, and scoring new and performing improvised music for and on them. He coaxed her into trying to improvise freely by having her play some traditional fingerings while changing the tunings to sound unexpected results. Later that day, she heard his live performance on the *zheng* with flutist Robert Dick and bassist Barry Guy, all improvising freely, on the 1997 CD *Gudira*. "My initial reaction was to feel unsettled," Han recalls. "Each individual pluck of the string was so focused and intense that the music was like an earthquake, almost too powerful to take in. Yet, at the same time, this power was so irresistible that it hit me right in my heart—a feeling that I never had experience with. I lifted my head and said, 'I feel free!'"[11]

Han's exposure to *Gudira* was, for her, most comparable to Kim's experience of finding the greatest resonance for her own texture-heavy and unmetered-rhythmic improvising in her engagement with African American players. In *Gudira*, Han found an interplay between, on the one hand, two of the most testosterone-driven virtuosi in the Western world of improvised music and instruments, and, on the other, Raine-Reusch's equally forceful handling of the *zheng*. My reading of her story and hearing of the recordings she made after that encounter with this CD lead me to hear her "individual voice" as that of a yin counterpart to the yang of relentless chromatic and extended-technical timbral-textural fireworks.

Han and Raine-Reusch married in 2001, and they have worked closely together abroad and at home in Vancouver's thriving multicultural creative-music scene since then. Her evolution as an improviser and arranger is documented in sound by a series of CDs with Raine-Reusch and as a soloist and leader of her own groups. These recordings span from her initial steps of improvising on clear patterns (ostinati, melodic phrases, measured rhythms) to her launch of free solo flights with a variety of tunings, melodies, motifs, and extended techniques. From her early *Distant Wind* (2001), a CD of original compositions designed to showcase her improvisations with Raine-Reusch on several Asian-traditional instruments and acoustic jazz bassist Laurence Mollerup, she turned to forays into Persian Jewish, Arabic *maqam*, Indian, and traditional Chinese material that featured improvisation in her *Road to Kashgar* (with Orchid Ensemble, 2004) and *Gathering* (with Red Chamber, 2014). She also turned to other plucked-string traditions, including American bluegrass, as with her album *Redgrass* (2008). *Outside the Wall* (2005), something of a more developed and signature improvisational statement, signals with its title its concept of escape from confinement. The title track, scored graphically by Raine-Reusch, leaves the choice of notes up to the player. "Bamboo, Silk and Stone," the CD's other fully improvised piece, consists of an electronic piece that Raine-Reusch and composer-synthesist Barry Truax made to spur improvisation.

Han's duo CD *Ume* (Japanese for "plum," 2006) with pianist Paul Plimley is her move to the high wire without a net. Like the *Gudira* event that first moved her, it is an open, spontaneous engagement of two improvisers without the training wheels of any prescribed patterns or concepts. Han's plucky runs meet their match, with surprise, in Plimley's staccato touch; her choice of notes and strums often suggest that so many contemporary pianists who play the inside of their instrument directly, with their hands, are only reaching for what she has in full. The influence of Asia on the piano, not least on jazz piano—an influence that has existed since the work of Claude Debussy and Maurice Ravel—is recalled in every one of these thirteen musical *haikus* (the artists' descriptor), as well as in the impressionistic lilt of the whole CD.

"For me, to be able to see the world in my way and to reflect it in my own music is the ultimate liberation . . . *Free improvisation has an expansive, almost imperceptible structure that allows unlimited possibilities.*"[12] My emphasis underscores the subtle key of improvised music that seems counterintuitive to the more obvious liberatory appeal it suggests: it is grounded in, not free of, a structure, just not one cobbled together artificially.

As the Western paradigm of freely improvised music helped Kim best access the Korean shamanist tradition that the West had also blocked her from, so it gave Han room to claim the Taoist balance between yin and yang that she saw in a deep Chinese tradition also so suppressed, by both Western and Chinese militarism, especially. The idea of the body and nature as form to inhabit and engage gracefully, not (like the male warrior/ascetic/dualist) as flesh and world to master and transcend into pure spirit, is claimed in her words about spontaneous improvisation and is sounded in her music.

Wu Man and Min Xiao-Fen (*pipa*)

So far my focus has been on techniques and aesthetics: Kim's and Han's extensions of their traditional instruments and theories to their work as improvisers and as composers/arrangers for improvisers. These aspects of their music's logoi are further evolved to serve its mythoi. That symbiosis sheds light on how improvisation moves from one context to another, changing the new context and its own soul and spirit even as it keeps its flesh, so to speak. The shifts in mythoi of the four artists discussed here are best displayed in the work of Wu and Min, who share improvisation-free backgrounds and overlapping yet also divergent experiences with free improvisation in the West.

Mythoi are imagined realities; some modern instances of mythos might include a "brand," or what lawyers call a "legal fiction." A mythos can be, by turns or simultaneously, both insular and permeable. An insular mythos is a world unto itself (a religion that claims universality over all others, for instance, or the notion of national sovereignty). A permeable mythos is one that allows movement: people can swim in and out of it, between it and other mythoi; they can merge it with those other mythoi syncretically, toggling from emic to etic perches at will. Mythos is also like theory or paradigm, a narrative or a trope. Modernism and postmodernism are mythoi, as are transmodernism, racism, colonialism, egalitarianism, feminism, and Whiteness. The metamythos underpinning all insular, open, hybrid, and newly generated mythoi is the understanding that the world includes them all, as patchwork quilt, melting pot, and salad bowl all at once. The mythic terrain resembles an animist's material plenum, or a pantheist's "great chain" of such imagined realities from the One to the Many.

The traditional *pipa* repertoire with which Wu Man and Min Xiao-Fen both started came with its own mythos. Both were well schooled on their common instrument from childhood; both enjoyed high professional success as young adults; both then worked in some of the same improvisatory genres and circles once in the United States and Europe; and (most useful here) both recorded, in their early years and since, some of the same traditional and contemporary Chinese material. The mythos of the original shared culture (the classical and contemporary canon) and those shared new contexts make for a richly informative baseline from which to assess how the two women have distinguished themselves as improvisers.

Born a few years apart, they were raised in the adjoining provinces of Zhejiang (Wu, in Hangzhou) and Jiangsu (Min, in Nanjing), in the eastern region of China, where the five historical schools of *pipa* are clustered.[13] Wu, who picked up her instrument at age nine, won entrance to the Central Conservatory of Music in Beijing at age thirteen. She spent most of her adolescence there, becoming the first recipient of a master's degree in *pipa* at her school and receiving first prize in China's First National Music Performance Competition, among many other awards. She recorded and performed throughout her twenties both traditional works and contemporary works by a new generation of Chinese composers exposed to Western composers. Min was born into a musical family and learned to play from her father, Min Ji-Qian, a professor and *pipa* instructor at Nanjing University. At age seventeen, she won first prize at the Jiangsu National Pipa Competition and began a decade-long tenure as *pipa* soloist with the Nanjing Traditional Music Orchestra of China. She, too, has recorded traditional and contemporary material on the international stage, to wide acclaim.

Among the classical works that both artists have recorded are "Ambush on All Sides" and "King Chu Removes His Armor," which appear on Wu's *Wu Man* (both songs, Nimbus Records, 1993) and on Min's *Spring River Flower Moon Night* ("King Chu," Asphodel Records, 1997) and *The Moon Rising* ("Ambush," Cala Records, 2010). Both works are programmatic, as is most of the Chinese classical canon, based on a historical battle between the Chu and Han kingdoms in 202 BC. "Ambush" is from the victorious Han perspective, while "King Chu" is from the defeated Chu perspective (the 1993 movie *Farewell, My Concubine* is based on the latter story).

Both Wu and Min have remarked often in interviews, including to me, that such traditional pieces in the *wu* (martial) style—right-hand-heavy techniques of percussive force and fast picking—share much with the dirty/noisy-timbral and pyrotechnic aspects of Western experimental and improvised music (from free jazz to electronica to other "edgy" genres). While those techniques are on full display here—mostly as depictions of the chaos and carnage of war—the whole is rich with equal portions of left-hand artistry, too, in sections reflecting the more lyrical *wen* (civil) style that evokes the tragedy of women undone and love lost to war.

Their *wen*-leaning versions of some equally venerable pieces suggest further points of interest. The common ground that the more feminine left-hand side of the tradition shares with creative music's palette is—like "blue" notes in jazz, Kim's Living Tones, or Han's *yun* craft skills—the reconception of a given pitch from fixed to fluid. Such a move liberates the pitch from its thrall to all other such fixed and tempered pitches in the Western paradigm of harmonic relations as the (potentially iron) heart and lung of music, releasing its potential as an expresser of emotion and signifier of meaning all by itself.

The original mythoi of the pieces (the wars won and lost, the women shattered by the patriarchal power plays) are—per the mythos called "the traditional canon," as in the West—re-created and revitalized, like sacraments in a religion, through each new generation of artists and audiences, their expressive and receptive skills and sensibilities laid down over theoretically endless time. The closest thing to individual improvisation serving the process is simply the balance between a performer's faithful conformity to her training and the score and her own nuances of energy, inflection, and personal sound.

Both women, firmly set on that stellar but conventional career track, decided that it was a gilded cage to flee. According to Wu, "I said, well, what am I going to do, play twenty or so traditional pieces for the rest of my life? When you're young, you have curiosity and a sense of more adventure than that. . . . The Chinese government opened the door to the West in the early eighties, and many of the younger generation of students then went to the West. . . . We were really curious about what the musician's life might look like outside of China."[14]

That generation included composers; Chen Yi, Bun-Ching Lam, and Tan Dun are among the most cosmopolitan, working in both Chinese and Western worlds. Both Wu and Min have also interpreted the same three compositions by them, some of which included some kind of improvisation, and all of which fed into their respective improvisational styles. The Chinese title (*Dian*) of Chen Yi's "Points" (on *Min Xiao-Fen with Six Composers* [Disk Union, 1998] and *Wu Man*) alludes to the eight different brush strokes of calligraphy and the rapid roll of all five fingers on one of the *pipa*'s strings, an action that simulates one sustained note. Min works as calligrapher and artist to adorn her CDs, suggesting the same kind of close association of the visual and audial found in much improvised music (such as, for example, Anthony Braxton's, Peter Brötzmann's, and Han Bennink's). Wu, who collaborated with the composer to develop the fingerings, brings a bright and forceful energy through both civil and martial techniques to her presentation. Both performances show how traditional styles, vocabularies, and techniques can organically expand in their new extensions to inform the improvised part of new-and-improvised music.

The mythos shining through these works is still that of Chinese classical music sounding in situ, but now it is in contemporary rather than historical moments. The mythoi of the individual pieces are more ludic than narrative/poetic, instigating and fostering (on the level of concept and structure) more creative agency in the performers than do the historical works. The mythos of this contemporary moment itself is of a Chinese music culture no longer cloistered and talking only to itself through iterations of its traditional canon, but hopefully adding to that canon engagements with ideas and influences, including improvisational strategies, from the West.

The next stage of these parallel paths to seasoned improvisational voices and styles beyond Chinese music covers the various collaborations each artist took on in the United States, outside of the Chinese American community, starting in the early 1990s. They ranged from featured guest spots to more cocreative roles in several different scenes—Asian American jazz operas and suites, African American jazz and free improvisation, White American bluegrass, various other ethnic traditions—each with its own set of mythoi merging with theirs out of China. The overarching mythos of such collaborations might be characterized as "world musicians abroad, hosting, guesting, and/or meeting in the middle," with Wu and Min taking on the latter two roles at first, often for their schooling in improvisation.

Through her connection with vocalist Liu Sola, a Beijing schoolmate who was active in jazz and blues genres, Wu worked with saxophonist-composer Henry Threadgill on Liu's *Blues in the East* (Axiom, 1994) and one of Threadgill's own big-band recording dates, *Carry the Day*, Sony Music Entertainment, 1995), Wu's "first experience with any kind of jazz." The duo CD *Posture of Reality* (Asian Improv, 2003) with bassist Tatsu Aoki (a Japanese expat in Chicago) indicates Wu's comfort and command with cross-cultural improvisation in the jazz idiom (as its guest), a command that could potentially flourish more broadly later (into the host role, as master of the idiom). It is a live concert, riffing on blues, root tones, and traditional Chinese tunes. Wu's improvising on the American gestures is artful, with no awkward reaches for half-rhythmic, half-baked melody lines to fit with chords. She is adventurous while maintaining command, revealing a refined sensibility for "noise" music and best timing for how to employ it, and her work exhibits unmetered rhythm within groove, the use of extended range and techniques to build lines and sculpt phrases, and give-and-take with energy and panache. All these qualities are on display in other recordings as well, such as the CDs *From a Distance* (Naxos Records, 2003) and, with Liu and American drummer Pheeroan akLaff, *Sola & Friends—Live Performance Recording from the 1999 Beijing International Jazz Festival* (Also Productions, 2000).

Some of Min's early collaborations in jazz and free improvisation similarly flowered directly into her own fullest fruits as a serious improviser of record, despite her initial doubts about that seriousness. Her first performance of free improvisation in public, with composer-trumpeter Wadada Leo Smith in the early 1990s, led to record dates with him (*Dark Lady of the Sonnets* [TUM Records, 2012]) and with the late violinist Leroy Jenkins (*The Art of Improvisation* [Mutable Music, 2006]), and to live gigs with Smith and others in the AACM/New York circle (Muhal Richard Abrams, Pheeroan akLaff). Her small guest spot in a John Zorn project (*Filmworks VIII* [Tzadik Records, 1997]) led Zorn to introduce her to British guitar magus Derek Bailey, with whom she eventually recorded two acclaimed CDs of freely improvised music (*Viper* [Avant, 1998] and *Flying Dragons* [Incus, 1999]) and toured in Europe.[15] Her collaboration with pianist Randy Weston on his CD *Khepera* (Verve International, 1998) musically explored the African roots of China's legendary Shang dynasty. Her treatments of jazz standards (by Thelonious Monk, Miles Davis, Duke Ellington, and Count Basie), mixed with some of their historical counterparts in 1930s–1940s Shanghai night-life repertoire, led her to be the first Chinese musician invited to perform in a Jazz at Lincoln Center program; her special interest in trumpeter Buck Clayton's visits to Shanghai in that time led her to craft and perform her 2014 program *From Harlem to Shanghai and Back*, which featured his music.

Both Min and Wu, separately, have also worked on collaborations that feature a special mythic resonance: the Asian *American* more-than-tinge. Violinist-composer Jason Hwang, saxophonist-composer Fred Ho, and pianist-composer Jon Jang have all brought the two into their projects; and Wu has also worked with saxophonist-composer Francis Wong. The host roles (leaders of those dates) are played by composers and improvisers well versed in their idioms, leading lights in the already-established Asian American more-than-tinge (and its mythoi) in the (mostly African American side of the) creative-music community. Their Chinese guests (Wu and Min) bring their sounds and ideas to the leaders' Asian American themes and styles.

From the Atlantic-world perspective, those leaders, too, are initially guests to African American hosts; their musical language derives from the jazz tradition, and their overtly activist themes of justice and full equality for people of color against White supremacy coalesce with and largely follow the lead of work from their African American counterparts. That said, their status as hosts suggests itself in how they have drawn from and expressed their more Pacific-world history and themes as composers and improvisers. That history, especially on the West Coast, is as deeply ingrained in their mythos within the jazz and art-music idioms as is the Atlantic world's history of slavery and anti-Black racism. This Pacific history includes the exclusion of the wives and daughters of the Chinese men let in to labor, patriarchal oppression of the women in their own land, and significant harsh treatment in America of the women when they were finally allowed in.[16]

These projects with Asian American musicians came at a time when activists and artists in the Asian American movement were branching out from their domestic coalitions and concerns to global ones, especially to the newly opened doors from China. The built-in musical chemistry between those hosts and those guests compares to that between the many "Black Atlantic" musicians who have combined their various local mythoi in collaborations.[17] That said, as with other such exchanges, including those Wu and Min had with African Americans, the Asian American scene/mythos would not be the final resting spot for either woman as improvisers sui generis.

Where Wu's attraction to improvisation produces the more signature results is twofold: her collaborations with composers-for-improvisers for their Chinese-cultural statements, and her cultivation of improvisation as employed by other world-music traditions to bring the *pipa*'s voice into them. The first kind of gesture stems from her earlier work as featured artist (guest) on pieces in which improvisation is variously orchestrated to serve a composer's concept. She assumes a more cocreative (hosting) role in later such programmatic projects, instilling her own Chinese themes, material, and visions in her improvisational toolkit. The CD *Immeasurable Light* (Traditional Crossroads, 2010) and the project *A Chinese Home* (2011) are two examples from her longtime collaboration with the Kronos Quartet. The former presents Wu's new pieces based on, and creative renditions of, notated *pipa* music spanning the eighth to the twelfth centuries; the latter uses a mix of traditional acoustic and modern synthesized and amplified sounds to suggest China's evolving identity through successive historical genres and styles.[18] As with Han

Mei's similar resurrections of early Chinese music, the governing mythos might be stated as (my words) "history holds buried treasure, which we unearth to revive and make new." Also reflecting Han's account, Wu says: "In the traditional Chinese music, improvisation is actually a big part of its history. But my generation lost out on that; we did not improvise. Everything was written out . . . especially in conservatory training, I never heard the word 'improvisation' in China. So basically I came here and relearned, rethought my own tradition."

These creative extensions of the composed art-music tradition bring Chinese history and culture to life beyond the ritual of rote recitation of scores. As improvisational events, however, Wu's forays into the music and mythoi of Chinese rural folk and of classical Uyghur musicians put her in direct, open engagements with these others in their respective milieux. Her attraction to the former (seen in the documentary *Discovering a Musical Heartland: Wu Man's Return to China*, 2016) visibly lies in its counterpoint of raw energy and joy to the schooled refinement and restraint of her formal training.[19] With the Uyghurs (CD/DVD *Borderlands* [Smithsonian Folkways Recording, 2011]), the adventure is of her own sophisticated classical tradition meeting its more highly improvisational and rhythmically complex counterpart on the latter's turf and terms. The payoff in that connection—sometimes surprisingly smooth, at other moments made only through half-blind leaps of faith—lies in bringing the *pipa* back to its pre-Han roots in Central Asia, roots it shares with the Uyghur music. "Every day I learn something from improvising. It makes me feel much more comfortable to just sit down with any kind of musician and say, let's play something together. I couldn't do that years ago."

Min's record as master over these various forms—traditional Chinese material, contemporary, hybrid Chinese and Western repertoire, engagements and collaborations with world music and (especially American) roots genres—is as strong and rich as the others', but her most-trod path has been through historical and contemporary jazz and in terrain of global post-jazz improvised music.

Han Mei has suggested a philosophy of music improvised with no prescribed mental map in speaking of a deep underlying structure that is not prescriptively orchestrated. Such koan-like, way-out-of-no-way allusions best describe the principle that Min's work also seems to embody. Indeed, on her website is this line from Lao-tze: "The name that can be named is not the enduring and unchanging name." Min has developed an improviser's idiolect that, whether or not she chooses to name names with it, stands stronger every day for and in the truth of that line.

Min's record *Dim Sum* (Blue Pipa, 2012), with Japanese percussionist-synthesist Satoshi Takeishi, reflects in her voice and language as much as her *pipa* the work she has done to forge that idiolect in her collaborations with other improvisers. *Dim sum* translates as "touch the heart." She writes in this CD's liner notes that its tracks 5 through 10 (also collectively titled "Dim Sum") are six musical dishes meant to touch the heart that sprang from sounds she heard as a child in Nanjing. Like distinct mushroom caps stemming out of the earth from their one common rhizome, the tracks sound their Taoist heart's voice. Invoking the ancient Tibetan/Indian improvisational sonic ritual of *rol mo* and Tang Dynasty material, drawing on bits of Miles Davis and John Cage, evoking a Mississippi blues sound on the *sanxian,* morphing into a heavy-metal thrasher on the electronic *pipa,* and vocalizing in a range from (Chinese) high and delicate to (Mongolian) low and guttural, the tracks raise the suggestion of childhood as of both nature and culture, both raw and refined, inseparably, and promising to remain so as it matures.[20]

* * *

Just as Jelly Roll Morton's "Spanish tinge" both mistook the source of the influence and identified it as something more like a seasoning than the core stock it was, so is the Asian/woman identity in these artists' work shorted if not given its rightful due. While "tinge" may suit some of their early work in the West as "guests," their less constrained "meet-in-the-middle engagements" with other improvisers, and their roles as "hosts" on the projects they conceived and led, have brought forth their deepest Asian-traditional roots to new musicalizations of ancient shamanism, Taoism, Confucianism, and Buddhism, joining Europe's more-than-tinges of Greek-modal, Judeo-Christian diatonic, and secular post-diatonic harmonic systems, and Africa's polyrhythmic, polyphonic dance and trance music. Those Asian mythoi, worlds, and histories join Pacific Rim to White and Black Atlantic as equally weighted ingredients in the creative-music gumbo.

As for the woman's face and voice, that too is more than a tinge. The work presented here argues well that the information it brings from Asia is on par with that brought from the Atlantic world; a more questionable assertion is that one gender is the primary bearer of that information. To suggest as much (as subjective portrait more than objective photograph) with some support, I thus turn to Kim's own version of this assertion. Her 1998 essay "Female Energy in Music" holds that human world culture, reflecting cosmic currents, is trending from a yang-exhausted to a yin-enlightening period, in the Taoist homeostat of such oscillations. Whatever one makes of such a claim, it is not controversial to paint with a broad brush historical Western music, American jazz, and Korean and Chinese classical traditions as male dominated, reflecting their histories/cultures, the many rich exceptions proving the rule. That said, the same brush is too broad to paint a present in flux and a future uncertain with the same confidently definitive stroke.[21]

I asked all four women why they thought that they, rather than four men, were having such marked success with this music in the West. Their answers ranged from parental pressure on girls (who are pushed to excel in music to enhance their prospects of professional success, unlike boys, who have been enjoying new and "better" options with the rise of a Chinese middle class; Min and Wu), to a general rise and liberation of women in all fields (all four); even to an unfortunate Orientalist phenomenon of Western preference for the Asian female (Han).[22]

What I notice is that even the best training, treatment, and recognition in Korea and China came with artistic, professional, and social limits, including some specific to women, that these artists were not willing to accept. Their moves to the West, and to improvisation once there, proved over time to be movement beyond those limits, movement that was effected with no guarantees, by dint of the women's own creative spirits and visions.

I also observe the contrast between their public personae as fully empowered, successful women and the not-too-distant, grimmer history of Asian immigrant women and its driving (Orientalist, anti-Asian, sexist) mythoi. None of these women are overtly political in their work, either reactively or proactively, yet their natural alliances and artistic gestures (Jin's Quagmire and No World groups, Wu's collaborations with China's ethnic minority and rural folk, the various projects of all with African and Asian American musicians and activist performances), along with their integrity and power as artists and people, add up to their own cultural-political statements.

Again, most of the "changes" of their sounds have been more about extending traditional techniques and aesthetics to new contexts of improvisation and mythos. One area where that observation is not true is their use of technology; all have made some use of electric amplification/distortion or computerized electronics on some of their projects (even there, the change is extension, not erasure or replacement). This timbral/textural aspect, in African American and much other improvised and experimental music, has often been the site where sheer sound has offended aesthetically or threatened socially—and their own work as cross-cultural improvisers and experimentalists has not been as well received in their home countries as it has outside them—but within the creative-music mythos itself, this aspect is just part of the palette.

These four snapshots are of a phenomenon that has happened throughout music (reflecting human) history: traditions that are by turns or at once cloistered within their own ways and open to engagement with their counterparts without (whatever "within" and "without" mean at a given moment). They may begin as "tinges" to each other—guests and hosts caught up in power plays, or in plays of mutual respect but also the safe distance of their respective borders—but down through the generations, they get closer, get intimate, intermarry their musical and other selves to bear new fruit. Like organs that evolve for one function to then prove useful for another, the logoi of musical technique, vocabulary, and aesthetics have tended to prevail and even strengthen and expand rather than get lost in such translations. Conversely, their natal mythoi do ostensibly recede, even dissolve, giving way to their new contexts abroad—but even that change looks more like the "death" of a seed bearing new life than of one being crushed, failing to sprout, or going unplanted. Improvisation in the West is not a stone against which "difference" has to reactively beat. It is power-of as much as power-over, and it can be made different by the proactive-beyond-reactive agency of another power-of. For scholars of the process, it may in fact be best understood as one that mediates the debate between those insisting on the incommensurability of cultures and those arguing for the reality of musical universals.[23]

The strong Asian presence in the Pacific Rim, North America, and diaspora more generally was not matched by the same presence at the creative-music party of improvisational (and predominantly yang) mixes and matches performed by the African, Latin, and later Asian Americans with the Europeans and Russians in the long twentieth century—but it is here now, and in a force and fashion that suggest an even longer (and yin-richer) party to come.

For complete and current details about the work of these musicians/ scholars, see these websites and Facebook.

http://www.jinhikim.com/
https://www.mei-han.com/meihan.html
https://www.mtsu.edu/chinesemusic/

http://www.wumanpipa.org
http://minxiaofenbluepipa.org/

Notes to Chapter 6

1. Daniel R. McClure's "'New Black Music' or 'Anti-Jazz'" covers both racial and gendered aspects of the historical ground under the improvisatory practice of the primarily Atlantic musical discourse that the women are engaging. Enrique Dussel's "Agenda for a South–South Philosophical Dialogue" offers a similar context for discussion of the women's own histories in the Pacific world, by virtue of his inclusion of China and Korea as part of the Global South. His call for a realignment of hemispheric relations in philosophical discourse to one of equals (South–South), beyond the history of Eurocentric dominance (North–South), resonates well with my move to assert the dynamic between these Asian women and this Western musical world as one of equals (a relationship that is more-than-tinge), in what Dussel dubs a *transmodern* exchange.

2. See, for example Dussel, "Agenda for a South–South Philosophical Dialogue," 12.

3. The more current spelling for *komungo* is *geomungo*, but I use the spelling from Kim's CDs and her quoted writings.

4. See Kim, *Komungo Tango*. Except where otherwise noted, all quotations from Kim are her own translations of passages from this Korean-language memoir.

5. Carter J. Eckert, Ki-baik Lee, Young Ick Lew, Michael Robinson, and Edward W. Wagner detail with some musical specifics the shamanist-animist primacy from prehistory through the Three Kingdoms period, prior to Buddhism's incursion in the 8th century AD. This volume is a rich corroborative source for the rest of the Korean history Kim presents, including the patriarchal suppression of female shamans, the shamanist aspects of the masked dance, and the current resurgence of shamanism in South Korean culture. See Eckert et al., *Korea Old and New*, 39, 121, 191, 409.

6. For a glimpse of the 1960s revival of Korean folk music, see Maliangkay, "The Revival of Folksongs in South Korea." Emma Franz's 2010 documentary film *Intangible Asset No. 82*, about Korean musicians Kim Seok-Chul and Kim Dong-Won, reveals how far Korean shamanist musicking has come, both at home and internationally, since the time Kim described.

7. Jones, *Black Music*, 77.

8. Heffley, 2000, 17.

9. Han, "The Emergence of the Chinese Zheng," 233.

10. Han, 235. Han is quoting from O'Dea, *Virtue or Virtuosity*, 16.

11. Han, "The Emergence of the Chinese Zheng," 234–35.

12. Han, 235, 238 (italics added).

13. The five "schools" (styles) arose through different collections of manuscripts interpreted through generations of masters and students. Wu describes the *Pudong* style she learned as more elegant and others as more dramatic. Heffley, interviews.

14. See Heffley, interviews, for this and all other quotes attributed to Wu.

15. *Viper* was named one of *Wire* magazine's 1998 Albums of the Year; *Flying Dragon* was *Coda* magazine's 2003 Album of the Year.

16. On the challenges and plights Asian immigrant women have faced in America over the last couple of centuries, see Lee, *Orientals*; and Chang, *The Chinese in America*. By happy contrast, see Zheng, *Claiming Diaspora*, for a better current picture, of which the three Chinese artists here are illustrious parts.

17. See Gilroy, *The Black Atlantic*. For a broader mapping of the Asian American music scenes and key actors, including those mentioned here, see Wong, *Speak It Louder*; and Waterman, "Improvisation and Pedagogy." See Jang and Wong, "A Conversation," for a detailed view of Asian Improv aRts (AIR) and its founders, Jon Jang and Francis Wong, around the time of their projects with Wu and Min. Fellezs's essay, "Silenced but Not Silent," examines the historical and still-problematic neglect of Asian American voices from the Atlantic-world discourse about jazz music. Fred Ho's collected writings, *Wicked Theory, Naked Practice*, constitute a wide-ranging counterdiscourse that is as "not silent" about the racial, gender, and political dynamics of Asian American jazz musicians as is their music itself.

18. See Wu's and ethnomusicologist Rembrandt F. Wolpert's liner notes on *Immeasurable Light* for how much freedom of interpretation such pieces allowed traditionally, and how much more freedom Wu took with them to bring them to new life. See also Wu, Harrington, and Chen, "Kronos Quartet and Wu Man: A Chinese Home," for video excerpts and programmatic details of *A Chinese Home*.

19. Samples of Wu playing with and talking about such collaborations with rural Chinese musicians were also showcased at the 2009 Carnegie Hall festival Ancient Spirits; for a clip, see Goñi, "Chinese Traditional Music."

20. See Ellingson, "The Mathematics of Tibetan Rol Mo," on *rol mo* (pronounced *römo*). This classical musical tradition dates back more than a thousand years through Tibetan Buddhist monastic ensembles to even older roots in Indian Buddhist music. It is a practice falling somewhere in between the regular and the irregular (à la fractal geometry).

21. Ellen Waterman suggests some cautions worth heeding about misconceiving and misperceiving the nature of improvisation, generically, under the "Asian" rubric, given the history of Orientalist sexism in Western thinking; see Waterman, "Asian Improvisation."

22. See Heffley, interviews, for the artists' thoughts on this question; and see Waterman, "Asian Improvisation," on this breed of Orientalism.

23. Peter Kowald and William Parker, two well-known improvisers from opposing sides of the Atlantic, have spoken to me in interviews about the process of "just playing"—freely improvising—across cultural/genre borders, beyond notions of power plays or mutual incommensurability of idioms. They are just two among many who have done so to fertile effect. See Heffley, Interviews. See also Gioia, "Face the Music," for an informed argument about music's capacity to evince universals even in its incommensurable expressions.

Works Cited

Chang, Iris. *The Chinese in America: A Narrative History*. New York: Penguin Books, 2003.

Dussel, Enrique. "Agenda for a South–South Philosophical Dialogue." *Human Architecture: Journal of the Sociology of Self-Knowledge* 11, no. 1 (2013): 3–18.

Eckert, Carter J., Ki-baik Lee, Young Ick Lew, Michael Robinson, and Edward W. Wagner. *Korea Old and New: A History*. Cambridge, MA: Harvard Korea Institute, 1990.

Ellingson, Ter. "The Mathematics of Tibetan Rol Mo." *Ethnomusicology* 23, no. 2 (1979): 225–43.

Fellezs, Kevin. "Silenced but Not Silent: Asian Americans and Jazz." In *Alien Encounters: Popular Culture in Asian America*, edited by Mimi Thi Nguyen and Thuy Linh Nguyen Tu, 69–108. Durham, NC: Duke University Press, 2007.

Franz, Emma, dir. *Intangible Asset No. 82*. Documentary featuring Korean musicians Kim Seok-Chul and Kim Dong-Won, with Australian drummer Simon Barker. New York: Kino Lorber Films, 2010. DVD, 90 min.

Gilroy, Paul. *The Black Atlantic: Modernity and Double-Consciousness*. Boston: Harvard University Press, 1995.

Gioia, Ted. "Face the Music." *Smart Set*. October 21, 2015. http://thesmartset.com/face-the-music/

Goñi, Ramón J. "Chinese Traditional Music Conquers New York." Posted October 28, 2009. YouTube video, 3:48. https://www.youtube.com/watch?v=NUlgmGGHFbc

Han, Mei. "The Emergence of the Chinese Zheng: Traditional Context, Contemporary Evolution, and Cultural Identity." PhD diss., University of British Columbia, 2013.

Heffley, Mike. "Anthony Braxton: The Third-Millennial Interview." 2000. Transcribed at https://www.academia.edu/2314587/Anthony_Braxton_The_Third_Millennial_Interview

Heffley, Mike. Interviews with Jin Hi Kim, Han Mei, Min Xiao-Fen, and Wu Man. 2007–16. Transcribed at https://wesleyan.academia.edu/MichaelHeffley/Interviews

Ho, Fred Wei-han. *Wicked Theory, Naked Practice: A Fred Ho Reader*. Edited by Diane C. Fujino. Minneapolis: University of Minnesota Press, 2009.

Jang, Jon, and Francis Wong. "A Conversation with Jon Jang and Francis Wong." By Nic Paget-Clarke. *In Motion Magazine*, February 1998. http://www.inmotionmagazine.com/jjfw1.html

Jones, LeRoi (Amiri Baraka). *Black Music*. Akashic Books, 2010. First published 1968 by William Morrow.

Kim, Jin Hi. "Female Energy in Music." *Festival Nieuwe Muziek*, 1998. Also published in *Evterpe Magazine* and *Logos Blad Magazine*, 1998.

Kim, Jin Hi. *Komungo Tango*. Seoul: Minsokwon, 2007.

Lee, Robert G. *Orientals: Asian Americans in Popular Culture*. Philadelphia: Temple University Press, 1999.

Maliangkay, Roald. "The Revival of Folksongs in South Korea: The Case of 'Tondollari.'" *Asian Folklore Studies* 61, no. 2 (2002): 223–45.

McClure, Daniel R. "'New Black Music' or 'Anti-Jazz': Free Jazz and America's De-Colonization in the 1960s." MA thesis, California State University Fullerton, 2007.

O'Dea, Jane. *Virtue or Virtuosity—Explorations in the Ethics of Musical Performance.* Westport, CT: Greenwood Press, 2000.

Waterman, Ellen. "Asian Improvisation: A Primer in the Politics of Recognition." *Critical Studies in Improvisation / Études critiques en improvisation* 1, no. 3 (2006). https://www.criticalimprov.com/index.php/csieci/issue/view/13

Waterman, Ellen, ed. "Improvisation and Pedagogy." Special issue, *Critical Studies in Improvisation / Études Critiques en Improvisation* 1, no. 3 (2006). https://www.criticalimprov.com/index.php/csieci/issue/view/13

Wong, Deborah. *Speak It Louder: Asian Americans Making Music.* New York: Routledge, 2004.

Wu, Man, David Harrington, and Chen Shi-Zheng. "Kronos Quartet and Wu Man: A Chinese Home." 2011. https://www.youtube.com/watch?v=stZqdOG UZ2E

Zheng, Su. *Claiming Diaspora: Music, Transnationalism, and Cultural Politics in Asian/Chinese America.* New York: Oxford University Press, 2010.

SEVEN | Upaj

Improvising within Tradition in Kathak Dance

MONICA DALIDOWICZ

Freedom comes from refined discipline with responsibility.
—Pandit Chitresh Das

Amid a lesson, kathak maestro Pandit Das stood before his students in a Berkeley, California dance studio and performed an improvised section of footwork, bare feet slapping rhythmically on the floor in a syncopated style of kathak free play. When he finished, he explained that this free-play footwork was *upaj,* something that his dancers must aspire to do. *Upaj,* a concept translated with the loose English equivalent of "improvisation," was for Das and his dancers the essence of kathak, especially in relation to a growing field of kathak dance that was trending toward choreography and recorded music. The true test of a dancer was on the stage, in a traditional solo, with live musicians, where unpredictability and the unknown reside, and the performer must be equipped with both the knowledge and the readiness to make it happen. *Upaj* as improvisation was a translation that made sense in the American context. In fact, a 2013 documentary that traced the production and tour of *India-Jazz Suites* (*IJS*), a cross-cultural collaboration between Pandit Das and tap dancer Jason Samuels Smith, utilized this translation as its title: *Upaj: Improvise.*[1]

Upaj as improvisation came to the foreground in new ways in the US context. In this chapter, I show how Das's work enabled a unique revisioning and heightening of improvisatory practices within kathak that complemented understandings and expectations of improvisation present in the United States. Das built on a narrative of "improvisation in tradition" to expand his audiences, to appeal to the growing South Asian diasporic population in the San Francisco Bay Area, and to provide a basis for cross-cultural performances. Narrated this way, *upaj* straddled the conceptual divide between the frequently opposed ideas of, on the one hand, novelty, innovation, and improvisation, and, on the other, tradition and authenticity. Cross-cultural elaborations like *IJS* epitomized the kind of novelty that could occur within kathak while remaining connected to tradition through strict adherence to aesthetic standards. *Upaj* was the perfect vehicle to demonstrate the coexistence of tradition and improvisation.

The hybridization of improvisational ontologies within North Indian kathak dance in new cultural contexts, and the crafting of a narrative of "improvisation in tradition," is an effective strategy that artists like Das have used to address the competing, simultaneous expectations to be traditional and to be modern. In what follows, I discuss the varieties of *upaj* that exist within a kathak solo and consider the importance of both novelty *and* accuracy within these variations. I then examine Das's engagement with *upaj* in relation to the US context and describe the different functions it performed. I return to a discussion of the critical role of rhythmic precision and timing and the ways in which rhythmic accuracy was used to realign the notion of *upaj* with a traditional framework. I end with a consideration of how the divine rhetoric attached to *upaj* enriched its meaning and experience in the diaspora and provided a culturally specific interpretive frame that pushed *upaj* beyond any monological understanding of improvisation.

Upaj in Kathak

Charlotte Moraga, Das's longtime disciple, explained, "*upaj* literally means, *from the heart*, but what it is . . . is improvisation."[2] In other North Indian musical genres, *upaj* has been variably translated as, for example, "grown out of" or "born out of";[3] "to render with connotations of invention";[4] "derivative phrases of a basic theme (*upajas*)";[5] or even "produce" or "product."[6] Ethnomusicologist John Napier explains that terms like *upaj* or those used to discuss what actually takes place in a North Indian musical performance carry rather different implications from the term *improvisation* and "describe general or specific processes of exposition or development, or they may refer to specific types of singing or playing."[7]

Das too used the term *upaj* in a variety of nuanced ways that extended beyond the limitations of the English equivalent of improvisation, for example in metaphorical phrases like "*upaj* is life."

Upaj in kathak is found in several places: in the production of rhythm through the feet; in the dance movements of the hands, arms, head, and entire body; and in the expressive elements of storytelling. Kathak dancers perform with *ghungru*, brass bells of 150 or more on each ankle, and they coordinate their actions toward the production of rhythm through the sound of their feet and bells rhythmically slapping the floor. In a traditional kathak solo, the lone dancer appears onstage with her musical accompaniment; this typically includes a tabla player on percussion, with the melody played by a sitar, sarod, or *sarangi* player (stringed instruments), and a continuous harmonic drone produced by the stringed *tanpura*. There is no score. Rather, all the performers play together, typically with limited or no rehearsal, within the recurring rhythmic time cycle, leaving the performance open to fluctuation, unpredictability, spontaneous additions, and *upaj*. Much of the unfolding of the solo occurs onstage. In this respect, the very nature of the solo as requiring in-process collaboration between musician and dancer is itself improvisatory.

Das's student Antara Bhardwaj noted of the kathak solo, "it is all *upaj* in some sense, because of the musicians, you do not really know what they will do."[8] The dancer acts as a conductor, ensuring smooth flow of the performance and coordinating the musicians. The dancer chooses the *tal*, or overarching rhythmic cycle, and then set its tempo. The soloist typically speaks throughout the performance and, during these interludes, indicates toward the musicians what was coming next. The soloist may also indicate gesturally or with her eyes when she wants a change. Since dancers typically recite dance compositions before they dance, vocalizing the rhythm in mnemonic syllables known as *bols*, this narration provides cues to the musicians as to what is upcoming. Each performer onstage closely attends to the others in order to sense changes and react accordingly.

Theoretically, the ideal of *upaj* is "to actually compose something on the spot," but introducing a true novelty in performance is exceedingly rare.[9] Improvisations in Hindustani music are, in fact, often described as variations or differing combinations of known compositions that "have in some way been pre-composed (though unwritten), often handed down by the teacher, and the word improvisation is only used there because there is a degree of recombination and a certain freedom of distributing."[10] The idea of improvisation is, in fact, quite alien to certain performers like the North Indian musician Ram Narayan, who associates the term with the deliberate attempt to transgress tradition.[11] Daniel M. Neuman, in his study of North Indian music, explains that "the improvisations themselves are usually made up of previously worked-out phrases, musical elements put together in unique ways for each performance."[12] Napier further expands on improvisation in his work on Indian vocal genres: "Most discussions emphasize that it is pre-existing material that is worked on in performance: compositions, stock phrases, and cadential devices such as the *tihai*, a thrice-stated phrase that concludes a section of performance with great accuracy of timing. Existing phrases are stretched or compressed, and the same may happen to motives from the phrases; further motives may be prefixed, infixed and suffixed. Phrases may be broken up or telescoped with others, and motives or phrases may be sequenced through different registers."[13] In kathak, dancers also employ such rhythmic-based *upaj*. Fellow dancer and ethnomusicologist Sarah Morelli describes this tendency as an "ability to work freely within the *tal* (*layakari*) which allows a dancer to improvise rhythmic phrases with footwork, and to produce something as complex as a *tihai* spontaneously."[14] Dancers rely on known rhythmic phrases, well-known footwork patterns, and rehearsed combinations of sounds from the feet.

Upaj also refers to movement-based improvisation in the rendering of known compositions. The dancer demonstrates *upaj* not only in the rhythms of her feet, but in the coordinated movements of her entire body. Dancers learn choreographed versions of kathak repertoire, such as *that*, *amad*, or the compositions known as *bol/paran*, but in all cases, the experienced dancer is expected to divert from the model and execute the composition in her own interpretive style with novel additions and individual flair.[15] Morelli explains that this movement-based *upaj* "involves the dancer building trust in herself, that the kinesthetic vocabulary of the dance form has been naturalized in the body to the extent that she can let go of a dependence on choreographed movement and move freely."[16] A dancer learns the basic rhythmic phrase but then learns to substitute other techniques within the same pattern, such as different footwork, *chakkars* or pirouettes, or a sequence of movements or gestures (say, a raised eyebrow or a crisp glance). *Upaj* in this sense refers to the spontaneous bringing forth of a known composition, a deviation from the learned model, and the unplanned nature of a presentation.

Upaj is evident in the dramatic storytelling elements of kathak. Das's dancers learned basic formats of a story and then learned to embellish on the characters, bringing their own expression forth to animate their character and evoke the right mood. In preparation for a solo, a dancer may loosely rehearse the *bhao* or storytelling segments with musicians in order to establish a shared frame; the dancer may, although not always, set up cues and give direction on significant moments in the storyline during which the music should escalate and punctuate the story. But for the most part, the interpretation of a story is produced in the moment of performance. This is the mark of a mature dancer. One line of a song can be enacted and expressed in many different ways; a character in the story can be portrayed with variation on each night of a performance.

Asked about the "improvisatory aspects of the solo," Das explained in an American radio interview, "you choose a rhythmic structure . . . a rhythmic cycle known as *tal*, a cycle of definite beats—*tintal* is sixteen beats, *dhamar* is fourteen, and so on. Then you start dancing. You can say it is choreographed, or you can take chances. Instead of taking pirouettes, you can just do footwork. Or you can just go into the nuances of *abhinaya*, which is showing facial expression, finishing the composition with the right eyebrow raised, something that was not in the original choreography, but you add to it."[17] All of a dancer's vocabulary—the rhythmic phrases, the known hand gestures or *hastaks*, arm positions, rehearsed stances, and so forth—may be brought forth in such moments of *upaj* and used within an existing choreographic structure. It is the assembling of known elements, and the spontaneity in which they are brought together, that is characteristic of *upaj*. Moraga has explained, "there are a lot misconceptions about Indian classical dance, that it is regurgitated, that you just perform the same thing over and over again, well in kathak, if you are performing in a very traditional and deep sense, you are never performing the same thing twice, because there is a lot of improvisation, there is a different environment, there is a different audience, and the dancer has to respond to all those elements."[18] From this perspective, tradition is improvisatory in execution and delivery, even in repetitions of known pieces, since the changing variables of the environment demand unrehearsed responses.

Additionally, some sections of the solo are left entirely unchoreographed. Improvised exchange between musicians and dancers is most apparent in the *sawal jabab* (question-answer) section of the kathak solo. During the *sawal jabab*, the kathak dancer produces unplanned rhythmic phrases with her feet, responding in a call-and-answer segment to the rhythmic phrases of the tabla. The *sawal jabab* is taken to be the section where the most freedom in recombination can be manifest and, subsequently, is most recognizable as improvisation.[19] The *sawal jabab* section of a kathak solo is "typically a favorite of Western audiences because of its ease of comprehension."[20] *Sawal jabab* is exemplary of *upaj* and is palpable for new audiences. It was thus the ideal way for Pandit Das to communicate the improvisatory nature of kathak.

Pandit Chitresh Das's Kathak Dance in America

Pandit Chitresh Das, a native of Kolkata, was a leading kathak maestro based in California since the 1970s. For over almost 45 years, he developed his unique style of kathak and taught at his Chhandam School of Kathak in the San Francisco Bay Area; by the 2000s, Chhandam was putatively the largest kathak school in North America. In the later years of his artistic career, he reignited his relationship with India and traveled there several times a year. In 2002, he reopened Chhandam Nritya Bharati in Kolkata, which had originally been established in 1948 by his parents, Nritya Acharya Prahalad Das and Nilima Das. For much of the year, however, he spent his time in California, a place that provided considerable inspiration for the developments in his artistic style. Pandit Das sadly passed away in early 2015; however, his students have continued to teach his style at schools in San Francisco, Los Angeles, Toronto, Boston, and Mumbai.[21]

Das's vision to create a "California *gharana*" or family of kathak in the United States was reflected in the development of his own distinctive style of kathak, defined by a proclivity for speed and rhythmic versatility in footwork and swift pirouettes or *chakkars*.[22] Such was his reputation for footwork, I was warned by his students in India, that when people learned that someone had studied with Panditji, they would look directly to that person's feet.[23] Morelli has extensively documented the changes in Das's style in the American context since the 1970s, explaining the push for speed, athleticism, and technical virtuosity in kathak as, in part, a response to the demands of the competitive dance field in the San Francisco Bay Area.[24] Das elsewhere explained his emphasis on athleticism as a response to the "tendency to look down upon Indian classical dances as a feminine trait . . . so I added the element of physical strength in it."[25] Subsequently, Das stressed the elements of *layakari* or rhythmic versatility and *tayari* or readiness, both of which were necessary to the kind of *upaj*-style performance required in a traditional kathak solo. Das's emphasis on *upaj* also pushed back against the growing trend toward recorded music and choreography, especially within India, where "modern kathak" was proliferating.[26] Das vigorously promoted the traditional kathak solo, whereby a performer must dance alone onstage with musicians, for up to two hours.[27]

Das was an innovator, but he still positioned himself as an exponent of traditional kathak; after all, he and other artists did not see tradition and innovation as opposing concepts. Das strongly emphasized long-term study in the *guru-shishya parampara* (master-disciple tradition), and in his later years of teaching, his adherence to traditional etiquette was definitive of his style. He positioned *Sadvyavahar aur tehzeeb*, generally translated as attitude and etiquette, as the most important element of a student's training. As Das frequently explained, "my guruji was more interested in how I walked into the dance class than how I danced."

This emphasis on tradition and cultural etiquette found a receptive audience among the burgeoning population of Indo-Americans in the Bay Area, for whom learning kathak served an important function in accessing Indian culture outside of the homeland. In later years, the demographic of Das's classes shifted from what he affectionately referred to as the "blondes and brunettes" who studied with him through the 1970s, 1980s, and even 1990s to an almost exclusively South Asian student body. Alongside these demographic changes came a stronger emphasis on maintaining Indian culture. With the rise of an affluent Indian diasporic population, especially in the South Bay, parents began looking for ways to educate their children on aspects of Indian culture. Teachers in California found themselves bearing the primary responsibility of transmitting "Indian culture" to new generations of diasporic Indians, many of whom were struggling with questions of identity. The growing anxiety around diasporic identity was best encapsulated in the common phrase "ABCD," or American-born confused *desi* (*desi* refers to someone from the Indian subcontinent). "ABCD" was used quite loosely to refer to Indians in the diaspora who seemed to be struggling with an unsettling sense of liminality created by their transcultural existence between two localities. Johanna Lessinger explains that "emigration inexorably involves loss of culture, a lessening of one's essential Indianness."[28] In response to the fear of a loss of Indianness, certain cultural practices were consciously reflected on, and retention of culture became an explicit objective. Das's version of kathak responded directly to this confusion and anxiety.

Das taught that kathak was "historical, mathematical, philosophical and spiritual," and he thus presented kathak as a dance form that could communicate the ideals and values of India. For Das, kathak was a source of pride in the diaspora. The ability for dance to communicate Indian values and to evoke a sense of India was a major incentive for families at Chhandam, as a local radio program reported about experiences of kathak in Das's school:

> JOURNALIST: One parent says kathak is something she is also dedicated to because it is an activity she can share with her children that reinforces traditional values. She has been taking kathak here for a year with her daughter. . . .
> MOTHER: I don't know if you know that Beatles song, "Get back to where you once belong"; it's like that. I know I can't go back, but the best I can right now do is to bring my India back here.[29]

Yet, it was not simply about bringing all of India back, or experiencing all aspects of India in America. Das presented his version of the best of India through kathak; in the process of migration, elements can be discarded and others amplified. Das's pedagogic and performative style must thus be understood as a wider artifact of migration, recontextualized and reimagined in a diasporic setting in which certain elements are brought into focus. *Upaj*—and the idea of "improvisation in tradition"— was vital in staking a claim to kathak's dynamism and its contemporary relevance.

Upaj Reinvigorated

Upaj provided Das with an important possibility for updating tradition and carving out a niche for kathak in the contemporary world. In kathak, as in other musical genres, improvisation was important for articulating "attitudes about . . . place in the modern world."[30] Furthermore, Das was able to tap into the wider American music and dance field and establish the possibility for cross-cultural exchange; the ability to collaborate and work cross-culturally shed some of the stereotypes of classical Indian dance as being fixed and rigidly structured. Such collaborations were also integral to drawing in new audiences; despite the formalities of tradition, kathak could still speak to other cultures and generations. *Upaj* was the very foundation for this kind of exchange.

Das emphasized *upaj*, in particular, through his collaborations with US tap dancer Jason Samuels Smith and Spanish flamenco dancer Antonio Hidalgo Paz. Improvised rhythmic play provided the ideal space for cross-cultural exchange, becoming the premise for the 2005–14 *IJS* and, with Hidalgo Paz, the 2014 *Yatra: Masters of Kathak and Flamenco*. For example, in *IJS*, the performance itself included individual solos for each performer, and a section where each dancer traded phrases with the other's musical trios: Das with the jazz trio, and Smith with the Indian musicians. The production concluded with a rhythmic *sawal jabab*–style exchange between Das and Smith. The show, originally called *Fastest Feet in Rhythm*, highlighted the rhythms of each style and, especially, the improvised collaboration between the two artists.[31] A *San Francisco Examiner* review described this rhythmic interplay through the jazz vernacular "as 'trading eights': one performer executes an eight-bar (or four-bar) 'break' and the next does the same, trying to match or outdo the first. It becomes a kind of dueling scat singing of the feet, accompanied by jazz and classical Indian music ensembles."[32] *Upaj* was the spontaneous, improvisational free play between performers. Das—and, following him, his disciples—introduced new pedagogical tactics into the classroom to cultivate this sort of free play.[33] For example, "cutting contests" were used in Das's classes to provide students with the chance to rhythmically duel with one another, exchanging a designated number of beats in which to improvise. Cutting contests have deep roots in African American expressive culture, and elements of Black culture were adopted through exchanges with tap dancers.

Of his collaboration with Smith, Das explained, "we do not mix the styles of kathak and tap dance and have no desire to do so . . . we perform in our own element together."[34] Das was at great pains to show that he and his art were still traditional in one sense, yet also evolving and appealing to a modern world. Both artists asserted the necessity of maintaining their respective traditions. "Don't call it fusion. It is a collaboration," explained Das. His disciple Charlotte Moraga explained further: "A collaborative performance is like a relationship between two artists. It is an understanding of one another's art. In fusion there is dilution, but in a collaboration, as Guruji puts it, there is evolution of two individual art forms."[35] Such discursive explanations asserted the legitimacy of this new work as authentic and traditional. Movements or dance techniques were not fused or exchanged; the collaboration simply occurred through rhythmic improvisation.

Das and Smith shared common ground: their collaboration facilitated an even deeper connection with their respective traditions. For both dancers, improvisation was at the heart of these traditions. Not surprisingly, Afrological jazz notions of improvisation shared with kathak an emphasis on tradition, the collective, and the use of the musical space as a platform for building identity.[36] A shared sense of difference and marginalization also connected some of Das's dancers to the African American artists with whom they collaborated, as dancers from both groups were members of visible ethnic groups in the US context. Das's experience of being an Indian kathak dancer in America and Smith's experience of being an African American tap dancer had much in common, even as they also diverged. Although in radically different ways, both artists and their respective communities experienced stigmatization on the basis of cultural difference and skin color, which contributed to the crystallization of a unique cultural identity that was outside white mainstream American culture. Das also tapped into American public culture flows and popularized notions of Black culture through his work with Smith. As artists, they shared a desire to build pride in cultural identity and to carve out a respected space for dance and musical forms that were outside the Western white hegemonic models. Improvisation was valorized for its ability to transcend categories of race, ethnicity, and gender. Smith commented: "culture is not a barrier, age is not a barrier, race is not a barrier, sex is not a barrier. The things that bring us together are more important. Rhythm and dance are those things."[37] This argument for the universality of such forms, like kathak or tap, also marked out an important space for these art forms in an increasingly racialized world.

Upaj was brought into the fore in new ways through this collaboration, but Panditji always reminded students that while the tradition must evolve, one must continue to work within the rules and attributes of the tradition.[38] *Upaj* was the ideal vehicle to show how tradition and improvisation could exist side by side, and how innovations could occur without radically altering the standards of the tradition. But how was the validity of this statement confirmed? And what was traditional about *upaj*? In the next section I return to the importance of the accuracy and precision of improvised renderings in asserting the authenticity of kathak performance.

Bringing *Sam*: Improvisations of Exactitude

Das taught that in kathak the freedom of improvisation is situated in relation to ideas of "refined discipline with responsibility" and adherence to tradition. Despite the Romanticist notion that true freedom emerges from a break with tradition, or the transgression of convention and rule-bound doctrine, in this case, freedom comes from systematic training, a deep understanding of the time cycle or *tal*, and the embodiment and memorization of a distinct repertoire.[39] *Upaj* relies on the mastery of rhythm and *tal.* Variation or novelty may be desired, but in performing *upaj,* rhythmic precision and great accuracy of timing are demanded.

The moment that the dancer concludes a rhythmic composition and resolves the composition on the first beat of the time cycle is known as "bringing *sam*" (pronounced "sum"). As Hindustani music is cyclic, the time cycle begins and ends on the same beat; all compositions must conclude definitively on this beat. The resolution on *sam* is one of the most distinctive and aesthetically pleasurable elements of a kathak solo: after a building progression of rhythm, intensity, and energy, the dancer arrives together with the musicians in a brief and unified moment of sudden stillness. Aesthetic enjoyment emerges from the development of the composition itself, but especially from the uncertainty of its resolution, the risk involved, and the eventual achievement of this rhythmic unison. Writing in 1973, Vamanrao Hari Deshpande described this key principle of musical aesthetics: "to build up the tension in the listener, to keep it mounting up to a point and then to resolve it, thus bringing the listener's mind to equipoise on the *sam.*" All North Indian music must aim at and land on *sam,* which, coming from "Saavastha—literally means a state of mental equilibrium or equipoise."[40] This moment of unison or equipose is achieved through great accuracy of timing and is vital to effective performance in Indian aesthetics. Effective performance of the composition relies, quite dramatically, on getting it right.

During a solo performance in San Francisco in 2009, one of Das's students presented a *bol* composition in a standard sixteen-beat cycle of *tintal.* With live musicians on the stage, the dancer set the tempo of the *tal,* or overarching rhythmic cycle. The dancer vocally recited the composition: all dance compositions are taught and remembered through corresponding rhythmic phrases made up of mnemonic syllables. She proceeded to dance the rhythm with her whole body. The composition lasted several cycles; the beginning of the *tihai,* a thrice-repeated pattern, foreshadowed the finale of the composition. With the imminent conclusion of the *tihai,* the dancer began a series of swift heel-anchored pirouettes or *chakkars.* The tabla player also began to play louder strokes, adding energy to the music, building toward this final resolve. At the precise moment of the conclusion of the composition, the tabla player accented the kathak dancer's arrival on the final beat of the time cycle, and then, a millisecond later, the dancer landed her last *chakkar* in stillness. But it was not in unison. She had missed the all-important conclusion on the final beat of *sam.*

Rather than trying to conceal her mistake and simply carry on, the dancer quickly indicated that she would do the same composition again. Contrary to the conventions of the proscenium stage, the mistake was not glossed over, passed by, or ignored; it was brought into full focus and made the subject of scrutiny for all involved. The soloist repeated the very same composition from start to finish. A missed *sam* is a glaringly obvious mistake. There is no in-between; one either lands on *sam*, or one does not. Although it is not a mistake that happens often, it certainly did happen on this stage, and it is something that I have witnessed several times in solo performances in both the United States and India. Even senior dancers make such mistakes; I was once told that a well-known dancer repeated a difficult composition eight times onstage before landing on *sam*. When a performer repeats a composition, dramatic tension is further heightened; the successful resolution on a repeated attempt is always met with even greater enthusiasm and applause.

"Bringing *sam*" makes the execution of known skills unpredictable. In a radio interview, Pandit Das explained the improvisational and unfixed nature of a kathak solo by describing the difference between balletic turns and kathak *chakkars*:

> In ballet . . . it is all fixed, but in Indian tradition, it is all improvising within the ring fence of a rhythmic structure—say sixteen beat, or 12 ½, or 5 ½ beat—and then you start improvising. When you take pirouettes, in ballet they take pirouettes on the toe, and that is very difficult—where in kathak we take pirouettes on the left heel, with five to seven pounds of metal bells wrapped around your ankles. And try to take twenty-seven turns, but it is within two sixteen-beat cycles. The mind is split because you have to be within the sixteen beats. You are not going with the musicians (because the turns fall off the main beat). The tabla player—they don't necessarily know what you will do, so it can mess you up. You have your ears to the drummer, your face to the audience, and you are taking pirouettes. Your pirouettes may not be centered, you may go a little to the side here and there. But the idea, is to bring it on the first beat. And right there is the major difference between the balletic turns and the pirouettes of kathak . . . in the ballet, they are not dividing sixteen into three equal parts. And with the drummer, nothing is fixed. There is no symphony there, there is just one drummer, and you just go on.[41]

In the United States, Das often used the contrast of ballet to communicate something of the intricacy of kathak; the difficulty of taking turns emerges because the dancer must perform her repertoire (in this case, *chakkars* or pirouettes) within the time cycle with live musical accompaniment. And the nature of this relationship with the musician and the time cycle is unfixed; musicians do not know what the dancer will do. The dancer must accomplish and improvise a kind of corporeal mathematics in the act of bringing the first beat, for example, laying twenty-seven turns evenly across thirty-two beats (or two sixteen-beat cycles of *tintal*). *Upaj* here relates to the difficulty of executing such corporeal mathematics, especially given the unfixed nature of performance and the unpredictability of the musicians.

The case of missing *sam* and the ensuing repetition onstage exemplify an important point: critical to successful performance is the act of getting it right. Aesthetic enjoyment emerges from the improvisatory risks involved in the rendering of something known and in getting it right, rather than in creating something totally new. *Upaj* in this case is found in the live relationship between musician and dancer, their unrehearsed performance, and the improvisations of exactitude required to "bring *sam*" when onstage. Live performance highlights the precision and accuracy required in the tradition. Individuality and personal style are certainly desired and appreciated, but they are not the sole mark of good performance. Accuracy and timing here trump variation and novelty. As Napier rightly points out, "valorization of a performance may depend as much, if not more, on the quality of the pre-composed materials, and on the accuracy of their re-presentation, than on the novelty and inventiveness of a performer in re-presenting them."[42] Whether in a fixed composition, a stylistically interpreted version, or an altogether new *tihai*, timing and precision remain the key measure of successful performance. In this regard, specific processes of exposition within the kathak solo may be understood by considering not simply the degree to which they are improvised but also the degree to which these elements succeed. The production of aesthetic enjoyment, in fact, relies on this ability to "get it right."

Divine Rhetoric and *Upaj*: The Felt Experience of Oneness

Dance so that you become one with everything.

—Pandit Ram Narayan Misra

Indian classical music and dance are not for entertainment, they are designed to elevate your consciousness.

—Sadhguru J. Vasudev

Successful improvisations are thus seen *and* heard. *Upaj* affords a particular felt experience for the performers and audience members, one that is given meaning within the interpretive frame provided by Indian aesthetics. *Upaj*, in its many forms, provides an important opportunity for aesthetic enjoyment, which, in a Hinduized version of Indian aesthetics, is itself an experience closely linked to the divine, transcendence, and an experience of the otherworldly.[43] Indian classical music and dance share with Hindu religion and philosophy the spiritual goal of higher consciousness, spiritual liberation or *moksha*, and a creation of oneness; through the experience of dance and music, one moves toward this goal. The aesthetic goal of creating oneness and achieving liberation emerged from a long historical and cultural tradition in which philosophy, religion, and aesthetics have been deeply intertwined.

Written in the tenth century, Abhinavagupta's commentaries on the Sanskrit texts of the *Natya Sastra* theorized that "in art the purified state of the undifferentiated experience was . . . a 'state of consciousness' akin to the bliss (*ananda*) of the enlightened, liberated soul."[44] For Bharata (author of the *Natya Sastra*) and the many commentators and aestheticians who followed him, the issues of performance, therefore, "were not primarily issues of entertainment as it is normally understood today," but rather a matter of "how performance might be the means to a very different experience."[45] Indian aesthetic theorist Kapila Vatsyayan has said that Indian art is not "religious in the ordinary sense, nor is there a theology of aesthetics, but the two fields interpenetrate because they share the basic world-view in general and the specific goal of *moksha* and liberation in particular."[46] But how does one attain such lofty goals in practice?

The Indian aesthetic theory of *rasa*, outlined in the texts of the *Natya Sastra*, provides a pathway. *Rasa*, most often translated as the savoring of aesthetic enjoyment, is the end goal of all Indian classical arts.[47] *Rasa* emerges through the shared experience between dancer, musician, and audience and is itself the production of a kind of divine bliss, providing an opportunity to move toward the goal of spiritual fulfillment. While Das did not dwell on the specifics of *rasa theory*, the creation of *bhakti rasa* was explained as the goal of performance; Pandit Das spoke often about "the goal of achieving pure *bhakti* through dance." *Bhakti*, or devotion, refers to "intense emotional outbursts of personal devotion to god" that are experienced in the act of worship, reflecting the ideals of the Bhakti movement of religious devotionalism that began in India in the sixth century.[48] Dance scholars have pointed out that kathak was in fact highly influenced by the Bhakti devotional movement, if not developed from its traditions.[49] The experience of oneness or temporary union that emerges in performance was thus often referred to by Das as *bhakti rasa,* or devotional sentiment.

Bhakti, I argue, is a feeling more easily translated and felt, especially in the US context, where Das's students and audiences often had little or no prior knowledge of the Indian arts. While perhaps not grasping the cosmological significance of the achievement of "oneness" through performance, his US audiences could still experience a sensuous transformation of feeling that conveyed something of *rasa. Bhakti rasa* was the perfect vehicle to reach the widest audience. The oneness achieved through successful moments of *upaj*—and through the precision of timing that *upaj* requires, especially in "bringing *sam*"—afforded an opportunity where this rhetoric of union made bodily sense. Pandit Misra's admonition to "Dance so that you become one with everything" did not just float off into idealism; these words were grounded in the lived experiences of the dancing body. *Upaj* creates opportunities for this felt experience of symmetry and alignment.

Das explained successful moments of performance, especially those that are unplanned, by saying "it was not me, it was the divine." Many Indian musicians and dancers speak of their playing as coming from a source external to themselves, as if they are vessels channeling this divine energy.[50] Creativity is felt, and thus explained, as being beyond the self, as "that curious feeling when music seemed to flow entirely by itself, propelling itself effortlessly, leaving the musician in utter astonishment, almost as a bystander."[51] Improvisatory moments in performance are thus explained as social and divine accomplishments, rather than individual ones, an explanation that resonates with other musical genres, such as the jazz tradition. David Borgo, for instance, describes the experiences of jazz improvisers: "Many free improvisers discuss spiritual, ecstatic, or trancelike performance states. Total mental involvement is cited by some, while others describe a complete annihilation of all critical and rational faculties. Musicians stress performance goals ranging from complete relaxation or catharsis to a transcendental feeling of ego loss or collective consciousness. Others describe a voluntary, self-induced form of trance—more akin to shamanic practices—as they guide the listener on a spiritual journey. Despite these diverse belief systems, a feeling of spirituality and reverence pervades many improvised performances."[52] The US context—with the prevalence of diverse cultural performance genres—offers a fertile space in which the social and divine nature of creativity makes sense.

The foregrounding of spirituality and divine explanations of improvisation as well as the emphasis on tradition and the collective found an audience, especially in California, where these ideas were already in circulation. As Bonnie Wade has explained, Eastern spiritual philosophies and cultural practices provided a viable alternative to many of America's disenchanted youth during the countercultural movement of the 1970s.[53] The San Francisco Bay Area proved to be a receptive site for Indian cultural practices. Yoga, meditation, and other alternative practices for health and well-being were (and are) commodified for consumption in the United States. Das's kathak also tapped into the wider market economy in non-Western therapies, which caters to an American public seeking authentic experiences of traditional cultures and reimagined ancient worlds.[54] Indian aesthetic theory provides the frame from which such culturally-specific interpretations of aesthetic experience are initiated, but these interpretations gain new meaning within the US context.

While the social nature of creativity provides one paradigm for experience, this is tempered with the quest for a "unique self that each musician should be able to express through his or her music."[55] Kathak carries with it the seemingly contradictory requirements of reproducing knowledge of its lineage as handed down through generations of gurus, along with the expectation that mature students develop their own artistic signature. Das was certainly an innovator, and during his forty-five years in the US, he succeeded in developing his own unique brand of kathak.[56] While personalization of authorship is not foreign to the field of Indian aesthetics, and not exclusive to the US, the US context certainly provided an environment in which individuality and unique artistic contributions became salient aspirations.[57] It was, in fact, the success of the great Indian musicians, Pandit Ravi Shankar and Ali Akbar Khan abroad that inspired his move to the US in the first place. Das joined a long list of earlier pioneers of Indian arts, music, and spiritual practices who had traveled to the West to share their traditions and practices. Das, in fact, saw his move as a chance to start anew, "to become rich and famous overnight."[58] The US context has certainly inspired and valorized a kind of heroic artist figure. While it did not occur overnight, Das did garner significant recognition within the San Francisco Bay Area and his legacy carries on through his disciples' schools in the US, Canada, and India.

Upaj in America: Improvisation in Tradition

The instabilities of living in an increasingly interconnected world and performing an art form that now exists between and across nations brought with it a new range of challenges. Nonetheless, Das found ways to negotiate the demands of remaining authentic yet relevant and contemporary in the twentieth and twenty-first century for different demographics of participants, audience members, and funders. The US context provided Das with a space to reimagine and develop his version of authentic Indian tradition, and *upaj* was at the center of that reimagining.

"Kathak is not choreography," students were reminded time and again. Authentic kathak was positioned in relation to *upaj*, the traditional solo, and the live interactions between the dancer and the musician. The belief that *upaj* represented a connection to the divine reinforced the conviction of dancers that it defined traditional modes of kathak. By assigning such a potent significance to *upaj*, Das and dancers in his lineage necessarily stigmatized any departure from it. The trend toward modern kathak, then—a dance based in choreography and recorded music—is associated with a decline in *upaj*, which thus endangers the "essence" of the form. The modern styles of kathak with recorded music and set choreography no longer rely on improvisation or an understanding of *tal* for successful performance, removing the element of risk and unpredictability implicit in traditional styles. A dependence on recorded music eliminates the need for adeptness and readiness to understand *tal* and improvise within it. Recorded music also reduces the possibilities for an experience of "oneness" and union, which are brought about through the uncertainty and improvisation of live creation with musicians. Das lamented that a large part of what defined kathak was moving to the margins; this jeopardized the meaning of a practice that gave an experiential sense of connection to divinity. His emphasis on improvisation, tradition, and spirituality can be understood as standing against secular materialism and the trend toward modern choreography. Such oppositional understandings are a further reflection of the emergent transcultural sphere—including India and the United States—in which the dance form has circulated.

Upaj offers a way to communicate the modern, creative, and fresh dynamism of the traditional arts. This objective was important to Das, as to other traditional artists in the United States (but also in India), where expectations for novelty and innovation prevail. The emphasis on *upaj* and its translation as improvisation serves a utilitarian purpose; the improvisational qualities of this traditional art counter erroneous assumptions about the tradition's irrelevance, its restrictions on freedom, and the stereotypes of Indian classical dance as boring. Das explained, "for many, the label of 'traditional' conjures up images of things stale, static, archaic on one hand or of things foreign and exotic on the other. These characterizations are one-dimensional and in the end obscure the depth, nuance and dynamism inherent in Indian classical dance . . . traditions are evolving. They must."[59] Traditional artists like Das have fought for recognition of their art form on the global stage; artists like Das have much at stake when laying claim to the innovative and improvisational elements of a strict traditional practice that, in the past, may have been perceived as limited in its creative possibilities. In a competitive artistic field where a modernist bureaucratic framework prevails, funding, sponsorship, and grants rely on presentation of novelty and innovation. Das's privileging of *upaj* as the essence of the form thus responded to these expectations for newness and innovation.

Upaj has also provided the perfect vehicle to communicate a new form of Indian identity for a generation of South Asian Americans struggling to define their place in between worlds. "Improvising in tradition" is an important part of defining a cultural identity that exhibits pride in traditional Indian culture and celebrates the imagined homeland, yet simultaneously makes claims to participation in the modern world. *Upaj* engages with a discourse on improvisation that is present in the wider field of music and dance in America, one that facilitates cross-cultural exchanges and the subsequent identification with ideas in American popular culture. *Upaj* thus provides an important platform to engage new audiences and generations. For a growing and affluent community of Indo-Americans in the Bay Area, *upaj* offers one response to being both Indian and American because its discourse on improvisation in tradition draws on both worlds for its expression.

While Das spent decades in America developing his art, in his later years, his brand of kathak found new appeal among Indian audiences. The production *IJS*, in fact, toured more extensively throughout India than the US, to considerable fanfare, as depicted in the film *Upaj: Improvise*. Das's unique style of kathak was born of an absence from India, which he explained as allowing him to "go deeper into the old school while adding new technique of my own."[60] This new technique and style were to become part of a return flow to India. Although I have not touched on this here, Das's version of kathak, his identity, coined by one of his students, as a "modern guru-in-training," and his conceptualization of Indian culture and tradition also appealed to new generations grappling with negotiating Indianness in contemporary India. Das's kathak gained growing legitimacy in India, through performances like *IJS*, which collapsed the distinction between traditional and modern, presented American popular culture in tandem with kathak, and sparked the interest of new generations of Indian youth.

Upaj, or improvisation, as it is commonly translated, was at the core of Das's philosophy. The translation of *upaj* as "improvisation" for US audiences was strategic and effective, up to a certain point, but the diverse experiences of *upaj* are easily glossed over in this translation. George Ruckert writes that the idea of improvisation is elusive and somewhat deceptive in Hindustani classical music: "those that relate improvisation in its jazz sense of reworking melodic patterns over a chordal harmony do not instantly grasp the compositional restrictions and elaborations suggested."[61] To apply a single Western concept with its own particular historical trajectory to diverse musical traditions neglects the diverse range of training, experience and meaning implicit in culturally specific aesthetic genres.[62] While Eurocentric notions of improvisation cannot be entirely divorced from our understandings of specific aesthetic genres like kathak in the global context of the twenty-first century, deeper digging into the culturally specific aesthetic processes and the particular contexts within which they are practiced provides us the space to widen our conception of what improvisation *is* and what it can *do*. By adopting a culturally situated understanding of what is required in these different forms of *upaj*, we can see how it *can* be "improvisation" and yet also how the ontological nature of these processes can extend beyond the limitations of this translation. Furthermore, improvisation itself cannot be reduced to any one specific cultural aesthetic form. Improvisation continues to be a multivalent social form that exists across cultures and traditions. Even within one cultural form like kathak, improvisation can take many different shapes, forms, and meanings.

Notes to Chapter 7

Research and writing for this book chapter were supported by a Social Sciences and Humanities Research Council of Canada (SSHRC) Postdoctoral Fellowship held at Carleton University between 2012 and 2014.

1. The film *Upaj: Improvise* premiered in the United States in 2013, with screenings to follow in Europe, Canada, and Australia; *IJS*, the collaborative project that was the subject of the film, toured extensively through the United States, India, and Australia. *Upaj: Improvise* was released on Amazon in 2019 in the United Kingdom and the United States. The official trailer is available on YouTube; see "*Upaj: Improvise* Official Trailer."
2. Moraga, "Interview with Charlotte Moraga," 4:05 (italics added).
3. Chandavarkar, "Composition and Improvisation in Indian Music," 99.
4. Napier, "Novelty That Must Be Subtle," 13.
5. Deshpande, *Indian Musical Traditions*, 30.
6. Clayton, *Time in Indian Music*, 94.

7. Napier, "Novelty That Must Be Subtle," 2.

8. Antara Bhardwaj, personal interview, San Francisco, CA, November 4, 2009.

9. From interview with Das's senior company dancer Seibi Lee, August 5, 2007, cited in Morelli, "From Calcutta to California," 178.

10. Meer, *Hindustani Music in the Twentieth Century*, 142.

11. Sorrell and Narayan, *Indian Music in Performance*, 113.

12. Neuman, *The Life of Music in North India*, 23.

13. Napier, "Novelty That Must Be Subtle," 5.

14. Morelli, "From Calcutta to California," 170.

15. For excerpts of a kathak solo from Pandit Das and his disciple Antara Bhardwaj, see Das, "Pt. Chitresh Das Performs in Kolkata"; and Bhardwaj, "Tale of a Kathaka."

16. Morelli, "From Calcutta to California," 170.

17. Das, interview with Mary Ellen Hunt.

18. Moraga, "Interview with Charlotte Moraga," 04:48.

19. For example, see Das, "Kathak—Lightning Speed Feet."

20. Morelli, "From Calcutta to California," 86.

21. Several of Das's prominent disciples opened kathak schools outside of California: Joanna de Souza in Toronto (1988), Gretchen Hayden in Boston (1992), and Seema Mehta in Mumbai (2010). Other disciples have carried on Das's work in California, teaching and performing his style.

22. On "California *gharana*," see Chakravorty, *Bells of Change*, 89. For an example of Das's penchant for footwork and pirouettes, see video of his company dancers: "JogKouns Tarana."

23. Although Das also emphasized *gat bhao* (storytelling), he was known for his rhythmic versatility, speed, and strength, in contrast to other well-known gurus, for example, Birju Maharaj of the Lucknow *gharana*, who was renowned for his grace, elegance, and expertise in *abhinaya* (expression).

24. Morelli, "From Calcutta to California," 70–71.

25. Quoted in Molekhi, "Yogic Twirls."

26. Indian dance scholar Leela Venkataraman suggests that in recent years the "depth and flowing ability needed to improvise" in a kathak solo has, in fact, been indirectly lessened by the structured formality of today's proscenium stage, which strikes at the very root of such open-ended presentations. See Venkataraman, "Kathak," 94. Recorded music is also positioned in opposition to the ability to improvise, since a fixed musical score further contributed to the fixing of entire solo performance, reducing the degree to which dancers can improvise onstage. Recorded music is steadily replacing live music, in part, because of the logistical difficulties and costs in securing live musicians. Pandit Das was a vocal proponent of the requirement of live music, having made it mandatory at an international kathak festival he held in San Francisco in 2006. The changes associated with modernity, then (e.g., the proscenium stage and recording technology), are also what contribute to a reduction of "improvisation" on the stage.

27. Although Das rigorously promoted traditional solos and live musicians, he also choreographed a number of ensemble pieces that used recorded music.

28. Lessinger, "Investing or Going Home?," 71. In India, Non-Resident

Indians (NRIs) and other returning members of the diaspora were often outside the definition of being an Indian; in America, their Indianness defined them as outside the majority. Questions on Indian immigrant identity were heard in the public sphere through the local Indian newspaper and Indian radio programs in the Bay Area. Johanna Lessinger has suggested that "both Indians and Indian immigrants in the United States are involved in endless discussion about what it means to be Indian as India itself changes what constitutes Indian-ness, and whether one can remain truly Indian outside of India. There is an ongoing attempt on the part of those groups involved in NRI investment to break with a narrow, nationalist definition of 'Indian' and to recast their identity in new, global terms. Meanwhile, people in India tend to see NRIs as no longer fully Indian, and to blame them for the social and spiritual dislocations inherent in the modernisation process itself. In some ways NRIs have come to stand for a whole category of India's urbanized, superficially Westernized 'new rich' who have flourished with modernisation." Lessinger, 57.

29. Kurwa, "U. S. Dance School," 03:36.

30. Ramsey, *Race Music*, 97.

31. For an overview of *IJS*, see Das and Smith, "Fierce Kathak & Tap."

32. Plfaumer, "A Dance Revolution."

33. Following Das's death, his disciple Seema Mehta carried on this collaborative work with tap dancer Jason Samuels Smith, touring in India, Canada, and the United States. In 2015, Das's disciples Rina Mehta and Rachna Nivas mounted a collaborative kathak and tap piece titled *Speak* with tap dancers Michelle Dorrance and Dormeshia Sumbry-Edwards. See Leela Dance Collective, "SPEAK Official Trailer."

34. Quoted in Jayakumar, "Shaking a Leg."

35. Quoted in Molekhi, "Yogic Twirls."

36. See Lewis, "Improvised Music after 1950."

37. Quoted in Dalidowicz, "Conversations in Rhythm."

38. Das, interview with Mary Ellen Hunt.

39. See also Wilf, "Rituals of Creativity"; and Hughes-Freeland, "Tradition and the Individual Talent."

40. Deshpande, *Indian Musical Traditions*, 31.

41. Das, interview with Mary Ellen Hunt.

42. Napier, "Novelty That Must Be Subtle," 5.

43. Explanations of "oneness" and transcendence of self through dance draw on both Hindu and Sufi cosmologies. Many of the elements of Muslim cosmology and Sufi heritage that suffuse different parts of India, however, tend to be suppressed in this version of kathak. The privileging of the dominant Hindu ideologies highlights a striking instance of the editing of tradition that occurred in the twentieth century.

44. Schwartz, *Rasa*, 17. The *Natya Sastra* (composed by the sage Bharata Muni somewhere between the sixth and seventh century AD) is one of the most elaborate treatises on drama and dance and is the earliest text on aesthetic theory in India.

45. Schwartz, *Rasa*, 13.

46. Vatsyayan, *Bharata*, 25.

47. *Rasa* theory takes emotions as central to performance. Bharata Muni's

Natya Sastra suggests eight primary emotions (or *sthaibhava*), plus the addition of a later *rasa,* collectively known as the *navarasa,* as explained by Chakravorty, *Bells of Change,* 104.

48. Chakravorty, 104–5. The Bhakti movement of religious devotionalism first took shape in Tamil country in the sixth century before gradually spreading northward. It provided individual worshippers with a direct line to access the divine, bypassing the interventions of the high Brahmin priests, effectively generating a new avenue to salvation. The ideals of the Bhakti movement were further embodied in figures like the sixteenth-century Bengali saint Caitanya and had particular pertinence for a generation of Kolkata youth, of which Chitresh Das was one. Caitanya, usually said to be the founder of Bengal Vaishanvism, "preached to all castes, and believed that all castes had the right to worship Krishna. He approved positively of breaking down caste barriers" (Dimock, "Doctrine and Practice," 119). As Chakravorty explains, the Vaishnava religion ran up against some opposition because of its progressive anti-caste and anti-Brahmin position and its emphasis on "the equality of the sexes [that] provided room for women from all segments of society" (*Bells of Change,* 37). Das's philosophy echoed the ideas of these early Bengali figures, especially in his goal of empowering women and his attempts to make dance equally accessible to students from all backgrounds.

49. Natavar, "New Dances, New Dancers," 7.

50. Sawyer, "The Semiotics of Improvisation," 283.

51. Chandavarkar, "Composition and Improvisation in Indian Music," 99.

52. Borgo, "Negotiating Freedom," 175.

53. Wade, *Music in India,* 8.

54. Lau, *New Age Capitalism.*

55. Duranti and Burrel, "Jazz Improvisation," 95.

56. Das's distinctive innovation, "kathak yoga," a practice of self-accompaniment in which the dancer sings and plays an instrument while dancing rhythms with his or her feet, came to mark his contribution to kathak. The discourse surrounding this innovation in tradition was elaborated in and drew on the US context, as discussed in Dalidowicz, "Crafting Fidelity."

57. Groesbeck, "Cultural Constructions of Improvisation," 23. Rolf Groesbeck has made this point clear in his study of improvisation in *tayampaka,* a solo Hindu temple drumming genre from Kerala, in which the "unique, dominant, prestigious, self-aggrandizing, autonomous individual" remains an important social category.

58. Morelli, "From Calcutta to California," 53.

59. Das, "Interview with Pandit Chitresh Das."

60. Morelli, "From Calcutta to California," 201.

61. Ruckert, *Music in North India,* 53.

62. Nooshin, "Improvisation as 'Other,'" 251.

Works Cited

Bhardwaj, Antara. "Tale of a Kathaka: Traditional Solo by Antara Bhardwaj." Posted April 28, 2010. YouTube video, 7:00. https://www.youtube.com/watch?v=SnZ4TFUXCu8

Borgo, David. "Negotiating Freedom: Values and Practices in Contemporary Improvised Music." *Black Music Research Journal* 22, no. 2 (2002): 165–88.

Chakravorty, Pallabi. *Bells of Change*. Calcutta: Seagull Books, 2008.

Chandavarkar, Bhaskar. "Composition and Improvisation in Indian Music." In *Aspects of Indian Music*, edited by S. Matatkar, 66–102. New Delhi: Sangeet Natak Akademi, 1987.

Clayton, Martin. *Time in Indian Music: Rhythm, Metre, and Form in North Indian Rag Performance*. New York: Oxford University Press, 2000.

Dalidowicz, Monica. "Conversations in Rhythm: Tap Kathak." *Indian Link* (Australia), November 2, 2010.

Dalidowicz, Monica. "Crafting Fidelity: Pedagogical Creativity in Kathak Dance." *Journal of the Royal Anthropological Institute* 21, no. 4 (December 2015): 838–54.

Das, Chitresh. Interview by Mary Ellen Hunt. *Up Front*. KALW 91.7, San Francisco, CA, September 26, 2008.

Das, Chitresh. "Interview with Pandit Chitresh Das." Traditions Engaged. 2010. Accessed July 19, 2014. Removed from the website by July 2020. www.kathak .org/traditionsengaged/about/about-festival/

Das, Chitresh. "Kathak—Lightning Speed Feet of Pt. Chitresh Das." Posted April 29, 2008. YouTube video, 1:02. https://www.youtube.com/watch?v=3SxWyvl i7es

Das, Chitresh. "Pt. Chitresh Das Performs in Kolkata." Posted February 16, 2020. YouTube video, 3:06. https://www.youtube.com/watch?v=MsvREisdbUA

Das, Chitresh, and Jason Samuels Smith. "Fierce Kathak & Tap—Pt. Chitresh Das & Jason Samuels Smith." Posted August 25, 2007. YouTube video, 6:08. https://www.youtube.com/watch?v=4sQn5bXbigo

Deshpande, Vamanrao Hari. *Indian Musical Traditions: An Aesthetic Study of the Gharanas in Hindustani Music*. Translated by S. H. Deshpande. Mumbai: Popular Prakashan, 1973.

Dimock, Edward C., Jr. "Doctrine and Practice among the Vaisnavas of Bengal." *History of Religions* 3, no. 1 (1963): 106–27.

Duranti, Alessandro, and Kenny Burrel. "Jazz Improvisation: A Search for Hidden Harmonies and a Unique Self." *Ricerche di Psicologia* 3 (2004): 71–101.

Groesbeck, Rolf. "Cultural Constructions of Improvisation in Tāyampaka, a Genre of Temple Instrumental Music in Kerala, India." *Ethnomusicology* 43 (1999): 1–30.

Hughes-Freeland, Felicia. "Tradition and the individual talent: T.S. Eliot for Anthropologists." In *Creativity and Cultural Improvisation*, edited by Elizabeth Hallam and Tim Ingold, 207–222. Oxford: Berg, 2007.

Jayakumar, Amrita. "Shaking a Leg, Fusion-Style." *Asian Age* (India), February 3, 2010.

"JogKouns Tarana—Chitresh Das Dance Company." Posted September 5, 2013. YouTube video, 1:21. https://www.youtube.com/watch?v=lXUDdTv5N5w

Kurwa, Nishat. "U. S. Dance School Imparts Indian Traditions." *The World*. Public Radio International, January 7, 2009. https://www.pri.org/stories/2009 -01-07/us-dance-school-imparts-indian-traditions

Lau, Kimberly J. *New Age Capitalism: Making Money East of Eden*. Philadelphia: University of Pennsylvania Press, 2000.

Leela Dance Collective. "SPEAK Official Trailer: A Kathak & Tap Collaboration."

Posted December 26, 2018. YouTube, 1:36. https://www.youtube.com/watch ?v=jLSBUptULJs

Lessinger, Johanna. "Investing or Going Home? A Transnational Strategy among Indian Immigrants in the United States." *Annals of the New York Academy of Sciences* 645 (1992): 53–80.

Lewis, George E. "Improvised Music after 1950: Afrological and Eurological Perspectives." *Black Music Research Journal* 16 (1996): 91–122.

Meer, Wim van der. *Hindustani Music in the Twentieth Century.* The Hague: Martinus Nijhoff, 1980.

Molekhi, Pankaj. "Yogic Twirls: Kathak Exponent Introduces the New Form of Dance." *Economic Times* (India), August 8, 2010.

Moraga, Charlotte. "Interview with Charlotte Moraga, Performing Diaspora Artist 2009." Posted by CounterPulse, August 18, 2009. YouTube video, 9:50. https://youtu.be/U1ZklGJHvCQ

Morelli, Sarah. "From Calcutta to California: Negotiations of Movement and Meaning in Kathak Dance." PhD diss., Harvard University, 2007.

Napier, John. "Novelty That Must Be Subtle: Continuity, Innovation and 'Improvisation' in North Indian Music." *Critical Studies in Improvisation / Études critiques en improvisation* 1, no. 3 (2006). https://www.criticalimprov.com/index .php/csieci/issue/view/13

Natavar, Mekhala. "New Dances, New Dancers, New Audiences: Shifting Rhythms in the Evolution of India's Kathak Dance." PhD diss., University of Wisconsin, 1997.

Neuman, Daniel M. *The Life of Music in North India: The Organization of an Artistic Tradition.* Chicago: University of Chicago Press, 1990.

Nooshin, Laudin. "Improvisation as 'Other': Creativity, Knowledge and Power— The Case of Iranian Classical Music." *Journal of the Royal Musical Association* 128, no. 2 (2003): 242–96.

Pflaumer, Andrea. "A Dance Revolution: Two for the Road." *San Francisco Examiner*, March 15, 2010.

Price, Sally. *Primitive Art in Civilized Places.* Chicago: University of Chicago Press, 1989.

Ramsey, Guthrie P. *Race Music: Black Cultures from Bebop to Hip-Hop.* Berkeley: University of California Press, 2003.

Ruckert, George E. *Music in North India: Experiencing Music, Expressing Culture.* Oxford: Oxford University Press, 2004.

Sawyer, Keith R. "The Semiotics of Improvisation: The Pragmatics of Musical and Verbal Performance." *Semiotica* 108, nos. 3/4 (1999): 269–306.

Schwartz, Susan L. *Rasa: Performing the Divine in India.* New York: Columbia University Press, 2004.

Sorrell, Neil, and Ram Narayan. *Indian Music in Performance: A Practical Introduction.* Manchester: Manchester University Press, 1990.

"*Upaj: Improvise* Official Trailer." Posted July 30, 2013. YouTube video, 1:43. https://www.youtube.com/watch?v=Sgoq9FVC9Jg

Vatsyayan, Kapila. *Bharata, the Natya Sastra.* New Delhi: Sahitya Akademi, 1996.

Venkataraman, Leela. "Kathak: Evolution of the Storyteller." *India Perspectives*, September–October 2009, 88–97.

Wade, Bonnie. *Music in India: The Classical Traditions in India.* Englewood Cliffs, NJ: Prentice Hall, 1979.

Wilf, Eitan. "Rituals of Creativity: Tradition, Modernity, and the 'Acoustic Unconscious' in a U.S. Collegiate Jazz Music Program." *American Anthropologist* 114 (2012): 32–44.

EIGHT | Ode B'kongofon

HAFEZ MODIRZADEH

Try to define me with words and these will become like nails in your own coffin,
for I do not know who I am, I am lucid confusion.

—Rumi

Prologue

The following cryptic verse, intended to be read aloud, moves with improvised flow through various streams, crossing phonemes— metaphorical, musical, theoretical, historical, cultural, natural— breathing B'kongofonic spirit from the saxophone, imbuing all with a sense of interconnectivity.[1]

Humming subtone, speaking subtext, singing subvoice—from the realm of intuitive certainty, a collective spirit rises through and out of saxophonic form. Invoked by name, the B'kongofon is born from those creational materials, humanly and earthly, underpinning an industrial revolution. As brass/woodwind, the B'kongofon projects *a gathering of sounds for a heroic people. kongo,* as "gathering," the historical homeland of a Central African people; *fon,* as "sound," the language of a West African people of the same name; and the occasional elision *B'* refers to all "peoples" on the resistance continuum. The B'kongofon also conse- crates those resources harvested by Congolese hands, exploited for the eventual production of one man's invention—the saxophone. This is the sound come-unity of ancestral memory imprinted within the horn's alloy, well below the surface engraving of the manufacturer, calling for an alchemic change of heart and mind, instilling the courage necessary for all oppressor/occupiers to make reparations at their own unconditional cost. Emanating from a saxophonic history of transnational proportion that has itself moved beyond militaristic origin, B'kongofonic song emboldens war cries to turn into love calls, rendering the host instrument with a musical and spiritual value befitting its own case—made here, rather than by enclosing the brass body in a proverbial wooden box, disclosing its soul by spoken word.

Body/Soul (part 1) introduces a complement of cosmic forces that generate earthly elements in all their organic beauty—human, mineral, plant, and otherwise. This theme is reiterated with Pulsivity/Resonance (part 7), which summarizes some concepts of practice gleaned from the overall Ode body, where fluctuating pulse is recognized for its broader effects on creative activity. Blood/Betrayal (part 2) threads history across borders of mind, time, and space, setting up Acknowledgment (part 3), which takes the reader through the experience of harvesting rubber and assembling saxophones; this, juxtaposed with humanity's desecration for the sake of such industry, invokes some common memory for moving forward.[2] The vindication finally reached with John Coltrane's *Africa/Brass* connects Resolution (part 4) and Pursuance (part 5), where a personal history of adapting Persian tones to saxophone in a polycultural context—hallmark of an Afro-diasporic heritage of syncretizing multiple systems of practice—opens a passageway for kongofonic utterance. Parts 3, 4, and 5 are borrowed from Coltrane's 1964 recording *A Love Supreme*, here signifying a realization process where resolution leads to pursuance, rather than the other way around. Song B'kongofon (part 6), then, arrives at a celebration of saxophonic experiences that join with a new family of fingerings to anoint, in sonic form, that spirit identified through this instrument. In closing, an epilogual improvisation sets all sound changes to an anthropomorphic liberation from every "ism," colonial and otherwise.

Ultimately, from crossing multiple focal points, portals open, thus illuminating axes intrinsic to double consciousness.[3] Such duality, in fluid, complementary terms, may lead toward a perception plurality that embraces myriad expressions while obliterating institutional repression in the process. As a composed improvisation, then,

Ode B'kongofon explores that split moment in the mind turning history on an ecstatic ear
where disparate thoughts, like constellations, are hyperactively interwoven,
where survival's buoyancy is more determinal than coincidental,
where, by orbiting the epicenter of those crown-spinning ghosts
dancing in our heads, we spin creative,
evaporating into creation Itself.

I. Body/Soul

fingers membrane
lining hollowed shells
sealing tones whole
with hands

this naqareh[4] mother-of-pearl
from ocean's ebb flows
our organic inorganic
resilient iridescent
mother of all colors

within your nacre shell
lunar gravity resonates
shorelines in pulsivity
sounding molecular strands
bonding in pairs at low tide
separating again at high tide
replicating spirits unhewn
while orbits vacillate distance
earth's rotation velocity
in fixed periodicity
with the sun

yet Sól embraces gah
the *se* of mi-to-Ra
brother fifth to mother third
mythrae earth from mah[5]
moving tonics as sister variates tides
transfers heat between poles while
climates oscillate
and speciation abounds
with every human
ancestral partials
plucked to atone
lone fundamentals

undulating
from this yellow brass
alloy body of
copper zinc
combined for strength resistance
in bones muscle liver
and respiratory systems
It breathes to us through us
smelted from the number turning all
3-tern-al

. . .

ore bodies of natural minerals native metals
born from high volcanic temperatures
coursing through hydrothermal veins
forming within magma chambers below Earth's crust
before copper ascends with heat rising to upper layers

and there, Elders with powers to extract ore
form a secret guild of "Copper Eaters"
along the Kasai River Katanga's *bwanga*
craft copper crosses from a sacred foundry
for currency of dignity and strength
handa

digging wells during months of drought
mined ore molten from high clay furnaces
ventilated with bellows from antelope skin
then refined and cast as copper before exported
far_____far from the southern coast,
to Europe . . .

II. Blood/Betrayal

Trees slashed open unleash horror
"beto febole yiwo"—rubber is death!
one ton a day harvested, otherwise
homes torched, people slaughtered
encaged, enslaved, starved
from the burned villages of Iteke, Yambi, Ilongo

Yambisi, Baurou, Yambumba, Likombe
Yamapete, Bokolo, Bikoro, Basoko
fleeing to the forest from death
"beto febole yiwo"!

. . .

Elsewhere,
"from the forest" Silvius Brabo appears
slaying evil incarnate from whom havoc is wreaked
crushing the wretched beast who severed hands, heads, feet
whose own hand now gets ripped off by the young soldier
and by casting it into river's mouth, immortalizes the battle
as Antwerp, delivered from such a reign, with a royal title
enshrines the hero's name, Duke of Brabant.

But neither "bold" nor "brave," this one duke,
reviled as a giant betrayer of humanity
deluded "soldier" of others' misfortune
lusting under the sheepskin of nobility
this bearded wolf reaping Congo booty
nourished an Industrial Revolution
while rubbering out lives in the process.

. . .

In 1890, as the equatorial peoples of Central/South America cultivated "cahuchu,"
from "crying wood," that sticky milky latex torn from trees of *hevea*,
rubberwood was being cut open in Equatorial Africa, under forced labor.
And as the *Mino*, women warriors of Dahomey, fought French encroachment into West Africa,
the Iranian people's Tobacco Revolt blocked their monarch's concessions to the British
while in the "Congo Free State," commercial exploitation of rubber befitted a Belgian king,
and from Congo Square in New Orleans, Black citizens challenged "separate but equal" doctrine.

For where in Africa America, memories of a Colonial America would have rather seen
pine trees set on fire than for their sap to have supplied naval yards with slave ship tar,
in Native America, a Paiute prophet named Wovoka, while cutting wood, had a vision
and was called upon to teach the Ghost Dance to his people, who by turning ecstatic
for white settlers to leave, dancing from the inside out for blessings, restoration
of peace and prosperity, personified Rumi's call to "dance in the middle of the fighting,"
where with Mowlana, "I stand up, and this one of me becomes a hundred of me" circling,

circling the widening hoop of our collective memory, envisioning the spirits of our dead
reunited with the living, a Ghost Dance continuum finally ending all foreign occupation.

The giant, then, is any hand that profits from human suffering and oppression,
whose unquenchable greed thirsts for the exploitation of natural resources,
at whatever the human cost. Worldwide trauma sustained from such crimes,
when left without reparations by the complicit, in/directly lays seed to far worse
at their own doorstep, the effects from which bear on us all . . .   Today,

copper for war shells uranium for bombs,
high profits from coltan in every cell phone
leaves an abuse continuum unhealed,
driving humanity into a forest unhinged,
where, beyond blood quantum or lineage,
Native partials dance in the balance.

All resistance then, in all forms,
binds all peoples to one resolution:
to rise, as copper to earth's crust,
to flow, as milk from rubberwood,
to pressure, from all directions,
interlopers' militaristic grip,
thrown into oblivion
by a handshake

With reeded shapes rattling from every spirit,
from the Ghost Dance to the Congo Basin,
through *Africa/Brass* . . .
breathing from saxophone
B'kongofon!

. . .

Where the Elder reed-warrior communes
with Sol and AACM, slaying 12-toned
imposters of the sacred bull, Hapis
heralding from hardened ebonite
through overturned Phrygian bells
a Mithraic soldier's call to Libertas:
"Now's the time to play like a mo****fu****! . . ."

Vulcanite forged by a Roman god of fire
with Mithra—Persian god of light, truth, order,
solar deity of integrity, harmony, and friendship—
from Achaemenid times turning patron god of soldiers
to convert a metal wooded military wail into matrimonial call
over millennia saxophones from *karna*.

Called cornet from scripture, blown straight, this double-reeded karna
of finite volume covering an infinite area of raised sonic soul, this horn's call
pierces deep, a shrill hollow tone curling inner ear's cochlea spiral,[6] calling
Sanskrit karna as "ear," said to have been born through that of his mother, Kunti,
mythical Karna, a great warrior lauded for his sacrifice, valor, and courage,
offspring of the Hindu god Surya, a sun deity mirrored in vedic Mitrá.

While Zoroastrian Mithra is rendered as *mehr* for kindness, mercy,
Roman Mithras wears the Phrygian cap for freed slaves, liberty.
Like the Phrygian mother of gods, Cybele,
this mediator born of rock shares the company of a lion,
yet sacrifices the lunar bull in tauroctony,
holding a sword in one hand, while she holds a frame drum,
reflecting together Ashanti adinkra for

                   blood_____drum_____spirit

. . .

Among Roman initiates into the Mithraic Mysteries stood Emperor Marcus Aurelius,
2nd century stoic philosopher, from les gens Aurelia, from whence Orléans evolves,
located along the Loire River, once inhabited by 5th century Iranian Alani people,
a center of thought during the 9th century reign of emperor Charlemagne,
and wherein the 15th century, troops of "The Maid of Orléans," Joan of Arc,
would deliver the city from siege for King Charles VII.

The kongofonic path unfolds seven "Charles"—each moving beyond "man," "king," or "warrior,"
with the first Charles [Marie de La Condamine], explorer of South America,
in 1731, sending samples of natural elastomer back to Europe, ushering in scientific inquiry;
the second Charles [Joseph Sax], father of Adolphe Sax, in 1814,
from Dinant—the old Belgian city of metalworkers—along with his son,
builds and supplies brass instruments for the King's army.

The same year Adolphe Sax patents his saxophone (1846),
Leopold II is named Duke of Brabant, then onto King of Belgium,
from 1865 until his last breath in 1909, the same year of Lester Young's birth.

Pres, a deity among saxophonists, was raised in New Orleans, a city named after
the French Duke of Orleans, maternal ancestor to the notorious Leopold.

By the late 18th century, code noir "relaxes" in New Orleans,
enabling markets by African descendants, in some Mithraic fashion,
to initiate just arbitration for the buying back of their own freedom
by donning price caps to cut off the profit limb of slave holders;
and by the 19th century, congregating at Congo Square, circling
that opening north of the French Quarter, African American
lifeblood pumps through the musical arteries of a Crescent City.

At the same time, before developing the Congo region for his employer—Leopold II,
Betrayer of Man—Henry Morton Stanley spends his formative years in New Orleans.
Then, with monarchial support in 1879, Stanley returns to Africa, spreading brutality,
building roads through forced labor, and eventually opens the lower Congo to commerce,
paving the way for the Belgian king's privately "owned" Congo Free State.

III. Acknowledgment

late 19th–early 20th century
The following is a juxtaposition of experiences transcribed from eye-
witness accounts—rubber harvesting, saxophone assembly, and detailed
human atrocities—preferably to be read in concurrence, dispassionately
(*optional silent reading for italicized portions that are particularly violent, potentially disturbing*).[7]

- **rubber harvesting: traveler's description while in Makala district, Congo**
- saxophonic roots: instrument production and instructions for assembly
- *kongofonic blood: accounts from the Congo Free State, which executed the state
  practice of cutting off the right hands of natives' dead bodies for unmet rubber
  quota; dismembered hands of men, women, and children were smoked to be
  preserved in baskets, routinely taken to officers, one amputated hand for each
  bullet cartridge spent; to account for missing cartridges, limbs were also cut
  from the living, their open wounds cauterized or burned closed.*

the natives usually go out in couples, build a little shanty in
the midst of the jungle and work in a circle around it

brass (from copper and zinc)
powered by water energy,
smelt, forged, cast,
hammered, flattened, rolled

dead bodies hanging from branches in the water . . . others strung up in the
form of a cross

climbing the rubber-bearing tree or vine, they slash the bark with two or
three V-shaped cuts, one below the other, and then arrange a broad leaf
underneath, so as to form a trough

on a long, tapered mandrel,
the brass tube is lubricated,
heated until malleable

gallows noose fixed rope twists and man writhes on ground, then shot in neck

the trough conducts the sap, which oozes out, about the consistency and
color of milk, ideally, into a gourd, or preferably, a gallipot, procured at
the station

steadily widening at one end,
its thickness is forged even,
soaked in sulfuric acid,
then bent curled at a shaping station

hands, heads, genitals of villagers—tied up hanging on a line fixed between two
sticks; up to four feet of blood squirted from the freshly amputated limbs

the rubber from trees and vines is mixed promiscuously—some vine
rubber is put with that from the trees, as it coagulates more rapidly—
the natives preferring to tap the latter, as they say it flows more freely

then water pressure forced through,
expanding, conforming to the walls of the die

a stake forced into her womb and then shot; to show they could kill men, sentries cut off and deliver testicles

returned to their hut, the gatherers pour the sap into an earthenware pot containing water, and then place it on the fire and stir it with a stick, which they call bosanga

the brass tube slipped on a steel mandrel,
a drill press lowered and threaded into a pulling ball, then raised

hand and foot cut off of a child, left in brother's arms; Ncongo (from Ikoko village) said: "one day they killed my sister—cut off her hands and feet (her name was Mobe)"

in about ten minutes the rubber, owing to the acid in the bosanga, begins to collect round the stick, and soon a mass is formed, then lifted out, and placed on a big leaf and rinsed with clean cold water

pulling the ball through and creating a hole with rim,
done with each tone hole in the shaft; and each can be drilled further
to sound less sharp, or filled in with shellac to sound less flat

fixed number of cartridges before a raid; to save cartridges, one bullet shoots through a line of heads

then, enveloped in leaves, it is kneaded for a minute or two with hands or feet, to press out the remaining moisture

then the body is coated with a clear lacquer finish
molten alloy into a steel die
keys forged soldered together polished

burning cobalt poured over a prisoner's head

now the rubber is cut up into rough cubes that are spread to dry on a little platform built over the fire

mechanical key stack assemblage with blued steel rods,
where nickel silver hinges pivot on screw pins,
for the needle and leaf springs holding keys in a resting position

whipped with "chicotte" whip made of rhinoceros hide dried in sun to rip the skin to shreds; mother and daughter flogged 200 lashes then their breasts cut off, left to die

here it remains for an hour or two, before it is packed in the loosely made baskets that the natives carry to the station

upper and lower octave keys,
left/right palm keys,
left/right thumb keys,
little finger keys on rollers,
while guards hover over keys

beat the boy's hands off with rifle butts against a tree (his name is Mola)

the rubber-laden caravan of men, women, and children, headed by the chief and the forest guard, wind their way from their village into the post chanting a chorus, while notes are blown on a kudu trumpet made from an antelope horn; long before the party reaches the post, this music, ever increasing in volume, heralds their approach to the official in charge, as he makes preparations to receive the rubber

pads of layered cardboard, felt, cork, or leather,
with a metal center to reflect sound,
are stamped then glued to each key

husband/father beheaded while looking in despair for his wife and child in the forest

he meets the laden caravan at the beam scale of the station where
the rough baskets are weighed, and the price paid in cloth, salt, bells,
soap, beads, and such coveted treasures. The payment over, off they all
rush . . . yelling and shouting at the top of their voices

keys are finished by being drilled and fitted with springs,
then mounted to the main tube and screwed onto small posts,
drilled to hold the key springs, then seated on the tone holes
with sealing tested and adjusted for airtightness

wives taken hostage (detained, tied together) by concession companies to be
released when enough rubber was collected by their husbands; the young ones
raped by sentries; husbands must wait for every 15 days when rubber is handed
in; public incest enforced for amusement

the rubber is then spread on platforms under large sheds, until the
women workers of the post have cut it into neat little cubes

buffers of felt, cork, leather, reduce friction, minimize noise from key
motion, optimizing keywork action for pad sealing, intonation,
speed, feel

one girl had her hand cut off and was alive; he recognized his young sister's
hand in the basket; the girl was hiding in the forest with her mother; mother was
killed, she was brought to mission and died some months later

meanwhile very neatly plaited baskets are being prepared from rattan
cane, into which the dry rubber will be packed, until every basket
weighs exactly 5 lbs

cork to line joints, keys watered, wax applied to joints,
crook attached to main tube, as well as mouthpiece

Tswambe said of the soldiers guarding the village of Boyeka: they took a large
net put 10 men inside, put large stones shoved the net closed into the water; in
another canoe, a basket was half filled with cut-off hands to give to officers

for three months the cubes have lain in layers on the platforms to dry—
turned once a fortnight until all the moisture has evaporated; during
this process some 25 percent in weight is lost

strap ring attached joints lined with cork and waxed so they fit together
smoothly; main body is stamped with the manufacturer's name and all
other finishing done

(In Baringa village) to punish her husband, a young woman (Imanega) tied to
a forked tree and chopped in half from left shoulder; sentry chopped through the
chest and abdomen and out to side

a tin label is attached to each basket, with the distinctive number and
place of origin, and they are then laid out in long rows, ready for
transport by porters, canoe, rail, and steamer to Europe

inspectors check for deformed parts, inadequate soldering,
check the physical dimensions of each part

From Bolima village, Chief Isekifasu's two wives and baby had been killed;
one woman sliced in half, another had her intestines ripped out; they had also
strung the child's entrails around the huts and stuck parts of his body on sticks

. . .

saxophone's tube as trunk,
rods as vines, keys as stems,
with fingers as three-lobed fruit
exploding with seeded ideas
blown through people's mouthpiece—
this vulcanite rubber
fired from white milky latex
carrying nutrients of high resistance
through pulsing memory
acoustical anatomic,
personifying kongofonic . . .

An anthroposonic system
of integral geometry
shaped by breath, signifying creation

where very small changes
effect tone sensation
determining the cavity's shape below the reed
facing and opening between tip and reed
vibration amplitude of wild river reeds, calling
from the chamber, shank, and baffle
to rails, window, beak, bore, and table,
for woodshedding chops on giant cane
bound ligature-tight, slicing air streams
through an aperture, to feel and hear
the redemptive pressure of Rumi's reed
a cry of separation from the Congo River Basin
empowering kongofonic spirit for reunification:

Children, mothers, fathers, sisters, brothers—you, who resisted the sufferings of
forced labor by defiantly cutting the landolphia vines, burning rubber harvests,
escaping to the forest, even choosing to depopulate yourselves rather than giving
in to being shot, captured, or maimed—

let your voices rise up and out
in righteous indignation,
from reed tip to brass bell,
whither vindication!

IV. Resolution

> *When I die, just hope someone's there to hold my hand . . .*
> —Grandma

Adolphe introduces his saxophone at the Paris Industrial Exhibition, in 1844,
the same year the third Charles [Goodyear] vulcanizes rubber to galvanize
an industrial production of hoses, tires, shoe soles, machine valves, seals, fittings;
then the fourth Charles [Gerard Conn], also born that same year, by 1875, patents
a rubber-rimmed mouthpiece for cornet, while marketing the "Wonder" model
that King Joe Oliver would go on to play in Chicago, most likely also played by
the New Orleans progenitor of jazz—cornetist, bandleader, cultural innovator,
the fifth Charles ["King" "Buddy" Bolden] (1877–1931).

By the late 19th century, Conn improves saxophone production in the US, supplying military
bands with brass instruments endorsed by J. P. Sousa; in New Orleans all kinds of brass bands
are employed for varying organizations' annual parades, picnics and dances, accompanying
radical political and social movements, laying groundwork for 20th century jazz.

With widespread availability of saxophones in the US by the turn of the century,
ragtime-playing brass bands with saxophones, along with vaudeville,
introduce the American public to the saxophone, and by the 20s, Sidney Bechet
and Coleman Hawkins establish the saxophone as a serious instrument,
setting the stage for a 20th century music revolutionary, descendent of the divine order of Lester
"Pres" Young, from Kansas City, the sixth Charles [Christopher "Yardbird" Parker] (1920–55).

Then, on June 30th, 1960, Congo would attain its independence,
yet with events set in motion by the US and Belgium, on September 14th,
Prime Minister Lumumba would be removed from office and assassinated on January 17, 1961.
Four months later, on May 23rd, John Coltrane would make his debut recording for Impulse!
Africa/Brass

sanctifying kongofonic blood at the saxophonic root
as **lib**erator of spirits, in equi**lib**rium, this strange fruit
within people, a primal drive to pour forth an offering,
as the river's bank rips the earth, cutting, tearing, growing
from trees leaves, inner bark—stripped, peeled,
parchment for written symbols, sounded in the mind,
become repositories for ideas, **lib**raries, pouring forth thought
eroding hardness, releasing **Lib**ertas over ethnos

. . .

At his home in Tangier, the agitated lull of Abdellah El Gourd's hajhouj revives
ships' creaking hulls, where voices to and from relatives separated over distant water
continue calling "Here I am . . . where are you . . . where . . . ?" And now,
in synesthetic friendship, from shared Sufi saints, Abdellah's wall-chart of
colors for Gnawan melodies parallel a chromesthetic for Persian melodies,
bonding psychoacoustics for both, and through time and beyond place,
Elvin Jones describes the colors flowing from his cymbals—reds and yellows circling,
blues and greens crashing, like the water, pushing forward, reaching back,
back to *Africa/Brass* from Rudy Van Gelder's studio

Eric Dolphy and McCoy Tyner's orchestrations, arrangements
for a brass ensemble with piano, two double basses, drums,
altogether seal soul from ten million Congolese, with
a creation of natural minerals informing the invention of
trumpets, euphoniums, horns, tubas, alto and baritone saxophones,
embodied by the spirituality of Trane's sound, raising hands towards
A Love Supreme

. . .

the saxophone's conical shape . . .
with upturned flared bell
hand-tooled key cups
forming each tone hole
opening each pitch
varied higher or lower
with the same fingering
generating overtone octaves
over finger buttons of
wood, abalone,
mother-of-pearl
. . . calls the inner B'kongofon
to release all voices heard healed freed

V. Pursuance

> *. . . we ought to pursue the mean between extremes . . .*
> —*Aristotle*

The original kongofonic link comes from a seventh [grader] Charles [Gaynes],
appearing momentarily in 1974, at Blackford Junior High, in San Jose,
when on the first day of band, Mr. Dunton goes down the line asking each of us
"what instrument do you want to play?"; and with the melodious answer springing up
"I want to play the alto saxophone!"—the same prompted here, repeating
without a second thought, "I want to play the alto saxophone!"
Charlie was gone after that, never saw him again . . .

. . .

Another entity named from the saxophone/hominid family of the alto/male variety,
born in Durham, North Carolina ("Charles" in feminine form), 1962—
by the summer of 1977, the sound of Bird's "Loverman" session on Dial
led to my hearing Sonny Simmons at the Eric Dolphy Festival, in San Jose.
Then, after seeking out Dolphy's 1963 *Iron Man/Conversations* with Simmons,
I watch Simmons' prayer ritual opening his horn's case
at the defunct De Anza Hotel on Santa Clara Street,
and with neck assembled, acerbic tones are heard searing perfect 5ths
with pearl-fitted fingers, wrapped vein-like vines, moving

with spider-like hydrostaticity, now becoming rhizomatic rootstocks,
releasing shoots stuck from the nodes of some subterranean plant stem,
creeping sonic buds, growing outward in planar extension, upward
with new shoots, these nomadic forgings, fingerings forging sonic interbeing,
embracing the origin of soul.

Now playing with Simmons and "Trumpet Lady" Barbara Donald, where/with
Smiley Winters' drumming lit soul under "Bud's Blues," and by Bud's blood,
between Kuumbwa's opening in 1977 and closing of Keystone Korner in 1983,
we play . . . kongofonic seed set in saxophonic form.

. . .

Then, the axial year of 1983 marked a *tetrapathic* linkage[8]
from Persian music studies with Mahmoud Zoufonoun
and composing with James Norton (in San Jose),
to saxophone studies with Joe Allard
and concept with George Russell (in Boston).

Allard's primary exercise was to match the sonic quality of overtones on the saxophone
with their real tones blown from the horn's full bore. With the lower lip gliding over the reed—
taking in more mouthpiece for higher partials than for lower ones—
fingers shift from closing all keys for the overtone,
to fingering designated ones for the matching real tone.

The order of overtones—which, paradoxically, decrease in distance from each other
while moving farther away from the fundamental—reach partials measuring
165 cents (11th), 150 cents (12th), and 138 cents (13th), precisely within
the range of the Persian intervals introduced to me by Mahmoud Zoufonoun,
master musician of wood and string—tar and violin—who awakened for me
new saxophone fingerings for what seemed like slightly flatted/sharped tones
respectively named *koron* and *sori* by Colonel Ali Naqi Vaziri,
and by such terms playing on his name, a kongofonic family is born,
spinning koron tones from quarter tones from the curved horn.

Compositional technique then developed with James Norton for the quartet Shiraz, where
saxophonal embodiment of an acoustical phenomenon like the harmonic series (Allard),
culturally harnessed with alternate fingerings for sounding non-European tones (Zoufonoun),
would combine with a harmonic concept based on the natural 5th (Russell)
to pursue sonic liberation in a systematic way.

George Russell's Lydian Chromatic Concept establishes the cycle of 5ths
as progenitor of the Lydian scale, demonstrating its raised 4th (from the first seven 5ths)
as a more justifiable basis than the major scale for parenting harmony.[9] As well,
his creation-mapping of Pres and Ornette as more horizontal, or "modal," based
on blues more so than the verticality of playing harmonic progression, had a lasting effect . . .
Combining intervals of the 5th and 4th (the first three overtones after the fundamental)
has been a foundational principle for tonal structuring since ancient times:
from Chinese pentatonic cores generated from sequences of rising 5ths and falling 4ths,
to Pythagorean tetrachords of two flexible inner pitches hinged on two fixed outer ones
4ths apart, stacked by distances of a whole step connecting octaves.

And now, a cycle can be generated for effectively splicing what become *tetramodes*:
the melodic activity prescribed to otherwise static tetrachordal structures; with inner tones
marked by an indeterminable "x," koron/sori accidentals can be applied to change all so-called
"half" steps into an infinite variety of "whole" step shadings, resulting in tetramodal linkage
around a cycle of 5ths. After all, tones, like humans, are all as qualitatively different as they are
whole creations, while the mindset that invented the idea of fixed "half-", or "semi-" tones,
also enabled a rationale for quantifying people in similar ways, as less than fully human.

B'kongofonic practice then, focuses on koron/sori intervals that
split the distance between 5th/4ths, resulting in 2nd/3rds
first tapped by Mansur Zalzal on oud in 8th century Baghdad; now
in transcultural context, sounding in between their major and minor
counterparts, these tones are mapped across time/space,
opening up octaves toward hyperextended resolutions,
liberating tonality from a "separate-but-equal" temperament
shaped by subconscious notions of chromatic supremacy.

With Pres' people having now found koron/sori finger members, joining
Yardbird's newly found changes on Cherokee from a Harlem chili house,
the changes of a chromatic neighborhood in 1939 still played here—
these "false" fingerings for the horn, like karna, once developed
for adding timbre, resonance, diversity—anchor koron/sori
to the chordal extensions of major and minor progression, stretching
toward a free-key melody, wherein:

C major, C sori (as a high 8ve) may resolve to B (as 7th) from D (as 9th), and in
A minor, C sori (as a high 3rd) may resolve to B (as 9th) from D (as 11th), for
sound rubbed rises like heat, raising consciousness, while

high densities of what Coltrane calls "ethnic stylization" fall,
and elementonal resultants re-enter a lingual Afro/Asian essential,
speaking gong and drum as one B'kongofon . . . Then,

Where a visceral sonic explodes B'kongofonic blood from saxophonic root,
fingers strike pearl coverings of hollowed tube, speaking from beyond
familiar veins, opening strange fruit. Later, adapting this approach to
Danongan Kalanduyan's practice of Filipino kulintang,
fingerings born from Persian tones become Maguindanao,
ultimately defining their existence by dissolving all systems
into sonic spectra tethered by braided hoops of transcultural unity.

And where within the tao splits,
swims therein a koron spirit,
turning **Saxophone tones . . .**
Africa/Brass blood tones,
Persian/Tar blood tones,
Maguindanao/Kulintang blood tones,
blood-tones from the Soul of All Tones
B'Kongofon

VI. Song B'kongofon

> *The instrument is just an invention, but you are a creation!*
> —*Ornette Coleman*

late 20th–early 21st centuries

- **description of experiences with people of the horn**
- prescription of kongofonic fingerings for right-hand (RH) and left-hand (LH)
- *musical examples with prescribed fingerings (accidentals carrying through)—the flag (koron) and hatched greater-than (sori) symbols, respectively, will lower or heighten their assigned pitches by approximately 38–65 cents*

While the fingers of Paul Contos would glide flute-like on a balanced action, those of Eddie Lockjaw defied logic, his phrasing so

personalized; and while blowing, **Pepper Adams** would squeeze a lit cigarette between F and E key fingers.

G koron
LH—closed; RH—both mid/side F# keys

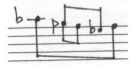

While Dexter's fingertips milked low-tone vibratos, John Handy's altissimo soared magically from unusual upper digits, seemingly from "Out of Nowhere."

F sori
LH—closed; RH—F#/D keys

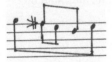

Joe Henderson embraced the horn with his fingers (could make it look like a feather, rising); after I asked him why my low B wasn't speaking, and after running it up/down with ears to the neck hole, he said: "well I'll be . . . I can't prove this in a court of law, but this is my horn!" Turns out the horn I had traded my balanced action for, with Jessica Jones (which she had acquired from a horn shop in NYC), was originally Joe's, he said stolen from him while at the Concord Jazz Festival. Now he would trade me his current Mark VI to honor the "return of the prodigal son." Putting it back in his soft bag, he said that the case shouldn't be closed too tight, that the horn "needs to breath."

F koron (E sori)
LH—closed; RH—F/D keys

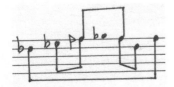

When Sonny Stitt moved his fingers over the keys, looked like brass and flesh were physically attached, like one was made for the other, grafted together; between sets, in an unhurried manner, he'd say "let me show you a fingering that Pres showed me for swingin' middle C," or "here's how to play the 4th C off the horn" (forking fingers on his left and right hands).

E koron
LH—high G, A/G keys; RH—closed

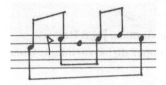

Stitt said Pres used to call the fingers "people"; in Lester's hands, the horn would levitate and almost seem to disappear, turning soul on sound.

D sori
LH—closed, side D# open; RH—closed

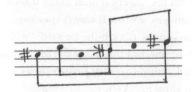

Ornette called Song X "a finger buster"; when going over it, he would change the ending every time we got there—said hearing the keys in another register on tenor would make his fingers play something else on alto; this reminded me of his saying, "I don't care about how many changes that go on . . . as long as it keeps going on."

D koron
LH—C, side D; RH—open

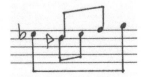

James Moody, after my asking what his fingers were doing—combining those pentatonics and 4ths that way: "that's a good question—if you're not doing anything tomorrow, come by the hotel, we'll practice together."

C sori
LH—C; RH—side C

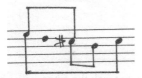

Eddie Harris would have his fingers so close to the keys you could barely see anything moving, like a statue; he'd make these wide leaps as if he weren't even breathing; once, he played a horn with diamond shapes he had cut out of the bell, said he liked experimenting with the sound.

C koron (B sori)
LH—closed; RH—side C

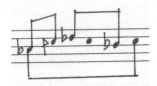

Joe Allard could defy gravity, playing scales going up while fingering down, and vice versa, demonstrating that personal sound comes from the throat, and how the mouthpiece and reed are stationed in the cavity of the mouth, where with/what the tongue was doing . . .

B koron
LH—B; RH—F (screw adjusted to leave upper pad half open)

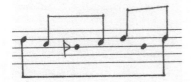

**Allard demonstrated physical mastery in lessons by wrestling the horn to
the point of singing any tone and then playing it in the extended register
with any fingers on any keys the student chose at random!**

A sori
LH—closed; RH—side Bb

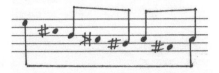

**Simmons (when asked about a lesson for how to work the fingers like he
does): "For one hundred dollars I'll show you how to use all the muscles
in your right hand, and for another hundred, I'll show you how to use
all the muscles in your left hand. [laughs] . . . But seriously, just practice
your 5ths."**

A koron
LH—B/A; RH—F/E

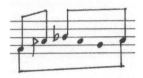

**Jimmy Heath, on Coltrane's fingers: "I was at the funeral. . . . I looked
at him in the casket . . . the only thing I recognized was his hands. He
had fingers that went kinda strange cause I mean lookin' at him . . .
that's the only thing that reminded me of Trane; you know, so that
wasn't him, he had passed on to the next place . . . his spirit was gone."**[10]

G sori
LH—closed, G# (posts altered or screw adjusted for pad to remain half
    open with RH closed); RH—E/D

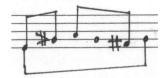

When Eulipia (now called Café Stritch) opened on First Street, in
San Jose, 1977, I was ready for news that Rahsaan Roland Kirk would
come by, but he died late that same year and never got to play there.
Blind, then paralyzed from a stroke, this patron saint of B'kongofonic
compassion defiantly kept playing multiple horns with one hand until
his last breath.

VII. Pulsivity/Resonance

A good traveler has no fixed plans and is not intent on arriving . . .

—*Lao-tzu*

Just as all planetary systems are bound to heliocentric orbit around the Sun,
the study of all human sound systems can be anchored to concepts
of fixed reoccurrence, or periodicity.

Yet just as the moon's tides have affected the development of life on Earth,
the infinitely nuanced effects of pulsation within the periodic determine
subtle variations of performance within each musician and musical practice.
Brother Periodicity then gets further defined by Sister Pulsivity, since
pulsivic embrace of performance practice enhances its quality,
and so by shaping the context of overarching periodic forms,
ritual space encompasses . . .

156–04

For example, inherent pulsivity in Persian poetic meter renders
a lyrical practice seemingly without metronomic time,
something generally discouraged in Western education
where fluctuating cyclic structures in music, as "pulse,"
are more often associated with derogatory notions of
"impulsive," "compulsive," or "repulsive"—
behavior in need of measured rationality.

Yet, the elasticity of poetic meter (as with Persian literary forms) helps
in balancing complementary fixed (periodic) and fluid (pulsivic) rhythmic recurrence
with improvisatory formulas composed for each musical artist's own pulse
to accelerate/decelerate, within a collective, in synchronistic harmony,
thus resulting in transient resolutions of unpredictable beauty.

Pulsivity practice focuses on shifting the silence between phrases,
where shorter/longer pauses are qualitatively felt more so than quantified,
and on shaping tones of variable length by combining pulse phrases,
or by undulating tones at variable speeds through pulse vibrato.

Another objective is to inspire our musical artists to express and interrelate
their own resonances, by exploring a more personal retuning of their instruments.
When expressed together, a rainforest of sonic modalities results, with familiar and
"foreign" tones interlocking incomplete ideas in infinite variety, ultimately
illuminating a potential for coexistence, finally, beyond the music itself.

The work of defining/applying categories of pulsivity and polytemperament
contributes towards a cultural sensibility relevant to issues of social equity,
where circles of learning stretch beyond any predetermined forms . . .
As a cup thrown into the ocean gets subsumed by its own fill,
periodic rims overflow with a pulsivity/resonance embrace, where
we naqareh shells get realized through our own will sounded.

With every person a fundamental
holding every ancestral harmonic
resonating a partial of humanity—
blood tones supreme
in dense and diverse proportion
without blood quantum
within beyond primary
secondary, tertiary—
tethering sympathetic
to all things,
these lines from
a saxophonic spectrum
light kongofonic expression
B'y
The Soul of All Things

*I played . . . until my heart turned into the same instrument. Then I offered this instrument
to the divine Musician, the only musician existing. Since then I have become His flute,
and when He chooses He plays His music. Now . . . to tune souls instead of instruments, to
harmonize people instead of notes . . . [for] in every word a certain musical value, a melody
in every thought, harmony in every feeling . . . every soul . . . a musical note . . . all life . . .
music.*

—Hazrat Inayat Khan

Epilogue

Once a bowl with warm food my companion, I was emptied upon my side and became a lute.
Now when the strings upon my neck are plucked, love consumes my core, resonating music.

—Mahmoud Zoufonoun

Horn's cylindrical trunk swells into a bottle-shaped base, flaring out into a bell
with keys and rods scrambling like vines over and around the tubed body
its brass color a shade of bark brown, and when ideas come to the player,
tones ooze out of this silky brass bark like blood latex freed into the air
with three leaflets of left- and right-side palm keys,
the left-side leaves spirally arranged
while the three right and left key finger-digits
sense membraned tips touching ellipsoidal pearl capsules,
exploding like tri-lobed fruit closing seeded tone holes
preparing to bear fruits of ideas bursting open when ripe.

When the idea-blood flows from the opening cut
in fluid form, exposed through an air stream,
it starts to thicken and become solid, undulating,
coagulating, into a coherent mass of tones and phrases.
Then as the flow is cut off, there is clotting and the bleeding stops,
and the wound heals in time for the next idea.

Meanwhile, as sound transfers to another mind/spirit,
in this way, it diffuses over a wider area, without claim.
Percussive seeds are then scattered from this human horn plant
as far as the sound will reach, and when growing among others,
a forest grows, ideas spreading like woody vine from horns of varying size,
their long-reaching stems filled with leaking life-blood damaged experience
and just as the ringed trunk of a rubber tree eventually divides into several stout stems,
so does the essence of an influential player drive others to either branch out or clamber
over their sound-host, Among the Trees.

And after the fruit of imitators has fallen, disciple-stems stretch into tendrils
wistfully spiraling around their host master to secure the great vine to its legend;
climbing to tremendous heights, others' interpretations of the original idea are propagated,
while shoots of fruit begin to flower at younger ages, feathering beats
even before life has grounded their sound.

Appendix—Images

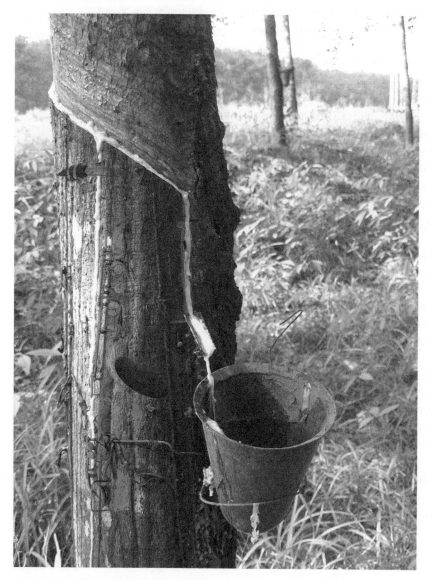

Fig. 8.1. B'kongofonic apparition from damaged rubber tree (Cameroon).

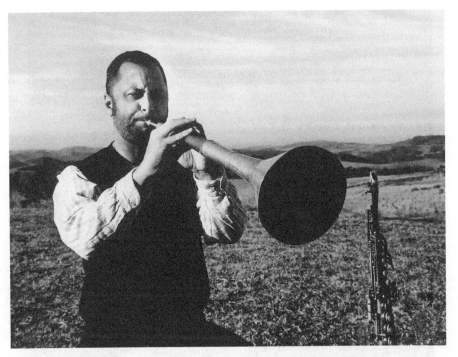

Fig. 8.2. Modirzadeh on the karna (Persian double-reed) at the Djerassi Foundation, during *Other Minds IV*, 1997. (Photo courtesy of John Fago.)

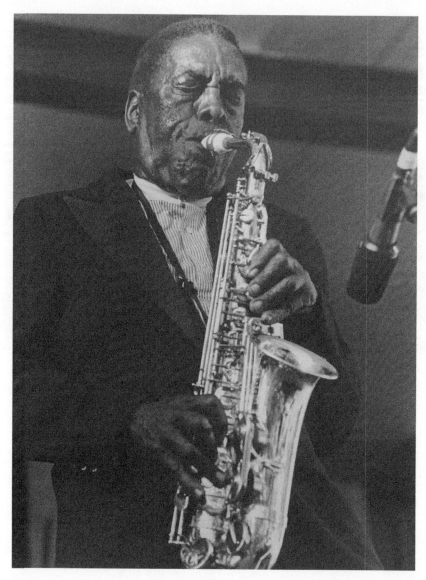

Fig. 8.3. Sonny Simmons at the 1995 Monterey Jazz Festival. (Photo courtesy of Andrew Nozaka.)

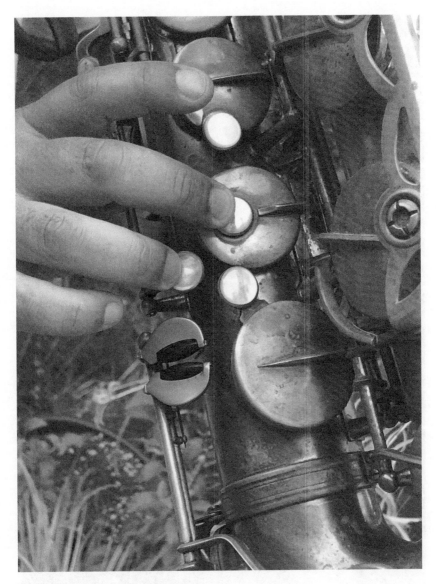

Fig. 8.4. Kongofonic fingering for G koron

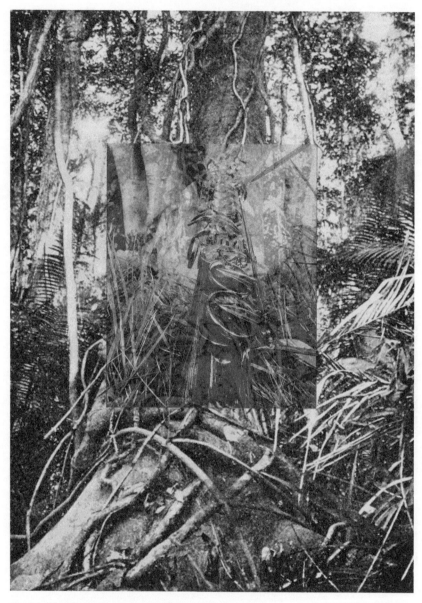

Fig. 8.5. Transformation from the base of a Mindoro rubber tree, into a straight B'kongofon (a.k.a. soprano saxophone).

Notes to Chapter 8

1. *B'kongofon* serves as instrumental companion to *Makam X*, a conceptual system discussed in an earlier work by this author, "On the Convergence Liberation of Makam X." Therein, transformative terminology is introduced as a creative word practice traditionally avoided in research writing, working as a portal toward realms of consciousness that can "turn thought ecstatic." By improvising various sound units across national and cultural boundaries, by recombining or reversing words' pronunciation, we may illuminate hidden meanings, signify anew, and unlock messages of personal relevance for each speaker/listener. This Ode (pronounced "owed"), then, is the attempt to capture on paper an imprint of mind and moment moving in multiple directions, with singular purpose.

2. Profound appreciation for saxophonist Kevin Brunetti's introducing me to a sordid facet of colonial history in connection with Coltrane's *Africa/Brass*, thus providing crucial impetus for the current work.

3. This double consciousness is directly inspired by Du Bois, *The Souls of Black Folk*.

4. From Arabic *naqr-*, meaning to "strike" or "tap"; this dual membranophone is of the kettle drum variety, which can also be related to oceanic nacre, that mother-of-pearl layer made into buttons for pressing down saxophone keys; as inner shells, tone holes are covered and drummed closed by a double-membranic force: pearl and fingertip.

5. Much of this Ode's encoding is left to the "enlightened madness" of each speaker/listener, where improvising on sound changes in such dense ecstatic order spins a frenzy of thought; this verse, for example, unravels a crux message in the following way: with the Norse sun goddess Sól referring to the fifth solfège degree, *gah* and *se* mean "place" and "three" respectively, in Persian (*segah* is an important mode throughout the Middle East, with tonic gravity positioned on the interval of a third); this gets reiterated as *mi* (third solfège degree), binding the bull's-eye center of Kemet's sun god Ra (also the fifth degree); and now from the Eye of Ra, "mi-to-Ra," sounds the Indo-Iranian sun god Mitra, or as the Zoroastrian divinity Mithra, is synonymous with Mehr (denoting kindness, and mutual contract). With love being as messy as it is transformative, intervallic distances get increasingly fluid: together, the first solfège degree *do* ("two" in Persian) and third degree *mi* (as *segah* tonicity, also saragam interval of *sagah*) give a tonic perspective embedded in both duality and triality (i.e., two-in-one and/or three-in-one), ultimately liberating all pitch (and peoples) from a fixed center, or hierarchical position, by realizing each as being/becoming the other; with plurality thus radiating from the fifth, Ra (also known as *Re*) refracts into a ninth (or second extended), illuminating saragam *ri*/solfège *re* as a fourth from *sol*; now with second/ninths circling fourth/fifths, Ra/*Re* emanates from itself, sealing Sól revolution in the Rumi exultation, "I stand up, and this one of me becomes myriad of me—they say I circle around you . . . nonsense, I circle around me, I circle around Me!" So, playing the sound changes here reflects a notion: that tonic positions of the "mother third" (as "mythrae" plays on "earth" turned "thrae" in reverse, pronounced "three"), while revolving around "brother fifth" (here, a sun deity turning male/female, a saragam *pa*/

ma, inverted fifth/fourth), are constantly variegated upon by sister *mah* (Persian lunar deity) in order to create all the partials resonating into life.

6. Here, a free-mapping of definitions bridge *karna* and cornet with cochlea and ear. Further description in Modirzadeh, "On the Convergence Liberation of Makam X," fig. 1, "The Harmonic Series."

7. This description of the *bosanga* method of rubber collecting is from Powell-Cotton, "Notes on a Journey," 8–9. The description of saxophone parts and assembly instructions are from How Products Are Made, "Saxophone"; and Wikipedia, "Saxophone." Congo Free State witness accounts are transcribed from Bate, *Congo*.

8. Tetrapaths are metaphysical constructs, mapping the interdependence that threads existence; like tetramodes in music, each is made up of three intervals between four points; in this 1983 case, the intervallic connections are from: (1) Zoufonoun to Norton, (2) Norton to Allard, and (3) Allard to Russell. These concepts are further discussed in Modirzadeh, "Chromodality and the Cross-Cultural Exchange of Musical Structure," 5, 123–28.

9. Russell, *The Lydian Chromatic Concept of Tonal Organization*.

10. Scheinfeld, *Chasing Trane*.

Works Cited

Bate, Peter, dir. *Congo: White King, Red Rubber, Black Death*. New York: ArtMattan Productions, 2006. DVD, 84 min.

Du Bois, W. E. B. *The Souls of Black Folk*. Chicago: A. C. McClurg, 1903.

How Products Are Made. "Saxophone." Accessed September 19, 2019. http://www.madehow.com/Volume-6/Saxophone.html

Modirzadeh, Hafez. "Chromodality and the Cross-Cultural Exchange of Musical Structure." PhD diss., Wesleyan University, 1992.

Modirzadeh, Hafez. "On the Convergence Liberation of Makam X." *Critical Studies in Improvisation / Études critiques en improvisation* 7, no. 2 (2011). https://www.criticalimprov.com/index.php/csieci/article/view/943

Powell-Cotton, P. H. G. "Notes on a Journey through the Great Ituri Forest." *Journal of the African Society* 7, no. 25 (1907): 1–12.

Russell, George. *The Lydian Chromatic Concept of Tonal Organization*. Brookline, MA: Concept, 1959.

Scheinfeld, John, dir. *Chasing Trane: The John Coltrane Documentary*. Meteor 17 Crew Neck Productions, 2016. DVD, 99 min.

Wikipedia. "Saxophone." Last modified September 19, 2019. https://en.wikipedia.org/wiki/Saxophone

Afterword

Sound Changes: The Future Is Dialogue

DANIEL FISCHLIN AND ERIC PORTER

No commodity is quite—so strange / As this commodity called cultural exchange.

—Iola Brubeck (*The Real Ambassadors*, "Cultural Exchange")

Improvisation Without End

Sound changes, as does the way we think and write about it. Improvised music, constantly anticipating the future of what sound might become, guides us to reconsider our perspectives on what we mean by sound, how we produce sounds, and how we listen. Long having shaped a creative-intellectual constellation of thought practice, improvisation continues to push us, centrifugally, toward a wider array of interpretive acts and social practices. Sometimes we lack the insights, experience, or cultural breadth to grasp what is being shown as it emerges. Work and play distract us as surely as do ossified expectations about what is aesthetically acceptable or thinkable. But as improvisers across the globe are becoming increasingly visible to, and interactive with, one another through physical movement (the product of privilege *and* precarity), emergent technologies, and venue and audience desire for musical "difference"— and as critical and aspirational writings about transcultural musical productions in which improvisation is a defining feature take form—we are pushed to examine our creative and interpretive paradigms, carefully.

As the editors of, now, three volumes collected and commissioned under the rubric of "sound changes," we have studied and cultivated essays addressing a continuum of iterative contexts that shape improvisatory cocreativity: from full-on specific cultural contexts wholly rooted in the local to glancing intercultural contacts to deep intercultural knowing brought on by years of connection, discipline, teaching, and learning. The vast flow of energies produced from such encounters is shaped in part by unique, culturally situated technological developments—from the premodern to the newly emergent—related to playing techniques and the instruments on which these are exercised. Technologies of sound production affect practice and the capacity of improvisers to generate previously unheard resonances. So does what Canadian composer and theorist R. Murray Schafer calls the soundscape, the fullness of contextual sonic events that occur situationally as the result of making sound in a specific environment.[1] And so unique sounds, cultural influences, and hybridizations unfold when Oji-Cree and Kitchi-Sipi Mi'kmaq First Nations artist known as Anachnid (Kiki Harper) blends indie trap, electropop, and neo soul using sounds derived from "rubbing bones, hoofs, and hides together to create samples," all the while weaving together "traditional storytelling and her Oji-Cree upbringing." Anachnid states, "In trap music, you have a snare, and in trapline hunting, you have a ground snare. . . . I am making the parallels between trap music and trapline hunting."[2]

The interface of cultural preferences, technologies, and access to various instrumentalities, the audient's position in relation to the full influx of sounds in a sonic environment, and the varying and often shifting social, political, and economic contexts that set the limits and possibilities of performance all give shape to what we might call the *intercultural soundscape*. And where it abounds, it is inextricably tied to aleatoric conjunctions, uncontrollable synergies and positionings. Relational sitedness, in which source contexts and audient positionings are determinative of what is being heard, conjoins with improvisatory and irreducibly complex arrays of interchange and production to generate new sounding possibilities that reflect on wider practices in which similar energies are unleashed. Improvisation without end, it might be said, is an unavoidable—at times vexing, at other times inspiring—outcome of our contingent relation to one another, to difference, and to the environments in which we act and sound.

Into and Away from the Abyss: Intercultural Translation

How best, then, to improvise, or to play analytically with this understanding of improvisation in mind, when contemplating its future and, by extension, our collective future? How do we, more specifically, at what appears to be a moment of crisis, following so many other such moments, begin to think through improvisation as a means of addressing what Portuguese legal scholar and social theorist Boaventura de Sousa Santos calls abyssal thinking, a fundamental component of global ecologies of knowledge(s). For Santos Western modernity is a "socio-political paradigm founded on the tension between social regulation and social emancipation," based on the invisible, abyssal distinction between "metropolitan societies and colonial territories."[3] Clearly, much improvisation sits on the other side of the line that separates regulatory and emancipatory forms of being. So how might improvisational practices that are rooted geographically and historically beyond the metropolitan—and that have a profound underlying principle of cocreative endeavor rooted in site-specific, diverse locales—potentially challenge that which regulates?

Santos proposes "intercultural translation" as the "alternative both to the abstract universalism that grounds Western-centric general ideas and to the idea of incommensurability between cultures. The two are related and account for the two 'nonrelationships' of Western modernity with non-Western cultures: destruction and assimilation."[4] Epistemicide and monocultural domination produce catastrophic assimilative and destructive contexts for encounters with difference, and they challenge the capacity to sustain diversity, biotic and otherwise. Improvisation's capacity for generative cocreation and the exploration, if not reconciliation, of supposedly incommensurate frames of knowing (and sounding) is a powerful resource that offers an antidote to abyssal thinking. The stakes, in other words, in what we make of improvisation as a way of sounding relational differences across cultural divides, are profound, and especially so in the era of the Sixth Extinction, where so many forms of being are vanishing as a function of biotic and cultural epistemicide.

We are well aware that distinct sounds central to improvisational practices develop within specific contexts as a function of instrumentalities available to creators (tools to create sounds), as a function of the use of music within those contexts, and as a function of techniques, aesthetic and ideological preferences, and inventive approaches to making sound that evolve in place-specific manners. Think the multiple finger, snap, and finger-ring techniques associated with the Persian *tombak*, as opposed to combined (strike and shake) hand *tamburello* (Italian) or split-hand *kanjira* (South Indian) techniques—all instruments from very different parts of the world that involve precise histories, contexts, sounds, and embodied techniques that have arisen out of specific circumstances. The *kanjira* alone conjures up the socioreligious world of *bhajan*, Hindu devotional music of no fixed form with a history that extends back to the Mughal Empire. And the intricate sounds of a *tamburello* thumb roll are as unique to its cultural contexts as are the extraordinary single split-hand techniques brought to their apogee in the *kanjira* playing of Govinda Rao Harishankar.

Indian ragas, described by Tanjore Viswanathan and Jody Cormack as the "foundation of melodic composition and improvisation in South Indian music," are similarly inseparable from the metaphysics that ground them.[5] Hazrat Inayat Khan, the Indian Sufi master and musician, notes that ragas derive from, among other things, both "the mathematical law of variety" and the "natural laws particular to the people residing in different parts of the land."[6] Variety and cultural location matter to this form, which makes extensive use of deeply improvisatory, instant-composition techniques. The provocative insight that variety is a mathematical law suggests that so too is improvisation, although it is clearly also tied to far-reaching metaphysical realities. Moreover, "Each Raga has an administration of its own, including a chief—*Mukhya*, the key-note; a king—*Wadi*, a principal note; a minister—*Samwadi*, the subordinate note; a servant—*Anuwadi*, an assonant note; an enemy—*Vivadi*, a dissonant note."[7] The congress of notes in this family points to wider practices of governance, of epistemic variety, and of assonance and dissonance, an improvisatory schema that lays out a way of conceiving sound that is pertinent to, if not emblematic of, wider social relations.

This connection to wider social circumstances is also found in Gamelan *gender wayang* ensembles, which use improvisatory practices in Bali, Indonesia. Gamelan master I Wayan Loceng observes how "Gender wayang, one of the most ancient musical ensembles existing in Bali, accompanies shadow theatre as well as tooth filings, cremations, and other religious ceremonies." Despite the ubiquity of this form of ensemble playing throughout Bali, "distinct regional styles feature divergent repertoire."[8] Loceng's comment underlines localized ubiquity but also particularity. South East Asian music scholar Nicholas Gray's research points to how microvariations are a "genuine form of creativity related to the kinds of changes involved in making a completely new piece."[9] Microvariations, in other words, are a form of improvisatory mutation that cumulatively produce new sounds, new compositions.[10] Such practices point to listening and playing strategies closely affiliated with, if not indistinguishable from, specific social and aesthetic practices in Bali. Here Bali is a geographic marker of multiple sites on the island, just as Bali and its musical practices sit within a much vaster Indonesian context where diverse gamelan, and especially *wayang*, practices abound.[11]

Yet, improvisational musical practices, like the cultures that produce and orient them, are well suited for—and even insistent on, given
their real-time reinventions—transformation. Cuban ethnomusicologist
Fernando Ortiz, discussing the variability of Afro-Cuban/Black song,
points to an underlying aesthetic based on the expectation of sonic
change:

> Un cantador negro, al pedirsele que repita un canto, con frecuencia
> lo hará inconscientemente con notas distintas de las que usó la prim-
> era vez. . . . Desgraciadamente, para la repetición, el músico no puede
> encontrar de nuevo ni el aire ni la canción por él creados, lo que
> constituye una dificultad más en el estudio de la música negra . . . los
> arpistas bakuba [improvisan] aires deliciosas y muy ajustados de tono,
> jamás pudo obtener de esos profesionales la repetición de los mismos
> aires. . . . No obstante, ni esta inconsistencia que difumina ciertas
> líneas tonales, ni el gusto por las improvisaciones y "floreos" que al-
> tera otros, destruyen la morfología básica de las canciones negras.[12]

> [A Black singer, when asked to repeat a song, will frequently do it
> unconsciously with different notes from those used the first time. . . .
> Unfortunately, when repeating the song, the musician won't repeat
> the tune or the song that he created again, which constitutes yet
> another challenge in the study of Black music. . . . Bakuba harpists
> improvise delicious tunes and very fitting tones,[13] yet one can never
> get these professionals to repeat the same tunes. . . . Notwithstanding,
> neither this inconsistency that blurs certain tonal lines, nor the taste
> for improvisations and flourishes that changes others, destroys the
> basic morphology of Black song.] (our translation)

Ortiz describes a consistent "morphology" in which constant improvisatory variation is a valued if not determinative feature. The variations and
microvariations that constitute these improvisatory practices are deeply
connected to site-specific practices and expectations that define a vocabulary and an embodied tradition. Sound changes, in the contexts Ortiz
is describing, reference variability within a localized set of sonic embodiments that are determined by contexts that are idiomatic. These idiomatic conventions that allow for change are themselves transposable to
wider improvisatory contexts, where variation, plurality, and unexpected
collisions of different sonic energies are valued and expected. The reality is that twenty-first-century transnational exchange only increases the

degree to which this scenario plays out the world over, an unstoppable flow of sonic interchange and movement deeply tied to how old sounds adapt to new circumstances.

That said, any diligent examination of musical practices that extend beyond North American and European models is bound to come into contact with autonomous improvisatory forms and practices that potentially serve as foundations for permutation and transformation outside of the original contexts in which they were conceived and practiced. Think the widespread instrumental improvisations of *taqsim* (usually melodic, nonmetric musical improvisations that introduce the performance of a traditional Arabic, Greek, Middle Eastern, or Turkish musical composition); Indian free-rhythmic *alaps* and composed-on-the-spot *ghazals* (based on a *misra* or initial line of poetry); Carnatic *niraval* and *svarakalpana*; Sufi *mashayikh* performing qasa'id and *muwashshaht*, with their blend of composition and improvisation; Turkish *makam*; Chinese Jiangnan *sizhu*, characterized by improvised ornamentations; Yoruban/Afro-Brazilian Santeria musical performances in which the mother drum (the Iyá, as in Cuban *batá* practices) improvises over polyrhythmic grounds; Bulgarian *chalga* musicians and their unscripted performances; Korean *pansori* traditions, lost during the postwar rush to industrialization in the country, and then recuperated and reconstituted by musicians like Bae Il-Dong and Kim Dong-Won; and the like. In each of these cases, musical practices that entail improvisation arising from particular sites and traditions have been the subject of permutations produced by intercultural exchange.

We say all this knowing full well that not all these exchanges are happy or productive: assimilation, appropriation, citational malpractice, and exploitation can just as easily be at work in intercultural translation as can be the genuine search for new forms of sounding that have affective power and present cocreative challenges to epistemic monocultures. Indeed, the sounds we associate with many improvisation-laden sites and creative practices, in the particularity of their contexts and epistemic realities forged out of cultural exchanges and collisions of short and long duration, point to asymmetrical social relations and the violence out of which they were wrought and also to strategies of surviving such violence in the past and present. The long history of transcultural, hybridized, musical interactivity across the African diaspora is, for example, also a history of improvisation's multiple emergences in contexts of slavery, colonialism, and attendant racisms. The hybridized rhythmic forms of Afro-Brazilian or Afro-Cuban musicking are unthinkable without a deep understanding of colonial and imperial encounters, the cultural practices and narratives that explained and helped people survive these encounters, and the ways that new people were created in the process. All continue to be heard in the actual sound of Candomblé or *batá* ensembles. In the Matanzas barrio of La Marina, home to one of the oldest continuous communities of Afro-Cuban culture, the experience of Afro-Cuban master percussionist and drum maker Gilberto Morales Chiong, part of the deep Matanzas tradition of spiritual and musical community making, shows that Chinese, continental African (Yoruban), and even precolonial influences can all be found alive within that culture.

El Indio (the Indian), as friends call him, embodies ethnic hybridity with a Chinese mother and a *prieto* father but also with hints that extend the family line back to preconquest Taino culture. The unique vocalizations and percussive techniques and polyrhythms deriving from Yoruban influences, contemporary *son*, hip-hop, and the hybridization of musical cultures specific to the La Marina community—with its extensive religious practices that involve music, its active street-life of *peñas*, and the public presencing of musical spectacle—are all embodied in El Indio's unique musical skills. El Indio's handmade *batá*, the sacred drums at the core of Afro-Cuban musicking, play a key role in conserving traditional knowledge within diasporic sites like La Marina. Crafted from handpicked trees cut when the moon is on the wane so as to make the wood more resonant because less moist, then hand-hewn and carved to specific calibrations that have been passed down for generations, these drums are highly prized for the unique tones that their distinctive mode of building generates. In other words, even as one can speak about the Matanzas community as diasporic and as embodying general qualities of African diasporic performance aesthetics,[14] to do so without attending to the sonic qualities coming out of this site would be to distort what that community produces.[15]

Narratives such as El Indio's are instructive. After having offered sustenance to the particular, aggrieved communities from which they emerge as extraordinary examples of long-term resilience, they insist to the world on the foundational presence of transcultural, improvised music of the Black diaspora. And the possibilities of emergence predicated on such survival are endless. Consider, for example AbdouMaliq Simone's compelling description of how an eruption of the music of James Brown—first, as sung loudly in the hallway by someone who had just watched a CNN documentary on the artist, and then, as played on as many as ten cassette players—produced not only a multistory party among African migrants living in a housing block in Dubai in 2008 but also a spontaneous expression of sociability stemming from mutual recognition of shared circumstance as migrant workers and racialized subjects.[16] Such stories offer inspiration to improvisation studies scholars in search of political possibility in the music and, by extension, concrete directed musical action for a world in crisis, defined in part by an anti-Blackness that shapes immigration laws, policing, social welfare possibilities, and sociability across the Global North and South.

Ultimately, as the contributions to *Sound Changes* and its partner volumes tell us, improvised music, whether geographically rooted or traveling, whether shaped most significantly by long-established, local, techniques and technologies or by outside influences, ask that we understand sound as more than a musical practice, more than an aesthetic. From an underground Mardi Gras parade in a midwestern US city to the collective occupation of a performance space in Greece,[17] from music education classrooms in the occupied West Bank to street concerts in post-Mubarak Egypt,[18] and from *las peñas* in Santiago de Chile in the 1960s to a kathak dance studio in San Francisco in the 2010s,[19] we learn how contextually specific yet interculturally shaped improvisational dialogues offer a capacity for practitioners and audents alike to negotiate their social and material circumstances and remake the substance of their lives.

This observation does not mean that improvisatory refashioning always happens, especially in the positivistic terms that so much writing about improvisation takes for granted. Improvisation in the social and political sphere—as evident in the real-time, unscripted actions of members of governments, militaries, and corporations—has made millions of people's lives much worse. Sometimes participation in musical improvisations can have no perceptible impact, and it may have a negative impact in terms of consciousness-raising or affect-transforming potential for participants (audents and performers). As has been well documented, improvising communities and encounters can be riven by the same social divisions (gender, sexual, ethnic, class, educational, age, political, citizenly, and so on) that shape the societies (singular or multiple) that produce them. And even the best-intentioned, carefully imagined exchanges can produce intercultural asymmetries, like those that occurred between Steve Coleman and AfroCuba de Matanzas in the making of the 1996 CD *The Sign and the Seal* (featuring the Mystic Rhythm Society). These asymmetries can creep in, even when they seem improbable. Coleman himself observes: "In Cuba, I found that the situation was more complex than I'd imagined; the people had preserved more than one African culture and these were mixed together under the general title of Folklore. There are the Abacuá societies (Ngbe, Ejagham), the various Arara cults (Dahomey), the Congo traditions (Nganga, Mayombe, Palo Monte) as well as the Yorùbá traditions."[20] Points of congruence—what Coleman calls "cultural transference"—undoubtedly occur at a certain level, but the iterative aspects of this musical encounter capture just as much the differential tensions between the two groups. Always underlying the encounter is the asymmetry of the intercultural exchange despite the apparent similarities and overlaps between jazz improvisatory soundings and traditional Afro-Cuban musickings.[21] And yet, the collisions with difference that Coleman describes present challenges and opportunities to learn. Santos argues that the "postabyssal experience of the sense is, above all, an experience of reciprocity: to see and be seen, to hear and to be heard. . . . It is frequently an asymmetrical reciprocity" that requires that the participants in the encounter strive to maximize the symmetry or minimize the asymmetry.[22]

A more radical position from within improvisatory ways of knowing might be that the constitutive tensions of asymmetrical relations provide the greatest opportunity, as well as the greatest challenge, for cocreative iterations of new knowledge. Achieving equality in such a situation can produce assimilation and appropriation effects, while, conversely, sustaining the very tensions and forms of knowing that can engender remarkable new iterations. The stretched feel of an underlying clave rhythm played in the Afro-Cuban contexts of La Marina is more about pulse than about mathematical precision, and percussionists from other contexts who try to erase that subtle reality from intercultural performances in the name of culturally determined notions of *precision* as opposed to *feel* do a disservice to the music and its sources. Santos notes that the "difficulties in defining reciprocities and equivalences result from the capitalist, colonialist, and patriarchal political economy of the senses and its specific inscription upon bodies" that produces inequality.[23]

In response, Santos calls for "deep self-silencing" as "the condition for listening to the voice of the inaudible."[24] Since silence is often a condition of resilience and of the sustainment of identity under threat of attack (with anonymity being a strategy for the preservation of identity when surveillance becomes the norm), improvisatory deep listening, which takes in silence as constitutive to cocreativity, is a critical element in intercultural translation and encounter. Santos talks about *corazonar* or the "warming up" of reason: "warm reason is the reason that lives comfortably with emotions, affections, and feelings without surrendering its reasonableness."[25] Music, which plays with the interlocutions of silence and sound, mediates the affect of knowing through resonance, echo, harmony, melody, rhythm, timbre, pulse, beat, and the like. Santos describes a situation in which "sequences and rhythms condition the contents or meanings of sound and soundlessness, of what is heard or not heard," suggesting that "some contents of meanings are traceable only in shared sequences and rhythms."[26]

The capacity to hear into these situational sounds reflects on the capacity to enter into the space of difference, which requires an improvisation of reciprocity as a function of *corazonar*. Sustaining what Barbara Tomlinson and George Lipsitz call "insubordinate spaces" requires listening in to the ways in which communities across the globe are constituting "new politics and new polities . . . through reciprocal practices of speaking and listening, asking and answering, teaching and learning."[27] These activities arise out of moments of encounter that always ask: "What next?" "How are we going to enter into a relationship with each other?" "What do you believe?" "What are we to make of and in this moment?" The responses to these and other questions require reciprocal improvisations and iterations, and they are deeply tied to Global South social justice struggles based on key concepts like "accompaniment, *konesans*, and *balans*," which "advance ideas about reciprocal recognition and cocreation everywhere as key components in the construction of new egalitarian and democratic social relations."[28]

Yet, perseverance, hope, and direct action persist and not merely through what may or may not happen within real-time sonic exchanges. Improvised music has the propensity to inspire "freedom dreams," to borrow a phrase from Robin D. G. Kelley, based on the lived experience and shared actions of its practitioners.[29] Again, we take a cue from Black music's generative potential, its impact on the critical thought of those who have listened widely and specifically to "the Music," as Amiri Baraka called it, with its sacred-secular, prophetic purpose and epistemological resonances, let alone its associations with directed actions against systemic oppression.[30] Think, to take one example, of the symbiotic relationship of Cecil Taylor's music and Black poetic thought. Ntozake Shange once said, "Many stories of mine seep out of the chords of Cecil Taylor's solos." She recalls, upon meeting Taylor, that "the cadence of his voice approximated the thundering chords, unexpected harmonies and rhythms I found in his music. The piano as battering ram, rebel shout, the fresh cicatrix of fast life in black space. When I need to feel whole, competent, daring, intricately evolving, I play Cecil Taylor."[31]

Poet-theorist Fred Moten has also engaged with Taylor's music and poetry. His book *The Feel Trio* is named after Taylor's ensemble (with Tony Oxley and William Parker), and he points to future engagements as he poses the question of how a writer best prepares "to play with Cecil Taylor." "The proper form," he suggests, is "perhaps the transcription of an improvisational blurring of the word; perhaps an improvisation through the singular difference of the idiom and its occasion; perhaps a calculation of that function whose upper limit is reading and whose lower limit is transcription—an improvisation through phrases, through some virtual head and coda. Taylor says to his interlocutor, 'I'm listening,' go on. Perhaps he will have said this to me or to the word: I'm listening, go on."[32] And many thinkers and dreamers do "go on," crossing a wide array of global cultural and social spaces, in dialogue with the many improvisers who inspire them to pursue their own graphic, visual, intellectual, political, meditative, emotive, and sonic expressions.

Improvising Transmodernity

But how, looking forward, might we move—if we even can—from small gestures of negotiation, inspiration, everyday acts of resistance, the modeling of new forms of sociality, and the accompanying *dreams* of deeper social and political transformation to an *actual* and *substantial* undoing of the regulatory structures that define twenty-first-century lives? How to achieve greater equity in a system governed by asymmetrical outcomes for differently positioned individuals and populations, from enrichment and status enhancement to social and actual death, across the globe? Might we, following the lead of the musical thinkers-improvisers across these three volumes, conceive of and implement an expansive intercultural dialogue with the potential to counter abyssal modes of thinking that privilege deeply acculturated norms? And, if yes, how might we do so without reproducing abyssal rethinking? For by engaging the music outside the line from a position inside the line (even when the political, social, or imaginative act is well intentioned; even when one's "insider" status is incomplete by virtue of linguistic, educational, or embodied modes of difference and marginality), we often reproduce the very epistemologies and cultural asymmetries that such acts seek to displace.

In his comments about a potentially emergent transmodernity, Enrique Dussel offers a potential way forward. Building from earlier comments that "peripheral culture—oppressed by imperial culture—should be the point of departure for intercultural dialogue" (a dialogue that, in turn, might contribute to a broader, liberatory politics), Dussel proposes "a future *trans*-modern culture," emanating from a somewhat differently conceived model of intercultural dialogue, as nothing less than the portent of a *new age of world history*.[33] Intercultural dialogue, however, is no easy feat given extant cultural asymmetries wrought by centuries of modernity's constitutive, incorporative exclusions (capitalism, colonialism, racism, and all the rest) and the illusions of cultural symmetry proposed by liberal multiculturalism. Such illusions obscure the workings of the multiculturalist state, as well as that of a conjoined transnational capitalism, which, while at times recognizing and even venerating cultures of the periphery, orients such intercultural dialogues to the cultural norms of the West and the needs of the market, ironing out putatively unassimilable expressions or values. Any productive intercultural dialogue must proceed instead from an awareness of how cultures "*inevitably* confront each other in all levels of everyday life, from communication, education and research, to the politics of expansion, and cultural or even military resistance." Within such confrontations, nothing is assured. Some long-standing practices and norms may persist or be transformed in unexpected ways, and some may not survive at all.[34]

Dussel instead imagines an intercultural dialogue emanating from "the shadows," from those cultural exteriorities across the globe that have "maintain[ed] an alterity with respect to European Modernity, with which they have coexisted, responding in their own way to its challenges." This intercultural dialogue, which can ultimately produce a "future *trans*-modern culture," must *not*, he insists, be substantially shaped by the "experts" of the academy or cultural institutions. Nor should it follow the lead of "cultural apologists" or fundamentalists who draw on recrudescent notions of culture when praising its virtues or defending it from critics. Rather, "it is, above all, a dialogue between a culture's critical innovators (intellectuals of the 'border,' *between* their own culture and Modernity). . . . But, additionally, this is not even the dialogue between the critics of the metropolitan 'core' and the critics of the cultural 'periphery.' It is more than anything *a dialogue between the 'critics of the periphery,'* it must be an intercultural South–South dialogue before [it] can become a South–North dialogue."[35]

Dussel's juxtaposition of critics from the "metropolitan 'core'" and the "cultural 'periphery'" calls attention to the asymmetries that have long arisen when those more or less in the core have venerated—but simultaneously diminished through an anthropological gaze—the cultural expressions from the outside when interrogating their own abyssal modes of thinking. And this is perhaps nowhere clearer than in many of the freedom-imagining writings about music that foreground real-time decision-making and kinetic movement, regardless of whether these writings are oriented toward the liberation of the embodied subject, the thinking subject, or the political subject. Yet, the gesture toward a transmodern culture forged by "critical innovators," situated in that hybrid space of intellectual borderlands, still speaks to a potentiality in improvised music, from the peripheries, to disrupt abyssal thinking through the exchange of sound and ideas in a global performance context that is defined by broader disruptions—through migration, travel, technological connectedness, and so on—of North and South.

In other words, contrary to so-called First World epistemologies that assume their privilege and centrality to all discourse, the rest of the planet is indeed the majoritarian world and sanctuary, if not harbinger, of multiple forms of knowing and being. And, what we have been witnessing in the context of shared improvisatory practices (among performers and audients in concert spaces and informal, neighborhood gatherings; in onstage and through-study interactions with recordings of past improvisations; via engagements with technology; and through all the other ways described in these volumes) is a remarkably resilient counternarrative to a modernity defined by industrial, imperial, and technological realities of subordination and alienation.

Such potential for disruption is rooted in many musical traditions, and access to these traditions can expand our understanding of what creative expression might accomplish at the epistemological and ontological levels. Consider the San people in southern Africa (Botswana, Namibia, and southern Angola), who are one of the oldest Indigenous peoples on the planet and under extreme threat of disappearance. The San notion of nǀom, the life force of creation, is intimately tied to improvisatory practices of community that empower "ecstatic healing" and spiritual connection through dance and music: "the openness and uncertainty fostered by improvisation helps us become more available to unexpected movement that is spontaneously choreographed by the felt interaction with mystery . . . nǀom takes us past improvisation [for] . . . Bushmen propose that they are danced by nǀom. Here the dancer is not improvising but is improvised by nǀom."[36] The notion of a life force that improvises an actant is culturally far removed from Western notions of discipline, technique, and virtuosity, in which individual creativity and technical autonomy operate on the instrument to produce improvisatory iterations.

A people like the San, reputedly able to hear the sound of the sun and stars, negotiate their imaginative, creative relations to sound in ways that cannot be separated from their sitedness and a set of deeply embedded cultural practices developed over millennia.[37] Some Aboriginal songlines in Australia are predicated on the notion that "the whole of Australia could be read as a musical score. There was a hardly a rock or creek in the country that could not or had not been sung. . . . The Ancients sang their way all over the world . . . wherever their tracks led they left a trail of music."[38] And as Jonathan Bate has shown, the "assertion that the Aboriginal sings the Ancestor's stanzas without changing a word or note is false; like all traditions of oral poetry, Aboriginal song involves a large measure of improvisation."[39]

Improvisation in such cases is a dynamic practice in which fixed realities dance with mutability and unpredictable shifts in the fabric of context, with consciousness being shaped in the process. It is also profoundly tied to earthborn realities of adaptation, survivance, and the capacity to negotiate differential landscapes and ways of knowing. As such, improvisation presents a remarkably resilient counternarrative to a modernity defined by industrial, imperial, and technological realities of subordination and alienation. By insisting on the intersections of human experience and the environmental and biotic realities on which humanity is contingent, site-specific improvisatory practices point to diversity, cocreativity, and community resilience as key markers of more extensive social practices.

The difficulty for broader challenges to abyssal thinking is how to avoid the West's capacity to incorporate such counternarratives into its hegemonic and economically exploitative cultural systems. And there are clearly no easy answers here, given the long histories of depoliticizing, assimilative, critically neutralizing, counter-cultural identifications with such counternarratives. The change begins, perhaps, with a recognition that anthropological frameworks that split between emic (cultural descriptions from a native to that culture) and etic (cultural analysis from a distanced, putatively neutral observer) reproduce abyssal thinking, figured as a form of asymmetrical knowing of the Other. Next comes, possibly, a turn to the insights of improvising intellectual-artists of the borderlands, individuals who are working through what may be to many of us unknown, or barely understood, ontologies and epistemologies, constituent parts of an emergent transmodernity emanating from

intercultural exchanges that occur on the peripheries of dominant epistemes. We have drawn from the insights of such figures already in this
afterword, while mapping some sonic foundations to this question, but
we must be attuned to the ethico-political perspectives they have generated as well.

The Korean traditional singer Bae Il-Dong, for example—whose
extraordinary improvisational vocalizations result from shamanic training that entailed living beside a waterfall for many years and learning
how to outsing it—suggests that experience and context produced the
unique constellation of realities he embodies sonically.

> Once time passes, it never comes back—the same for a beat, too.
> That's why . . . the movement of music is the same as the movement
> of the universe. If you think about it . . . music itself is improvisa
> tion. Just like time passing. In the universe, time and space pass by—
> in music, beat and melody pass by. This continual movement itself
> is music. Also, if you look at the meaning of the word *jukhung* (the
> Korean word for "improvisation"), *juk* means the current (now) and
> *hung* means the pleasure that comes from your immediate situation/
> environment or landscape [Bae uses the word 정경情景, which means
> a scene or a landscape that brings in an emotion into your heart].

Yet such embodiments shift with context and through intercultural interactions. "If I go to Africa tomorrow," he continues, "I will meet Africans,
and their emotions and my sentiments will meet, and we'll experience
that 'hung.' That immediate emotion is *jukhung* [improvisation]."[40]

Here, Bae is at considerable pains to point out the situatedness of
music in a "scene" or "landscape"—that is, a context associated with
affect, what Santos discusses as *corazonar*. Context matters because it is
tied to affect. Moreover, the ephemerality of the beat is singular, never
to be repeated again in precisely the same moment. Improvisation is
closely tied to this movement of concatenated ephemera that generate
affect, much like the notion of duende, which Spanish poet, playwright,
and director Federico García Lorca called "the most ancient culture,
of spontaneous creation."[41] Being in the moment allows for "hung" to
happen and, by extension, for affective contact to take place with others.
In a 2018 tour of Canada, singing traditional *pansori*, Bae encountered a
number of situations where he performed with improvisers from without
his traditional formation. His remarkable ability to enter into immediate
dialogue with these musicians had a great deal to do with the notion of

"hung," the capacity to engage affectively with the immediacy of whatever is one's context, even as that capacity is firmly grounded in a site-specific notion of sonic production.

Such an emergent creative space born of intercultural encounter can be thought of in relation to French improvising percussionist Lê Quan Ninh, who appeals to improvisers to "search out other locations where the geography of the playing space is not already so defined, a territory upon which we can explore its hidden nooks and crannies without risking a repatriation by those default codes and signs . . . a space without geography, in no way carved up by criteria for membership: an atopy capable of welcoming all languages."[42] Sound changes along this continuum of specific geographies, moving toward Ninh's utopic "atopy capable of welcoming all languages." Such a continuum of sound changes implies a politics of respect for the contingencies that produce difference, as well as the desire, via improvisation, to elaborate narratives of encounter that point toward cocreative communities of engagement.

This ethical frame, then, animated by sound changes, is perhaps the germ of an improvisationally motivated component of a broader challenge to abyssal thinking. Ninh's appeal to avoid musical gestures that are easy defaults via an encompassing attention to differences, to keep moving through the "hidden nooks and crannies," aligns with writer, producer, and curator John Corbett's notion that "freely improvised music is the first thoroughly transnational musical art form, its identity inflected by the various intersections and cross-pollinations engendered by all this migration."[43] These intersections and cross-pollinations, of course, are products of the pasts and presents of globalization's asymmetries, but they remain the potential terrain of a dialogue that might just disrupt these imbalances.

The Ongoing Coda

The epigraph to this chapter cites Iola Brubeck's lyrics to "Cultural Exchange," a piece from *The Real Ambassadors,* a composition written (and revised) over several years in the late 1950s and early 1960s by Dave and Iola Brubeck, recorded in 1961, and performed just once, at the 1962 Monterey Jazz Festival. In this performance, the artists figuring most prominently were Louis Armstrong, members of his and Dave Brubeck's bands, the vocal group Lambert-Hendricks-Ross, and vocalist Carmen McRae. *The Real Ambassadors* was, as Penny Von Eschen astutely discusses, a commentary on the contradictory politics of US State Department–

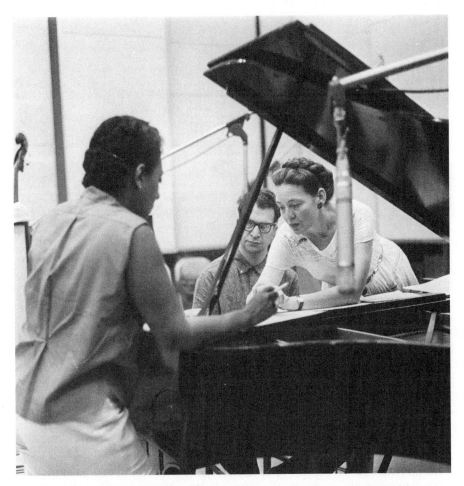

Fig. 9.1. Carmen McRae and Dave and Iola Brubeck, recording *The Real Ambassadors*, Columbia Recording Studios, New York, September 1961. (Photo Credit: Burt Goldblatt.)

sponsored overseas tours of jazz musicians and other cultural workers at this moment. The composition referenced directly the irony that African American musicians were being asked to serve as representatives of American democracy while still having to contend with Jim Crow conditions at home, and the critique of "cultural exchange" voiced across its constituent pieces drew from the insights of tour participants who recognized that "they had deliberately been sent into the front lines of major foreign-policy crises" and were, in a sense, being asked to give legitimacy to the United States' Cold War escapades in Eastern Europe and across the Global South.

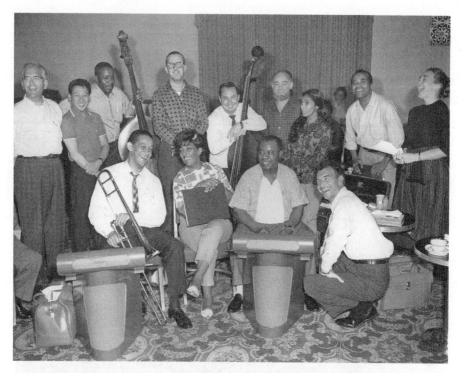

Fig. 9.2. Full cast of *The Real Ambassadors*, rehearsing for Monterey Jazz Festival, at the St. Francis Hotel, San Francisco, 1962. (Photo Credit: V. M. Hanks.)

The Brubecks drew on their own experiences from a 1958 State Department tour of the Middle East and Eastern Europe and were inspired as well by Armstrong's privately sponsored tour of Ghana in 1956 (just before independence that was praised by the US government) and, more recently, by his 1960–61 State Department–sponsored tour of newly independent nations and colonies across Africa. *The Real Ambassadors* also built on a tour Armstrong refused to do. In 1957 he pulled out of a State Department tour of the Soviet Union and South Africa as a protest over President Eisenhower's tepid response to Arkansas governor Orval Faubus's calling out the National Guard to prevent Black schoolchildren from desegregating Central High School in Little Rock. At an early 1960s moment, when he was being chastised for not speaking out more forcefully on civil rights and being compared unfavorably to younger artist-activists, the Brubecks "recovered [Armstrong's] submerged militancy and paid homage to him as a political actor."[44]

Gilbert Millstein's liner notes to *The Real Ambassadors* underlines the connection of the musical's main plot to the bandleader's recent history.

The musical places "Armstrong and his band in an unspecified African country newly arrived at independence, and its essence is simply that the kind of diplomacy coming out of the bell of his horn is apt to prove more efficacious in winning the United States friends than the official kind." Armstrong, as Millstein notes, had himself stated that "My public, they ain't thinkin' about politics when they call me Ambassador. They thinkin' about that horn and them notes and that music and them riffs." Iola Brubeck had been "struck by Armstrong's reception wherever he went, particularly on his 1960–61 African tour. In Leopoldville [now Kinshasa] men of the Baboto, Ekonda, and Nkongo tribes painted themselves violet and ochre in Armstrong's honor and bore him aloft into the city's stadium on a throne improvised from a canvas and metal tubing chaise lounge."

Yet, Brubeck, Armstrong, and the other performers voiced a critique as well. Brubeck's lyrics to "Cultural Exchange" open by referencing Dizzy Gillespie's 1957 appearance in Greece as part of the State Department's first goodwill jazz tour: "The band's last stop was Athens, where students had recently stoned the local headquarters of the United States Information Service in protest of Washington's support for Greece's right-wing dictatorship. Yet many of those same students greeted Gillespie with cheers, lifting him on their shoulders, throwing their jackets in the air and shouting: "Dizzy! Dizzy!"[45]

> From reports on Dizzy Gillespie
> It was clear to the local press, he
> Quelled the riots in far-off Greece
> Restored the place to comparative peace
>
> That's what we call, cultural exchange
> That's what we call, cultural exchange
> That's what we call, cultural exchange
> That's What We Call, Cultural Exchange!
>
> When Diz blew, the riots were routed
> People danced and they cheered and shouted
> The headlines bannered the hour as his
> They dropped their stones and they rocked with Diz!
>
> That's what we call, cultural exchange
> That's what we call, cultural exchange

That's what we call, cultural exchange
That's What We Call, Cultural—Exchaaaaaange!

Yeeeeeeeah, I remember when Diz was in Greece back in '57.
He did such a good job we started sending Jazz all over the world.

The State Department has discovered Jazz
It reaches folks like nothing ever has
Like when they feel that jazzy rhythm
They know we're really with 'em
That's what we call cultural exchange

No commodity—is quite so strange
As this thing called cultural exchange . . .[46]

Millstein underlines how "The nature of *Cultural Exchange* is probably best indicated by its gently sardonic tag, actually an improvisation hit upon during rehearsal by Armstrong and his fine trombonist, Trummy Young. 'And if the world goes really wacky, / Well get John to send out Jackie.' At this point, Young interpolated, 'You mean Jackie Robinson?' to which Armstrong responded, above the explosion of laughter that resulted (and that was retained for the recording), 'No, man I mean the First Lady. / That's what we call Cultural Exchange!'" So even as the song and its lyrics seem to hint at progressive ideals associated with jazz and improvisatory Black musicking, the musicians themselves point to the rifts and "strange[ness]" of the commodity of cultural exchange, as the state appropriates jazz to its own propagandistic purposes. What, after all, is the meaning of Dizzy Gillespie ostensibly quelling (through music) riots that were protesting American support for a right-wing government?

Iola Brubeck's lyrics discordantly point to the use value of jazz as a US commodity, while the musicians performing the piece spontaneously improvise ironic responses about the racial divide (Jackie Robinson for Jackie Kennedy) and perform the sarcastic notion of cultural exchange as a trope for state self-interest, even as the music itself signals its own power to interpret and cross cultural divides. This contradiction is more tragically illustrated off record by Armstrong's own interpretation, in retrospect, that his 1960 concert appearance in Elizabethville, in the Congo's Katanga province, put a temporary truce to the armed conflict over the region's attempted secession so that members of both sides could hear

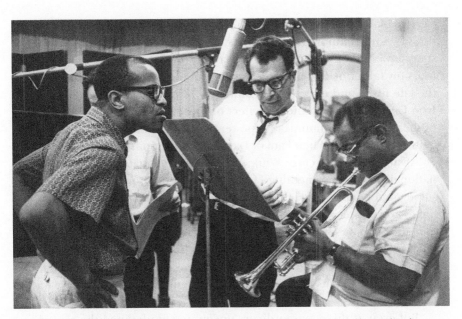

Fig. 9.3. Jon Hendricks, Dave Brubeck, and Louis Armstrong, recording *The Real Ambassadors*, Columbia Recording Studios, New York, September 1961. (Photo Credit: Don Hunstein.)

him play. What Armstrong did not realize was that his own government, along with Belgium, supported the secession movement because of US designs on Katangan mineral deposits, including uranium, and dissatisfaction with recently elected prime minister Patrice Lumumba's socialist and nationalist vision. And he could not have known that shortly after his Congo concerts in October and November 1960, Lumumba would be deposed, imprisoned, and murdered over the course of December 1960 and January 1961 (while Armstrong's band was still on the continent), with the approval of the Eisenhower administration and assistance of the CIA.[47]

Traveling across the abyssal divides of cultural difference and indifference, "Cultural Exchange" cannily underlines the dangers of appropriation even as it performs its own critical response via the very strategies of improvisation that make Black musicking so powerful. Iola Brubeck's contributions to the liner notes for the 1962 vinyl album observe how "Louis embodies in magnificent proportions all the elements of jazz we wanted others to understand. . . . The music that pours from [his horn] contains magic even the magician does not fully comprehend. Anyone who has been caught in Louis' spell can really believe that if he were to blast three times 'round, the walls of hate would come tumbling down!" Sonic empowerment here is in uncomfortable apposition with state power. Matt Brubeck, son to Dave and Iola, comments how "the tours my father made under the auspices of the US State Department in the late fifties and early sixties (India, the Middle East, and behind the Iron Curtain) had a profound effect on Dave and Iola's understanding of the universal communicative power of music. It was a *lingua franca* of cultural exchange. When Paul or Dave quoted Chopin during a solo, the Polish audience went crazy. While one could argue that this response was nationalism, I feel something far deeper was going on. The Poles, as a subjugated people, may have recognized that someone was really listening to and appreciating their musical culture. When Joe Morello [drummer in the Dave Brubeck Quartet] jammed with Pazhani Subramania Pillai (mridangam and kanjira virtuoso Trichy Sankaran's teacher) very few words were exchanged, but it was evident from the head shaking of the Indian musicians and Joe's smile that something extraordinary was taking place."[48]

But even as these extraordinary encounters underlined the remarkable power of music to generate cross-cultural dialogue and understanding, the Brubecks "also spoke of their frustration that they could not find the financial backing for the show [*The Real Ambassadors*] to have a New York run at that time. As I remember, even with Louis agreeing to be the centerpiece, the show was considered 'too political' for the producers with whom they met. As Dave recalled in the Columbia Jazz Masterpieces CD reissue, 'We weren't supposed to have a message . . . we couldn't lecture the American public on the subject of race.'"[49] Further, Matt Brubeck observes, "The State Department may have thought that jazz musicians represented the USA. Musicians, however, represented something far more important than the nation-state. Jazz musicians represented African American musical culture. They demonstrated a way of cocreating music spontaneously and, perhaps most importantly, engaged with musicians of various cultures by listening deeply and intently to what they had to offer. Improvisers have always had the power to reach across cultural divisions. I think that this is one of the central themes of *The Real Ambassadors*."[50]

Indeed, writer and musician Chip Stern's liner notes to the 1994 Columbia remastered reissue of the album remind listeners that Dave Brubeck was "a lifelong foe of racism, [his] steadfast refusal to perform for segregated audiences or to replace his quartet's black bassist cost him many a television appearance and college tour. . . . When Dave and

Iola Brubeck first conceived the idea for *The Real Ambassadors*, America was at the end of a bitter historical cycle. The festering inequities of American apartheid—built into law by the framers of the constitution and adopted into the social fabric of everyday life after the American Civil War thanks to the Jim Crow laws—were often enforced at the end of a rope in socially accepted pogroms. . . . American society was separate and unequal, and even the subsequent passage of a Civil Rights bill [1964] proved too little and too late."[51]

In *The Real Ambassadors*, then, Brubeck's use of "exotic" scales and multiple musical forms, the diverse voicings of musicians who had emerged from very different contexts, and the incisive lyrics written by Iola Brubeck all imagine an alternative vision of how to encounter difference, how to learn across the abyssal divides smothering intercultural dialogue in the name of alienation, sustained racism, and inequity. Hybridized musical forms that invoke improvisation, that cross borders, that inspire respect across divisive and asymmetrical power relations, and that do so while also demanding reciprocal engagements are as much at stake in *The Real Ambassadors* as are critiques of how these powerful forces can be subsumed to other uses. In the sounding of its changes, improvisatory dialogue and play reveal other ways of knowing, other ways of being in the world that engender humor, understanding, critique, and action in the name of generative cocreation. The future, or ongoing coda to the historical contingencies we have arrived at in this moment, resides in the improvised dialogues yet to be made across the differences that sustain new ways of knowing the magic that "even the magician does not fully comprehend."

Notes

1. Schafer, *The Soundscape*, 7.
2. Greenway, "Wakefield's Anachnid Wins SOCAN Prize," 9.
3. Santos, "Beyond Abyssal Thinking," 46.
4. Santos, *Epistemologies of the South*, 212.
5. Viswanathan and Cormack, "Melodic Improvisation," 219.
6. Inayat Khan, *The Mysticism of Sound and Music*, 161.
7. Inayat Khan, 162.
8. Southworth and Ziporyn, "Gender Wayang by I Wayan Loceng."
9. Gray, *Improvisation and Composition*, 127.
10. Traditional Hindustani ragas, too, depend on microvariations that arise from *shruti*, "a very subtle note intonation, a microtone or micro-interval, defined always in relation to the tonic," with some theorizing a "division of the

octave in 22 microtones." In his discussion of master *bansuri* player and impro-viser Hariprasad Chaurasia, Henri Tournier notes that the "utmost virtuosity can be expressed in this art of variation of compositions; they are never sung nor played twice identically." Tournier, *Hariprasad Chaurasia*, 18, 24. Such music blends composed and improved articulations and relies heavily on improvisatory artistry to achieve a balance between tradition and innovation.

11. A mark of the often-contradictory challenges of intercultural understand-ings of improvisation is R. Anderson Sutton's work on Javanese gamelan music in a "broad intercultural perspective" and his conclusion that "Javanese musicians improvise, but Javanese music is not really improvisatory." See Nettl, introduc-tion, 17.

12. Ortiz, *La africanía*, 261.

13. Here, Ortiz references the music of Bakuba and the eight-stringed *enanga* harp. The Bakuba, Kuba, or Bushongo was a precolonial kingdom located in Central Africa that thrived from the seventeenth to the nineteenth centuries.

14. See, for instance, C. S'thembile West's summary in "African Diaspora Performance Aesthetics": "African aesthetic qualities—namely rhythmic dyna-mism, antiphony (call and response), repetition, improvisation, wholism, asym-metrical balance, coolness, and syncopation—link African Diaspora communi-ties to Africa" (32). The specifics of such linkages point to multiple differential practices across a wide spectrum of sites.

15. Here, we align with José Luiz Martinez's argument that "To consider merely what might possibly be known about a musical culture, it is necessary to include cultural history in the equation. . . . Perhaps as wrong as the idea that music is a universal language, is to think that music in non-Western cultures does not change." See Martinez, *Semiosis in Hindustani Music*, 10.

16. Simone, *City Life from Jakarta to Dakar*, 268–70.

17. Fischlin and Porter, "Improvisation and Global Sites of Difference," 5.

18. See the essays by Daniel Fischlin and Darci Sprengel in Fischlin and Porter, *Playing for Keeps*.

19. See the chapters by Kirstie Dorr and Monica Dalidowicz in this collection.

20. Coleman, "The Sign and the Seal."

21. Michael Dessen writes, "Whereas [Derek] Bailey's 'non-idiomatic category links experimental improvisation to an allegedly culture-free space, the model of experimentalism at work [in the AfroCuba de Matanzas / Coleman collabora-tion] does not seek to avoid cultural traditions so much as to bring them into dia-logue . . . while speaking of African culture, overall, [Francisco Zamora] Chirino [leader since 1957 of AfroCuba de Matanzas] also emphasized that this work was very much grounded in the traditions specific to the Matanzas region. He took care to differentiate the traditions of Matanzas from those of nearby Havana, and even within the context of Matanzas he emphasized his own group's distinctive *sello* [seal or 'group sound']." See Dessen, "Improvising in a Different Clave, 182.

22. Santos, *The End of the Cognitive Empire*, 167.

23. Santos, 168.

24. Santos, 177.

25. Santos, 14.

26. Santos, 178.

27. Tomlinson and Lipsitz, *Insubordinate Spaces*, 8.

28. Tomlinson and Lipsitz, 14–15. Tomlinson and Lipsitz specifically situate *konesans* and *balans* in relation to "discussions of the metaphor and practice of accompaniment articulated by Archbishop Oscar Romero in El Salvador . . . that fueled Father Jean-Bertrand Aristide's *lavalas* movement in Haiti" (15):

> Mastery of *konesans* requires that people not only place proximate events in a broader perspective . . . but also acknowledge the pull of the past on the present, recognizing the lifetime of indebtedness that individuals have to suffering, struggle, and sacrifice of ancestors and elders. . . . People cannot "will" themselves to be outside of history . . . or to escape the responsibilities it requires. By itself, however, *konesans* is not enough; it needs to be infused with the quality of *balans*.

> *Balans* holds that everyone has a part of the truth, that people's weaknesses come from many of the same sources as their strengths, and that the truth and the lie—or the right thing and the wrong thing—are often not mutually incommensurable opposites but instead different poles of a dialogically and dialectically connected unity. (Tomlinson and Lipsitz, *Insubordinate Spaces*, 40–41)

Intercultural encounter necessitates improvisations in which *konesans* and *balans* are critical ways of enacting contingency, cocreative relations, and reciprocity in order to achieve accompaniment.

29. Kelley, *Freedom Dreams*.

30. See especially Baraka's "The Changing Same," in *Black Music*, 180–211.

31. Shange, "The Writing Life."

32. Moten, *In the Break*, 45.

33. Dussel, "Transmodernity and Interculturality," 33, 43.

34. Dussel, 37, 40–41.

35. Dussel, 42–43, 48 (italics in original).

36. Keeney and Keeney, *Way of the Bushman*, xxviii. Even San notions of their own demise and precarity are figured in musical terms, as in Stephen Watson's poetic distillation of San narratives from the Bleek-Lloyd collection of interviews: "Because / of a broken string, / because of a people / breaking the string, / the earth, my place / is the place / of something / a thing broken / that does not / stop sounding / breaking with me." Skotnes, *Sound from the Thinking Strings*, 152.

37. Van der Post and Taylor, *Testament to the Bushmen*, 153.

38. Chatwin, *The Songlines*, 13, 73.

39. Bate, *The Song of the Earth*, 241.

40. Il-Dong Bae and Dong-Won Kim, personal interview with Fischlin, Guelph, Ontario, 2014.

41. García Lorca, "Play and Theory of the Duende," 49.

42. Lê Quan Ninh, *Improvising Freely*, 79. A question one might ask of Ninh's notion here, as with Derek Bailey's now well-rehearsed notion of "non-idiomatic

improvisation," is: when does the non-idiomatic become idiomatic? In other words, at what point does ossification in so-called non-idiomatic practices that conform to specific cultural contexts make improvisatory iteration a parody of itself? See also Bailey, *Improvisation*.

43. Corbett, *A Listener's Guide to Free Improvisation*, 16.

44. Von Eschen, *Satchmo Blows Up the World*, 59–68, 79–82, 85.

45. Kaplan, "When Ambassadors Had Rhythm." For more information on the antigovernment and anti-American student protests in Greece in 1957, see Stefanidis, *Stirring the Greek Nation*, 104–8.

46. Lyrics cited from Sambson, "Lambert, Hendricks, Ross & Armstrong."

47. Von Eschen, *Satchmo Blows Up the World*, 66–68.

48. Matt Brubeck, email message to Fischlin, July 9, 2019.

49. M. Brubeck.

50. M. Brubeck.

51. Stern, Liner notes to Brubeck and Brubeck, *The Real Ambassadors*, 5–6.

Works Cited

Bailey, Derek. *Improvisation: Its Nature and Practice in Music.* Ashbourne, England: Moorland, 1980.

Bate, Jonathan. *The Song of the Earth.* Cambridge, MA: Harvard University Press, 2000.

Brubeck, Dave, and Iola Brubeck. *The Real Ambassadors: An Original Musical Production by Dave and Iola Brubeck.* Produced by Teo Macero. Columbia Records OL 5850, 1962. LP.

Chatwin, Bruce. *The Songlines.* New York: Penguin Books, 1987.

Coleman, Steve. "The Sign and the Seal." *m-base.* Accessed February 2, 2016. http://m-base.com/recordings/the-sign-and-the-seal/

Corbett, John. *A Listener's Guide to Free Improvisation.* Chicago: University of Chicago Press, 2016.

Dessen, Michael. "Improvising in a Different Clave: Steve Coleman and Afro-Cuba de Matanzas." In *The Other Side of Nowhere: Jazz, Improvisation, and Communities in Dialogue,* edited by Daniel Fischlin and Ajay Heble, 173–92. Middletown, CT: Wesleyan University Press, 2004.

Dussel, Enrique. "Transmodernity and Interculturality: An Interpretation from the Perspective of Philosophy of Liberation." *TRANSMODERNITY: Journal of Peripheral Cultural Production of the Luso-Hispanic World* 1, no. 3 (2012): 28–59.

Fischlin, Daniel, and Eric Porter. "Improvisation and Global Sites of Difference." In "Improvisation and Global Sites of Difference," edited by Daniel Fischlin and Eric Porter, special issue of *Critical Studies in Improvisation / Études critiques en improvisation* 11, nos. 1–2 (2016). https://www.criticalimprov.com/index.php/csieci/issue/view/204

Fischlin, Daniel, and Eric Porter, eds. *Playing for Keeps: Improvisation in the Aftermath.* Durham, NC: Duke University Press, 2020.

García Lorca, Federico. "Play and Theory of the Duende." In *In Search of Duende,* translated by Christopher Maurer, 48–62. New York: New Directions, 1998.

Gray, Nicholas. *Improvisation and Composition in Balinese Gendér Wayang: Music of the Moving Shadows*. Burlington, VT: Ashgate, 2011.

Greenway, Trevor. "Wakefield's Anachnid Wins SOCAN Prize." *Low Down* (Quebec), June 5–11, 2019.

Inayat Khan, Hazrat. *The Mysticism of Sound and Music*. Rev. ed. Boston: Shambhala Editions, 1996.

Jones, LeRoi (Amiri Baraka). *Black Music*. New York: William Morrow, 1967.

Kaplan, Fred. "When Ambassadors Had Rhythm." *New York Times*, June 29, 2008. https://www.nytimes.com/2008/06/29/arts/music/29kapl.html

Keeney, Bradford, and Hillary Keeney, eds. *Way of the Bushman: Spiritual Teachings and Practices of the Kalahari Ju'hoansi: As Told by the Tribal Elders*. Rochester, VT: Bear, 2015.

Kelley, Robin D. G. *Freedom Dreams: The Black Radical Imagination*. New York: Beacon Press, 2002.

Lê Quan Ninh. *Improvising Freely: The ABCs of an Experience*. Translated by Karen Houle. Guelph, ON: PS Guelph, 2014.

Martinez, José Luiz. *Semiosis in Hindustani Music*. Delhi: Motilal Banarsidass, 2001.

Millstein, Gilbert. Liner notes to Dave Brubeck and Iola Brubeck, *The Real Ambassadors: An Original Musical Production by Dave and Iola Brubeck*. Produced by Teo Macero. Columbia Records OL 5850, 1962. LP.

Moten, Fred. *The Feel Trio*. Tucson, AZ: Letter Machine Editions, 2014.

Moten, Fred. *In the Break: The Aesthetics of the Black Radical Tradition*. Minneapolis: University of Minnesota Press, 2003.

Nettl, Bruno. "Introduction: An Art Neglected in Scholarship." In *In the Course of Performance: Studies in the World of Musical Improvisation*, edited by Bruno Nettl and Melinda Russell, 1–23. Chicago: University of Chicago Press, 1998.

Ortiz, Fernando. *La africanía de la música folklórica cubana*. Havana: Letras Cubanas, 2001. First published 1950.

Sambson. "Lambert, Hendricks, Ross & Armstrong—'Cultural Exchange' Lyric (from *The Real Ambassadors*)." *Obsessed with Jazz* (blog). June 24, 2015. http://obsessedwithjazz.blogspot.com/2015/06/lambert-hendricks-ross-cultural-exchange.html

Santos, Boaventura de Sousa. "Beyond Abyssal Thinking: From Global Lines to Ecologies of Knowledges." *Review* 30 (2007): 45–89.

Santos, Boaventura de Sousa. *The End of the Cognitive Empire: The Coming of Age of Epistemologies of the South*. Durham, NC: Duke University Press, 2018.

Santos, Boaventura de Sousa. *Epistemologies of the South: Justice against Epistemicide*. London: Routledge, 2016.

Schafer, R. Murray. *The Soundscape: Our Sonic Environment and the Tuning of the World*. Rochester, VT: Destiny Books, 1994.

Shange, Ntozake. "The Writing Life." *Washington Post*, March 31, 1996.

Simone, AbdouMaliq. *City Life from Jakarta to Dakar: Movements at the Crossroads*. New York: Routledge, 2010.

Skotnes, Pippa, ed. *Sound from the Thinking Strings: A Visual, Literary, Archaeological and Historical Interpretation of the Final Years of \Xam Life*. Cape Town: Axeage Private Press, 1991.

Southworth, Christine, and Evan Ziporyn. "Gender Wayang by I Wayan Loceng." Translated by Maria Bodmann. *Gender Wayang* (website). Archived April 23, 2008. https://web.archive.org/web/20080423021748/http://www.genderw ayang.com/gender.shtml

Stefanidis, Ioannis D. *Stirring the Greek Nation: Political Culture, Irredentism, and Anti-Americanism in Post-War Greece, 1945–1967.* Aldershot: Ashgate, 2007.

Stern, Chip. Liner Notes to Dave Brubeck and Iola Brubeck, *The Real Ambassadors,* 5–9. Digitally remastered, Columbia Jazz Masterpieces, Columbia Legacy CK 57633, 1994. Compact disc.

Tomlinson, Barbara, and George Lipsitz. *Insubordinate Spaces: Improvisation and Accompaniment for Social Justice.* Philadelphia: Temple University Press, 2019.

Tournier, Henri. *Hariprasad Chaurasia and the Art of Improvisation.* Paris: Accords-Croisés, 2010.

Van der Post, Laurens, and Jane Taylor. *Testament to the Bushmen.* New York: Penguin, 1986.

Viswanathan, Tanjore, and Jody Cormack. "Melodic Improvisation in Karnātak Music: The Manifestations of Rāga." In *In the Course of Performance: Studies in the World of Musical Improvisation,* edited by Bruno Nettl and Melinda Russell, 219–33. Chicago: University of Chicago Press, 1998.

Von Eschen, Penny. *Satchmo Blows Up the World: Jazz Ambassadors Play the Cold War.* Cambridge, MA: Harvard University Press, 2004.

West, C. S'thembile. "African Diaspora Performance Aesthetics." In *Encyclopedia of the African Diaspora: Origins, Experiences, and Culture,* vol. 1, edited by Carole Boyce Davies, 32–33. Santa Barbara, CA: ABC CLIO, 2008.

Index

Abdul-Malik, Ahmed, 25
Abhinavagupta, 188
Abrams, Muhal Richard, 165
abyssal: divides, 253, 255; post, 241; thinking, 12, 46, 235, 243, 245–46, 248
Adams, John, 154
Adams, Pepper, 219
Africa/Brass (Coltrane), 201, 205, 214, 218
African American musicians, 6, 8, 155–56; collaborations with Asian American musicians, 159, 164–66, 169; collaborations with continental African musicians, 15–16, 18–20, 26–27, 29–30, 33, 35; and experimentalism, 18; and hip-hop/rap, 90, 95; as hosts in improvisational settings, 166; as representatives of American democracy, 249
African Cookbook (Weston), 24, 37n36
African diaspora. *See* diaspora: African
African Rhythms Quintet, 28–29. *See also* Weston, Randy
AfroCuba de Matanzas, 240, 256n21
akLaff, Pheeroan, 165
Alarcón, Rolando, 52
Allard, Jean-Philippe, 27
Allard, Joe, 216, 221–22
Alvarado, Elena, 59
"Ambush on All Sides," 162
American Society of African Culture

(AMSAC), 24–25. *See also* US State Department, the
Amman, 9, 82, 85, 87, 92, 95; downtown, 79–80, 94
Anachnid, 234
Aoki, Tatsu, 164
appropriation: in improvising collaborations, 116–17; of transcultural practices, 92
Arabic music: Cairo Congress of, 145, 147n24; classical forms of, 131–32, 135; Hassan Khan and, 127; hip-hop/rap and, 90–92, 95–96; improvisational traditions of, 126; popular forms of, 135; traditional tropes of, 84. *See also* Shaa'bi music
Armstrong, Louis, 12, 248–54
Arts and Humanities Research Council, the (AHRC), 76
Asian American musicians, 10–11, 165, 172n17; collaborations with African American musicians, 159, 164–66; use of electronics by, 169–70
Association for the Advancement of Creative Musicians (AACM), 155, 165, 205
Atlantic, the: "Black Atlantic," 166, 168; slave trade and, 5, 150; and transdiasporic collaboration, 8, 16, 26; world context of, 151, 166, 168, 172n17
"audiotopia," 67

jazz (*continued*)
by Asian American musicians,
164–67; Latin, 116, 119–20; in New
Orleans, 150, 213; as nomadic, 101;
pan-African, 28; piano, 160; use in
the *India-Jazz Suites* stage show, 183;
Western, 116, 119–20; "white," 120
Jenkins, Leroy, 165
Jewel (Hassan Khan): as an active
immersive reality, 144, 148n47;
creation of, 128–29, 140, 142–43;
description of, 139–140; dance in,
143–44; and *Dom Tak Tak Dom Tak,*
125, 127–29, 132 142–45; and phonochoreography, 142–43, 145; symbolism of angler fish in, 140–41
Jiménez, Ernesto, 59
Jones, Elvin, 214
Jones, Jessica, 219
Jones, LeRoi. *See* Baraka, Amiri
Jordan, 9, 76; and cultural constric-
tion, 89–90; English in, 91; French
cultural identity in, 81–83; hip-hop/
rap in, 77–78, 84; refugees in, 78;
social stratification in, 93–94; youth
in, 79, 82–84, 95–96
Jordanian State, the: cultural sonic
preferences of, 78, 84, 95–96
jukhung, 247–48. *See also* improvisation

Kafka, Franz: minor tradition and, 120
Kaiser, Henry, 155
Kapchan, Deborah, 16
karna, 206. *See also* saxophone
kathak, 10–11; and Afrological jazz,
183–84; Americanization of, 180–
81, 190–91; athleticism in, 180–81;
vs. ballet, 186–87; and the *bhakti*
devotional movement, 188–89, 191;
choreography in, 178; as communi-
cating Indian values, 180–82; and
cross-cultural exchange, 182–84;
the divine in 188–91; mistakes and
resolutions in, 185–87; "modern,"
180–81, 191, 194n26; *sawal jabab* section of, 179–80; solos, 177, 179, 183,
185–87, 191, 194n26; storytelling in,

178–79; tradition of, 175–76, 179–81,
184; *upaj* in, 175–80, 193; yoga, 190,
196n56
Kelley, Robin D. G., 242
Khan, Ali Akbar, 190
Khan, Hassan, 10; on "the conditioned self," 129–30; development
of practice, 129; on "engineered
cultural spaces," 127; on the "invisible audience," 126; use of Shaa'bi
music, 125–126, 128–30, 133–34,
136–37, 139–40, 142–43, 147n25. *See
also* individual works
Khan, Hazrat Inayat, 236
Khlyfy, Abdelkador, 32
Kibwe, Talib, 28, 30–31
Kim, Hyelim, 112, 115–16
Kim Dong-Won, 171n6, 238
Kim Jin Hi, 150–51, 159, 160–61, 163;
discovery of African American
music, 155–56; improvisational style
of, 156; "Linking," 154; and "Living
Tones," 154–57; personal/cultural
history, 152–54; on traditional
Korean folk music, 153; on transcultural improvisation, 156–57
Kindred Spirits, Vol. 1 (Shepp), 16, 32,
38n58, 38n62
"King Chu Removes His Armor," 162
Kirk, Rahsaan Roland, 26, 223
komungo, 152, 171n3; electrification of
the, 155; and gender, 153–54; Kim
Jin Hi on the, 153
kongofonic, 212; blood, 207, 214;
expression, 224; family of instruments, 216; fingerings on the
saxophone, 11, 218, 229; path, 206,
215; spirit, 213; utterance, 201. *See
also* B'Kongofon
Korea: history of, 152–53; social limits
of, 169; traditional music of, 153,
155–56, 171n6
krkabas, 17, 22, 28–30
Kronos Quartet, 154, 166

Laing, R. D., 125–26
Lake, Oliver, 156

ness of, 144; transcendent potentialities of, 140

Shaa'bi Music, 10; as a collectively
produced genre, 127; commercialization of, 138–39; electronic
instrumentation in, 131; and *fasaaha*
(clarity of enunciation), 131–32;
genesis of, 130; in Hassan Khan's
practice, 125–26, 128–30, 133–34,
136–37, 139–40, 142–43, 147n25; and
improvisation, 125–26, 128, 130, 135,
138, 143; and *moulids*, 130–31; New
Wave, 129, 131–32, 138; and street
dancing, 138–39

Shakry, Omnia El, 139

shamanism, 152–53, 168, 171n5, 189; in
the music of Kim Jin Hi, 155, 160

Shange, Ntozake, 242–43

Shankar, Pandit Ravi, 190

Shepp, Archie, 8, 26; collaborations
with the Gnawa, 16, 31–35, 38n62;
Kindred Spirits, Vol. 1, 16, 32, 38n58,
38n62

Shouly, 90

Siddall, Gillian, 6

Sigimse (intonation), 154. *See also* Kim
Jin Hi

Simmons, Sonny, 215–16, 222

Simone, AbdouMaliq, 239–40

Simone, Nina, 25

slavery, 33; in the Congo, 200, 204–
205, 207–13; master-slave relationship, 104–105, 113, 119; in New
Orleans, 207; trans-Atlantic, 26–27,
111, 150, 166, 242; trans-Saharan, 15,
21, 26–28

Smith, Jason Samuels, 175, 182–84,
195n33

Smith, Wadada Leo, 165

Smokable, 91

social movement scholarship, 44–
45

"Song X" (Coleman), 220

Sousa, John Philip, 213

South Korea. *See* Korea.

space, "insubordinate," 242; nomadic
vs. sedentary, 102, 104, 113, 121; sed-

entary, 106–109; smooth vs. striated,
104, 121

spirit possession: 17, 34–36. *See also*
Gnawa, the

Spirits of Our Ancestors, The (Weston),
16, 38n50

Spirit! The Power of Music (Weston), 15,
28–31, 38n54

*Splendid Master Gnawa Musicians of
Morocco, The* (Weston), 15, 27–28, 31

Stanley-Niaah, Sonjah, 45–46

Stern, Chip, 254

Stitt, Sonny, 220

Stover, Chris, 101, 103, 120–21

Stroman, Scoby, 25

Stuart, Alejandro, 64, 68; on *peñas*, 58,
63, 69; role in operating La Peña
del Sur, 59–61

Subramania, Pazhani, 254

Sufism, 15, 130, 146n15, 195n43, 214

Sukran, Nasser-El (Nassar the Drunkard), 131

Synaptik, The, 9, 77, 81; on ciphering, 86; early career of, 94; on
improvisation, 83–84, 87–88, 93–94;
and Palestinian tradition, 87; on
refugeeism, 87–90, 95–96; use of
language by, 90–92

Tan Dun, 163

Taoism, 152, 158, 160, 168–69

Tarab: dance, 139–40; music, 131, 135,
147n24

Taylor, Cecil, 136, 145n8, 155, 242–43

territorialization: and gender, 115; in
improvisation, 103, 120; and "lines
of flight," 108

Threadgill, Henry, 164

tihai: in Hindustani music, 178, 185,
187

Tomlinson, Barbara, 242, 257

Touati, Noureddine, 32

trance: the Gnawa and, 17, 34, 36n10;
and improvisation, 189

Trance of Seven Colors, The (Sanders),
15, 21, 35, 37n23

transcultural: collaboration, 151; dif-

Printed and bound by CPI Group (UK) Ltd, Croydon, CR0 4YY

09/06/2025

14685668-0001

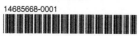